The Patient and the Plastic Surgeon

The Patient and the Plastic Surgeon

Second Edition

Robert M. Goldwyn, M.D.

Clinical Professor of Surgery, Harvard Medical School; Head, Division of Plastic Surgery, Beth Israel Hospital; Senior Surgeon, Brigham and Women's Hospital, Boston; Editor, Plastic and Reconstructive Surgery

Little, Brown and Company
Boston/Toronto/London

Copyright © 1991 by Robert M. Goldwyn
Second Edition
Previous edition copyright © 1981 by Robert M. Goldwyn

All rights reserved. No part of this book may be reproduced in any form or by any electronic or mechanical means, including information storage and retrieval systems, without permission in writing from the publisher, except by a reviewer who may quote brief passages in a review.

Library of Congress Catalog Card No. 90-64046

ISBN 0-316-31978-3

Printed in the United States of America
HAL

To my wife, Roberta

Contents

Preface to the Second Edition — *ix*
Preface to the First Edition — *xi*
Acknowledgments — *xiii*

1. *Antecedents* — *1*

2. *The Initial Consultation* — *9*

3. *Plastic Surgery: Reconstructive and Esthetic Surgery* — *51*

4. *Types of Operations and Types of Patients* — *113*

5. *Stages in the Professional Life of the Plastic Surgeon* — *277*

References — *306*
Appendix — *321*
Index — *351*

Preface to the Second Edition

Significant changes during the past decade, not only in the concepts and procedures of our specialty but in the social and medical milieu, have prompted the second edition of this book. Today's plastic surgeon is buffeted by increasingly critical and insistent patients, some even hostile, and besieged by unending and expanding bureaucratic demands. One wonders whether the massive machinery would continue to whir and regurgitate paper tasks even in the miraculous absence of disease and doctors.

We physicians are obviously less in charge and more on the defensive than we would like to be, to a degree that we never thought possible during our medical school and residency years. The fear and reality of litigation, the increasing cost of malpractice premiums, the flourishing of advertising, the prevalence of health maintenance organizations, the intrusiveness and ultimate power of third-party payers, and the more-than-occasional adversarial relationship between patient and physician have transformed not just plastic surgery but all of medicine. For those of us who were once the honored heirs and heiresses of Hippocrates, there is no eye of the storm in which to take refuge.

This book addresses these issues in addition to numerous others in an attempt to give a perspective and some help to plastic surgeons who take care of patients. Although the reader will find idealism in these patients, he or she will also discover that it is well tempered with reality and, sometimes, I fear, with a milligram or two of cynicism based on my own observations, mistakes, and hard lessons learned in daily work with patients over the past 30 years.

R.M.G.

Preface to the First Edition

I have written this book to share my observations and thoughts with other plastic surgeons. It is a personal statement about taking care of patients, not a manual on office procedure or an encyclopedia on the doctor-patient relationship. Library shelves already buckle from the latter, which recently have come mostly from nonmedical authors. Of physicians writing on this topic, few have been plastic surgeons. Although what transpires between patient and plastic surgeon has many similarities with other doctor-patient relationships, there are differences that are crucial to recognize and to act upon. I hope this book will aid in the care of patients by increasing the awareness of the dynamics and subtleties in the interaction between patient and plastic surgeon, particularly during the initial consultation. For most of us, helping people was the stimulus that prompted our choosing medicine as a career, that buoyed us during the troughs of medical school and residency, and that still occupies most of our waking and working lives.

By examining the role of the doctor and the patient, this book emphasizes the actions and reactions of each and the effects and consequences for both. As a physician, I was conscious of the temptation to confine my sights mostly to the patient. This narrowness of focus, however, has been the defect of other writings on this subject. We must not forget that when we do something to a patient, we are doing something also to ourselves and the patient is doing something to us.

Medicine has survived because humankind is subject to disease and death. That one person has a problem and that another might have a solution is the immutable crux of the singular alliance between doctor and patient.

Finally, for humility and balance, we should remember that we who are physicians will eventually become patients. While it may be impossible to establish the priority between chicken and egg, it is certain that there was disease before there was medicine, and there were patients before there were doctors.

R.M.G.

Acknowledgments

Readers will recognize the influences of many in this book. I have recorded consciously and unconsciously the experience and wisdom of past and present teachers, colleagues, friends, and, particularly, patients. To all of them I am grateful.

In doing this second edition, I have continued to benefit from the support and skills of the staff of my publisher, Little, Brown and Company. In particular, I wish to thank Susan F. Pioli, Executive Editor; Karen M. Feeney, Production Editor; Michael A. Granger, Production Supervisor; Wendi Schnaufer, Copyeditor; Phyllis Coyne, Proofreader; and Julia B. Figures, Indexer.

To Ruth Anderson, who did the typing, I am very appreciative.

You must begin with an ideal and end with an ideal.
Frederick G. Banting
Codiscoverer of insulin

The Patient and the Plastic Surgeon

1

Antecedents

6:45 P.M.: Surgeons' dressing room.

On the other side of the lockers, two senior residents in general surgery are talking without realizing that I am listening:

"Another long, helluva day and it's not over yet for me. More drudge work to do, more patients to see. If only someone had told me this before I applied to medical school, I could have saved myself a lot of aggravation—and money—$55,000 in the hole now and rising."

"About the same with me," his companion replies, "and it's going to get worse because my wife will be leaving her job when our baby comes in a couple of months."

"Is it really worth it?" the first resident queries; they both leave without answering the question.

Had they asked me, my response would have been that it is worth it; it has always been worth it, but I am 60 years old and have been in practice almost as many years as they have been alive. When I entered the premedical steeplechase, doctors still generated admiration and respect; a career in medicine was to be envied, not avoided or scorned. I finished medical school and five years of general surgical residency as well as two years of plastic surgical training during what in retrospect were the "good and grand" old days. By usual standards, I have been as successful and happy in my work and life as one can reasonably expect.

Any physician, unless he or she were in a space shuttle, must have noted that things were changing in our profession about 10 to 15 years ago, and I am not referring to scientific advances. Patients were becoming more demanding and critical and less tolerant of honest errors. They did not seem to realize, even though they had been informed, that medicine in general, and plastic surgery in particular, could not guarantee only excellent results. Quiet and not so quiet grumbling and complaining rapidly escalated into the legal realm. Malpractice threats and fears became the tenor of the times. The grateful patient, once the usual, was soon the unusual. From the public, which was receiving the best care in human history, came hostile protests about the inadequacy of treatment and the greed of doctors. The media reflected and reinforced this trend [43, 155, 156]; soon it would be rare to see an article in the lay press, and even in medical journals, in praise of medicine. The fashion was and still is to criticize and chastise the physician and organized (really disorganized) medicine.

Although I enjoy my work and have never been bored, my peers talk of early retirement and are angry because they feel unappreciated, overworked, and underpaid. If I point out to them that their annual income is in the upper five percent of all wage earners in the United States, they counter by saying that they labor longer, take more personal risk and responsibility after having studied and trained far longer and harder than any other group, especially those most vociferous in condemning medicine. They believe—and who can dispute?—that medicine is not what it used to be. So earnestly do they hold their views that some of my colleagues have discouraged their children from becoming doctors. This attitude, as well as the perception by the public that a medical career is not as lustrous as it was, has led to a decline in the number and quality of applicants to medical school.

I admit that I never thought I would witness such despondency in physicians, who traditionally exemplified buoyancy of spirit. Medical students with whom we work sense the disaffection among their

1 Antecedents

mentors. In fact, some physicians go out of their way, maliciously I think, to tell them that they should have chosen another career—law, business, or "anything else." This attitude worries medical educators who have urged the faculty to be more enthusiastic about our profession in our interaction with students. But how can one evince and maintain an emotion without truly feeling it? And many of my colleagues feel just the opposite; that practicing medicine is causing them more displeasure than pleasure, and that if they could do something else (but still generate the same income), they would willingly do so.

That all this is likely to change I hope and expect, but I do not believe that the year 2000 will reproduce what it was like being a doctor 40 years ago [164, 174, 180]. But even if such a miracle happens, we who are doctors now must deal with today's reality.

My father, a neuropsychiatrist, was in practice for 55 years, even until six months before his death at 84. He loved his work (and his family) and considered it a privilege to be a doctor, to be able to work every day helping people, and, as he said, being well paid for being engaged in such interesting, useful activity. I hope my attitude is as good and lasts as long as his.

Before the plastic surgeon and the patient ever get together, much has already happened in society and to them to structure that relationship. Nothing could be truer with respect to their future interaction than the saying that the "past is prologue." This does not mean that what has happened determines everything that will happen, but it does mean that both the plastic surgeon and the patient bring into the relationship his or her expectations, stereotypes, prejudices, and fears based on what he or she has already experienced, learned, or heard about—whether it be rumor, fact, or fantasy. A 1990 Gallup poll survey undertaken for the American Medical Association disclosed that about 70 percent of respondents believe that doctors spend insufficient time with patients; about 60 percent believe that doctors fail to explain things well; 75 percent object to waiting much too long for doctors; about 70 percent feel that doctors are too interested in making money; and about 60 percent think that "doctors don't care about people as much as they used to"—the last a disappointing commentary on a profession that is supposed to be a "caring" one [37, 156].

In the relationship between the doctor and the patient, there is no *tabula rasa;* the blackboard is never completely erased when the next lesson begins.

A critical element that both the patient and the plastic surgeon bring to their relationship is vulnerability. The patient obviously is vulnerable to his or her condition, real or imagined, and to his or her fears that the physician may not provide sufficient skill and empathy; the surgeon is vulnerable because of fears that his or her performance may be insufficient to cure or palliate or to satisfy the expectations of the patient and the family. A major problem in medicine today is the lack of recognition on the part of both the physician and the patient of their mutual vulnerability. How the patient and the plastic surgeon handle this fragility as well as their strength will significantly affect their relationship, even the treatment, and perhaps the outcome.

SOURCES OF PATIENTS

The question of where patients come from is not only interesting but important. What a patient expects of the plastic surgeon and what the plastic surgeon expects of the patient depend to some degree on how that particular patient reached that particular surgeon. For example, someone who chooses a plastic surgeon by asking friends and physicians is a different kind of patient from the one who simply looks in the yellow pages and on that basis alone makes an appointment. In both these instances, however, there is a latitude of choice. The patient who may be in a prepaid health plan and is assigned to that organization's sole plastic surgeon or, perhaps, a panel of several plastic surgeons has limited choice.

The fact that the patient enrolled in a Health Maintenance Organization with fixed referrals already differentiates that individual from others who want to exercise their options in picking their doctor. This distinction is not simply economic, in that prepaid health plans are generally less expensive for the subscriber than individual health plans that allow free choice of physicians; some people, well or ill, are more individualistic than others.

The following list, by no means complete, gives sources for patients to find doctors. Each possibility is not necessarily exclusive, since many patients may use several approaches in finding a plastic surgeon.

> Library research (e.g., *Directory of Medical Specialties*).
> Recommendations from friends who may or may not have been former patients of a specific plastic surgeon.
> Recommendations from a physician, nurse, or administrator financially independent of the plastic surgeon, i.e., not employed in the same Health Maintenance Organization.
> Assignment within a Health Maintenance Organization.
> Local medical society.
> National society (e.g., Executive Office of the American Society of Plastic and Reconstructive Surgeons, Inc.).
> Media (e.g., a program on television or an article in a newspaper or magazine).
> Yellow pages.
> Advertising by the plastic surgeon.
> Assignment under urgent conditions (e.g., in the emergency room where a plastic surgeon is called to attend a patient unable to choose).

Data from the membership of the American Society of Plastic and Reconstructive Surgeons indicate that 43 percent of patient referrals come from other patients; 41 percent from other physicians; 8 percent from yellow page advertising; 3 percent from state or regional societies; 2 percent from the American Society for Plastic and Reconstructive Surgeons; and 3 percent from advertising and public relations [5].

One should remember, however, that no matter how the patient selects a plastic surgeon prior to the initial consultation, every patient expects at least competence. Nobody knowingly chooses an incompetent physician or plastic surgeon.

A significant antecedent, therefore, in the relationship between the patient and the plastic surgeon is the pattern of referral. The interaction between patient and plastic surgeon starts before it actually begins.

SOURCES OF PLASTIC SURGEONS

The emphasis of the preceding few pages has been on the provenance of patients. The obverse, important also, are the sources of plastic surgeons. I am referring here to board-certified plastic surgeons, although I realize that much plastic surgery, both good and bad, is done by those who are not board-certified plastic surgeons. Also, certification per se does not guarantee that the plastic surgeon is competent with regard to the specific operation contemplated. Moreover, even if he or she had the morals of a saint and the skills of a Gillies, operative results might still be imperfect (see Chap. 3).

As we know, plastic surgeons differ in where and how they practice: solo (private), group (within a Health Maintenance Organization or clinic); affiliated or unaffiliated with a university; part- or full-time; geographically based or not. Several combinations of these categories are possible. A 1987 survey of 3,443 active and candidate members of the American Society of Plastic and Reconstructive Surgeons as well as applicants showed that 61 percent were in solo practice; 23 percent in group practice, 6 percent in a multispecialty group, and ten percent were "academicians" [5].

Unlike what medicine was a couple of decades ago, factors beyond the individual plastic surgeon and patient significantly affect how the patient and plastic surgeon will eventually meet and interact. This does not mean that today's patients and plastic surgeons are simply puppets, controlled and manipulated by unseen powers, but it does mean that the complexities of medical care and its cost have decreased physician choice and patient selection.

DOCTOR, PHYSICIAN, SURGEON, OR PLASTIC SURGEON?

When the patient meets the plastic surgeon for the first time, whom is he or she meeting? Does that plastic surgeon think of himself or herself as a plastic surgeon only, as a physician also, or simply as a doctor [111]? I am conscious of these choices whenever I must declare myself, for example, when registering at a hotel. What haunts me is that, perhaps apocryphal, epitaph: "Here lies _____. Born a Man, Died A Gastroenterologist." It would be interesting to survey the approximately 4,000 board-certified plastic surgeons in the United States, asking what they considered themselves primarily to be—doctor, physician, surgeon, or plastic surgeon. The question is not trivial, since each response likely reflects differing attitudes about what they think of themselves and their relationship to the patient. My concept is that I became a doctor when I graduated from medical school, but I am first a physician and second a plastic surgeon. Somehow, despite my five years of training and board certification in general surgery, I do not picture myself primarily as a surgeon in the generic sense, but as a hybrid—a physician–plastic surgeon. Our professional self image determines to a significant degree the way we conduct our consultation with the patient and our subsequent treatment. If the plastic surgeon considers himself or herself a plastic surgeon in the narrowest sense, that person's vision of the patient will likewise be constricted because he or she will not want to "burden" himself or herself with "extras"—some of which are relevant and consequential, as, for example, stresses in the patient's life, such as previous response, both psychological and physiological, to past operations, and to work or marriage. The broader our self image is as professionals, the broader our involvement with the patient will be from the moment we meet him or her to the end of the treatment, and the less likely we are to think of the patient as a mere seeker of and payer for an operation; however, the daily demands of taking care of a large number of patients influence our view of ourselves as well as that of the individual patient. So complex has the edifice of medicine become that the cornerstone, the interaction between patient and doctor, tends too often to become hidden if not forgotten. Talking about the physician and the patient and their interaction is usually reserved for graduation day, generally in speeches given by those who do not have their own patients and do not directly have the responsibility of their daily care.

2

The Initial Consultation

> Medicine always meant service; therefore at all times certain qualities were required of the physician—readiness to help, knowledge concerning the nature of disease, and skill in curing the sick man. However, the medical ideal was a very different one in different periods of history, determined by the structure of the society of the time and by its general conception of the world.
> Henry E. Sigerist, M.D.
> *The Physician's Profession Through the Ages*

BEING A PHYSICIAN AND BEING A PATIENT

He was a 20-year-old African-American from Mississippi; he had left the state that summer for the first time to attend the Harvard Health Professions Program, which enables minority students to view firsthand the workings of medicine. After a morning with me in the operating room and a long afternoon at the office, he exclaimed enthusiastically to his weary mentor, "It must be wonderful having people come to you for help and being able to take care of them." With the brilliant insight of the ingénue, he had captured the essence of medicine, which too often is lost in the process of doctoring. What this young man just beginning his arduous medical journey had not realized was that the patient with treatable ills and the physician with ample skills do not necessarily equal a happy outcome. When and why things go right between a patient and a plastic surgeon and when and why and what to do when they go wrong are what this book is about.

It all begins and ends with the doctor-patient relationship. That phrase, albeit worn, still denotes a special interaction. Although it has been called a "two-party contract," it contains much that is noncontractual—intangibles that cannot be guaranteed in any legal agreement between two persons [60, 69, 78, 83, 173, 201–203]. Indeed, the confusion in the doctor-patient interchange relates to those impalpable but critical components of concern and compassion. In general, patients desire more than having a service performed. Seneca, the Roman statesman and philosopher, wrote: "If, therefore, a physician does nothing more than feel my pulse, put me on the list of those he visits on his rounds, instructing me what to do and what to avoid without any personal feeling, I owe nothing more than his fee because he does not see me as a friend but as a client" [236]. Seneca had in mind this quality of caring on the part of the physician, not just technical competence meted out perfunctorily. It is interesting that recently hospital administrators urged all physicians and medical personnel to call patients "clients," as if that implied an equality that truly existed. As far as I am concerned, that type of thinking is token democracy, without substance but loaded with ambiguity. Illness has been called a "parenthesis in ordinary affairs," but if it is severe, it could be a period to life [134].

A point that too few doctors remember is that the word *patient* is derived from *pati,* Latin for "to suffer." In addition to pain, illness generally has another dimension, a subtle but potent one that relates to the "perceived hierarchy of body parts," as Blacher [26] has phrased it. Cultural and idiosyncratic factors as well as physiological and anatomic considerations determine this ranking, which generally puts the brain and heart at the top of the list and gives precedence to the breast over the gall bladder. Which part of one's body is affected will determine not just the treatment but the attitude of the physician, family, and society in general.

Human beings have endured pain and disease so long that all societies have developed specific expectations of behavior from those who are ill and from those who are supposed to treat them. Being sick has its role requirements, as does being well [161, 228, 241, 247]. Patienthood, however, is a state of being that most of us would like to avoid but almost by necessity must at some time endure.

Patienthood involves duties as well as rights [241]. In all cultures, the one who is ill has a responsibility to help himself or herself get better with guidance from the healer, who is a physician in our society. Although sickness is allowed, under most circumstances it is not praised or perpetuated since no society could function effectively or survive if most of its members were unable to perform their tasks, such as gathering food, bearing children, and defending the community. Furthermore, the sick person has the added responsibility of getting better as quickly as possible in order not to strain the resources of the society in caring for that individual.

In general, a patient consults a doctor in our culture because of a problem, real or imagined, and the need for help. Few patients have the confidence to make a medical decision or the means to implement it. They are likely to be under strain—emotional, physical, or both—and may even have pain. Patients hope that their problem is not serious, that their recovery will be rapid, and that medical care will be available and affordable, the latter not always possible within the United States.

Siegler and Osmond [241] state that

> The art of patienthood lies in being medically prudent, which means steering a well-plumbed course between the Scylla of medical piety and the Charybdis of skepticism and self-treatment. . . . One cannot take a rigid stance, but rather, one must engage in a continuous dialogue between oneself and the doctor, between oneself and oneself: "How much can I expect from the treatment this doctor has to offer? How much will be demanded of me? Am I willing to carry out my part of the bargain? Does this doctor have my best interests at heart? Is he a good doctor? How much is known about my illness? Am I better not treated at all? Am I prepared to live with myself if I don't treat it and it gets worse? Am I prepared to live with myself if I *do* treat it and it gets worse? What price am I willing to pay for putting myself in this doctor's hands? If I feel things are going badly, or if I have had enough, will he listen?"

Being a good patient does not mean being a totally compliant, unquestioning patient. The patient, if possible, must be alert to his or her treatment and should exercise some degree of critical evaluation. The sticky point comes when the doctor interprets, perhaps correctly, the patient's assessment of the care being received as "complaining." The patient then falls into the category of "difficult" and may soon be on the way to being shunned or shunted.

As Siegler and Osmond [241] have observed: "A sick person at home is like an animal in its natural habitat; a sick person in a hospital is like an animal in the zoo. At home, the patient and family draw strength from being in their own territory, with its familiar surroundings and comforts. In the hospital, the patient lives in an alien and frightening environment, while the family skulks in the corridors, without a territory and so almost without a status."

Some patients react to being totally dependent on a foreign environment by becoming more demanding; others, by turning mute, give up, and enter a state of resigned passivity. The good physician, whatever he or she may be in addition, such as a plastic surgeon, must be able to perceive the patient's predicament and act promptly to ameliorate it.

The honor that is accorded every healer in every society carries also an onus [242]. For the privilege and power bestowed by the culture, the healer has definite responsibilities to the sick. These include being available, maximally using his or her skills to help the patient, and behaving with concern, compassion, dignity, and honesty [249]. The healer must not exploit the patient sexually, financially, or in any other way, such as making the patient undergo a clinical trial of a new technique or medication without having sufficiently informed the patient and the family if the patient is a minor or is unable to comprehend the risks and alternatives of treatment.

In a world with so much mistrust in general and now with mistrust of the medical profession, it is reassuring and even surprising to witness how most patients will reveal confidences, allow examinations (and in plastic surgery even photographs) of parts of the body usually not seen by strangers, entrust their lives to a person known to them perhaps just a few minutes before and then only by name; sometimes, as in an emergency, even that is unknown. The success of this process is due not just to the performance of that doctor or that patient but to centuries of successful doctor-patient interaction [85]. Any erosion of that trust has consequences not just for that particular patient and a doctor but for future patients and physicians. Faith in proper enactment of roles is not unique to medicine in our society or our times. It has existed whenever and wherever living has become sufficiently complex to require different tasks of different people. In small, primitive societies, entrusting one's life to an unknown human being is rare. In our culture it is commonplace. We allow restaurants with unseen cooks to prepare our meals, and, as air passengers, we put our lives in the hands of pilots who we have never met, and we trust machinery that we cannot comprehend. Even the most cynical among us expects an event to turn out as expected according to probability. When, in fact, a plane mysteriously explodes, our vulnerability is thrust on us and we become overtly fearful and anxious. Most people who become patients and most people who become doctors expect that when each meets the other, if the medical condition is not serious and the treatment is uncomplicated, the outcome will be satisfactory. We know, of course, that the result could be otherwise, disastrously so, but we usually suppress or repress that dire intruding thought.

Not every person is born to be an excellent patient, as if endowed by nature. A person can improve as a performer in his or her patient status through the exigencies of the medical situation, submitting without fuss when there are few if any alternatives, with proper instructions from the doctor and appropriate support from family and friends. The role of the patient requires dependency, with which all adults, even those seemingly most independent, are familiar, primarily because they were all once infants and children. But some patients have great difficulty acknowledging that dependency, which illness and disability intensify. For them, denying their deep desire to be cared for has been an important mechanism for achieving independence. The discerning physician should be alert to the basis for the behavior of those who "protest too much" about accepting patienthood.

Selfishness and Altruism in Medicine
To think of the physician and the practice of medicine as being "altruistic" and some other activities in our society, such as business, as being "selfish" would be naive and incorrect. Parsons noted "the seeming paradox . . . that it is to a physician's self-interest to act contrary to his own self-interest, in an immediate situation, of course, not 'in the long run' " [201].

Physicians, therefore, conform to their social role by putting the welfare of patients above their own—at least they should, for example, by being available for emergencies, by working long hours, by reducing or omitting fees, the last more in the past than present. In return, physicians generally receive respect, are addressed in the United States not as Mr. or Mrs. but as Dr., and earn a higher average income than most people and most professionals; in short, "from whom more is given, more is expected," a Biblical aphorism frequently expressed by Dr. Albert Schweitzer.

> *Only He Who Is A Good Person Can Be A Good Doctor*
> A. Nottnagel

The validity of this quote from the renowned nineteenth-century physician, Nottnagel, initially seems obvious; yet on reflection, the "good person = good doctor" equation is simplistic. A kindly person should and may be a kindly doctor, yet that person might not be a competent doctor. Moral probity is not necessarily synonymous with job capability. In fact in certain fields, such as politics, these attributes may be mutually exclusive. Some physicians, moreover, are excellent professionally yet cheat on their income taxes and on their wives. Human beings can compartmentalize their behavior in the fulfillment of their different roles.

Drane, in trying to assess the place of virtue and character in medical ethics, concluded that

> doctors should also pay attention to the tradition, with its emphasis on individual virtues and character. The realities of character and habits of heart are important to becoming a good doctor. And so, too, are commitments to solving public medical issues and public policies and helping the needy get adequate medical care. The medical tradition includes public commitment and objective norms as well as character development and medical virtues. If doctors do not pay attention to their tradition, which moves in both of these directions, they will become more and more like the rest of us in American culture: preoccupied with facades rather than substance. The phony or selfish doctor, however, turns out being uglier than the similarly distorted lawyer, politician or businessman: more repulsive, more offensive, and more of a scandal. Maybe this tells us something about what makes a doctor different [62].

As Drane also notes, talking about virtue these days approaches the laughable since the topic seems too pious and self-righteous to the usual person. Furthermore, even if one could talk about virtue freely, would the discussion necessarily generate virtue? How does one teach virtue? By example? But most of us know of people whose parents, as far as we can determine, were highly ethical but they turned out differently; we recall physicians who had studied with the most ethical in their field, yet inexplicably emerged with a moral flaw, which likely had always been there but with time became evident.

I would define a good doctor as somebody who not only knows what to diagnose and treat with regard to the patient's medical condition both technically and psychologically—but also has an implacable personal commitment to the patient and to his or her well-being. I believe that one cannot learn that sense of responsibility in or after medical school; it has to be present much earlier in life. However it gets there, a sense of personal responsibility for the patient is the necessary hallmark of a good physician. Although admittedly some people learn to dissimulate their selfishness and can even force themselves to put the interests of the patient above their own for the short-term, the cover-up usually does not last long: That person's true self will be more visible as he or she gets older and achieves the status desired, and becomes more lax about commitment to others. This does not mean that egocentric people cannot enter medicine; it does mean that to be a good physician a narcissist must include others, such as patients, within his or her sphere of self-interest.

Genesis

The relationship between the patient and the plastic surgeon must begin at some point. As I have mentioned, antecedents to the initial consultation bring the patient and the surgeon together through a variety of reasons and a variety of ways: from a formal introduction in a hospital to an unplanned meeting at a cocktail party.

Many years ago, at one of the meetings of the American Society of Plastic and Reconstructive Surgery, I took a rhinoplasty course from the doyen of that subject, Dr. Gustave Aufricht. His first words were: "Of course to do a rhinoplasty properly, you must have a patient." To those of us starting in practice, his observation had a painful cogency. I am now fortunate enough to have many patients, but sometimes I am amused and surprised by the circuitous course of referral. In most urban areas of the United States, patients, unless in a plan that assigns them to a specific plastic surgeon, have a choice.

Although certain types of patients may gravitate to certain kinds of doctors, based on a personality characteristic, this phenomenon is probably less seen in plastic surgery than in other medical areas where the doctor-patient relationship is protracted, such as internal medicine, general practice, gynecology, and psychiatry. For many patients, their interaction with a plastic surgeon will be short-lived, and they might overlook a lack of empathy and sympathy by reasoning that "it will be over soon." Admittedly, this would be far from an ideal doctor-patient relationship, but it might still be workable. Later if that patient wishes additional plastic surgery, he or she may try to find another plastic surgeon. With more choice available now than even a few years ago, the patient at the outset does not need to feel constrained to accept an unsatisfactory situation with a doctor who is irascible, uncaring, or possibly incompetent.

The physician—specifically for our purposes, the plastic surgeon—also chooses his or her patients to some degree. As economic pressure increases because of greater competition, however, the plastic surgeon who once favored a particular referral pattern will become less choosy and even grateful when patients arrive at his or her office. Yet plastic surgeons still select patients in various ways. A surgeon who does only esthetic operations will not see those who require reconstruction. Hand surgeons will not treat patients with head and neck tumors. High fees for consultation and operation may eliminate the relatively poor. Some plastic surgeons dislike "minor" procedures such as the excision of lesions, and these patients either will not receive an appointment or will be given one so far in the future that most of them will seek another doctor. Some surgeons and patients do better with those of the opposite sex or with a different personality. One patient may feel secure with an authoritarian doctor whom another might find arrogant. A surgeon's sense of humor will relax some patients but annoy others. Race and ethnicity may influence a patient's selection of a plastic surgeon. More African-Americans and Asian-Americans are seeking esthetic procedures that they may want performed by someone of similar background with whom they may feel more comfortable. Today, compared to just a decade ago, the spectrum of plastic surgeons in the United States includes every race and almost every ethnic group. Many factors, therefore, influence the choice of doctor and of patient; however, as noted earlier, many patients are being assigned to plastic surgeons just as they have been assigned to other doctors within a prepaid medical plan.

THE SETTING

I have alluded to the setting earlier. The usual places for a plastic surgeon and a prospective patient to meet are a private office, a private clinic, a clinic at a teaching hospital or a nonteaching hospital, an emergency room, or the patient's bedside.

In general, the patient who has an appointment with a private plastic surgeon already knows at least the name, if not the reputation, of the person who may perform the operation. In many clinics, especially at a university hospital, the patient generally does not know beforehand who will be the surgeon. The reputation of the hospital or the medical school, not that of the individual surgeon, is what brings many patients to the clinic. The Leahy Clinic and the Mayo Clinic are spectacular examples of patient magnets. Care there, in a clinic of lesser repute, or at a university hospital may be better or worse than it would be with a private doctor; what is certain, however, is the fact that the settings and the circumstances differ.

Patients may fear that in a private office they will be exploited for financial reasons; in the university setting, they may fear they will be used for teaching purposes. Even in a private office patients frequently ask, "Who is going to do the surgery?" The specter of the "ghost surgeon" is strong. The patient's questions should be answered clearly and honestly. One should remember that the patients in a doctor's office, wherever it may be located, or in a hospital bed, are isolated from their usual environment. They are on somebody else's turf. If a member of the family accompanies the patient, you may gain some idea of the family dynamics, but only at a distance and only partially. On a few occasions I have made a house call, usually for a patient with a decubitus ulcer for whom a visit to the office or hospital would be a great inconvenience. One then has the opportunity to see the patient in his or her own surroundings, among their pictures and photographs and interacting with *their* family. The doctor thus observes the patient in vivo. Yet, even in a home, we fail to see the patient in his or her usual role, healthy or at work; thus our knowledge of that person is still partial.

The Hospital

The hospital is a phenomenon among institutions and within our society. It is so commonplace today that we seldom remember that its birth and development required centuries. We physicians are so accustomed to the hospital and its vagaries that we forget the fear that it evokes in a patient, the family, and even in visitors. Although the hospital may be a familiar setting for television dramas, the viewer who becomes a patient will experience different emotions. He or she will certainly not feel simply entertained.

A hospitalized patient's perspective of the world changes, not only because illness and fear of death reorder priorities, but literally one becomes horizontal while the rest of the world is vertical [222]. A few hours ago the patient was a participant, and now he or she is out of the game, a relatively powerless observer of the ongoing scene.

Although patients entering a hospital may be handed a Bill of Rights, now a popular and regular feature in many hospitals [23, 51], they will seldom be completely reassured [23]. They are likely fearful and anxious not primarily because of the possibility of death but because of the uncertainty—uncertainty, in fact, being the only certainty. A patient realizes that events will be soon beyond his or her control, just as his or her illness is. Once proud of their individuality and accomplishments, patients generally come to the unpleasant realization that they are "just like everybody else." Tagged with a hospital number and entered into the hospital's inexorable, bewildering routine, dressed in a tasteless unisex garment, they have become almost nameless among the minority of the sick. Even the most caring of physicians and nurses as well as ancillary personnel cannot totally dispel this feeling of loss of control [223]. One of my patients summed it up nicely: "Going into the hospital for me was like going into the army: You realized that there was little you could do about anything and to make the best of it, you simply had to lie back and let events sweep you on—toward what you were never sure." Although a patient may feel that he or she has been treated humanely, hospitalization inevitably entails dehumanization. A woman, for example, admitted for operation that day must relinquish the clothes that she purchased with great care, the jewelry and rings that have commemorated important events in her life, the makeup and nail polish that she may have just applied with such punctiliousness—all this in the name of safety and under the edict of routine. Even though she may realize that these measures are for her ultimate good, that is an abstraction; the tangible feeling is being helped but helpless on a therapeutic assembly line.

The reasons for doing things in a certain way in a hospital are usually known and are unambiguous to the staff but not always to the patient. Moreover, the patient in pain or under medication may be even more bewildered and feel more helpless.

As someone who has been a patient for relatively minor problems—a kidney stone and an umbilical hernia—I can assure you that being the doctor, despite the long hours and stress, is far preferable. When we are on the giving side of the bed, we usually think that we know what we are doing and what will happen [26]. The patient, in contrast, is never quite sure even though he or she may have been well informed. Every day that I go to the hospital as a surgeon, I never think that I may not emerge alive or intact. Not so with the patient. Even the most rational will have an irrational thought that may dominate a brain that on most occasions is the essence of pure reasoning. As an example, one of my relatives, a skilled businessman, had severe anxiety when his surgeon told him, in response to his query, that the chance of his dying from the operation was "1 in 500,000." The "1" far outshadowed the other 499,000.

In the hospital, time becomes the supreme factor [289]: admissions, operations, medications, tests, and procedures are scheduled; the staff walk briskly, even running in an emergency. Today's work must be finished today only to begin again tomorrow. The hospital has little randomness. Not much is left to probability except the outcome of treatment, which, after all, is the principal concern of the patient.

Stephen Vincent Benet described this abnormal world within the world:

> As he often did when he waked up, he had a sense of the whole big mechanism of the hospital, cut off from the rest of the world, yet self-sufficient, like a boat or a train. That was a hang-over from the dreams after the operation. But it made an amount of sense. There was a routine, with fixed stops, and you saw a great deal of people you would probably never see again. Sometimes you didn't even see them—just knew them as you knew his name or, No Visitors, from a card stuck in a door or in a radio heard through the wall. . . . So it was all modern and scientific and well-arranged. You could die very nearly as privately in a modern hospital as you could in the Grand Central Station, and with much better care [17].

In comparison to the patient, the physician in the hospital has the power. Yet, this past decade has seen its waning.

Gamble, president of the Hospital Council of Southern California, recently wrote:

> When the doctors on your medical staff start working for the nurses, how will you cope with the management challenges? [He was addressing hospital administrators.] A convergence of factors is irreversibly changing the power structure between physicians and nurses in the hospital, and hospital management is caught in the middle. For a century, convention has held that only a medical doctor can practice medicine, and a nurse is the physician's handmaiden. Now, however, it appears that convention does not match reality. The public's image of the ideal physician—who is kindly, capable, caring, and reassuring as Dr. Marcus Welby of television fame—is more often embodied by a nurse. The demarcation between the roles of physician and nurse is rapidly blurring. And while the nurse wants management to support the changes, the physician expects management to preserve the status quo. . . . Medicine has divided up the patients into episodic visits among its various specialists. In contrast, nursing has honed the skills of understanding, monitoring, and caring for the whole person around the clock. The physician may be legally 'in charge' of the patient, but the nurse in the indispensable mechanism for managing most of the healing process—which often involves knowing whether and when to call in the physician's specialized expertise. . . . The science of medicine, with its spectacular cures, has made crisis care the physician's treatment of choice, leaving the art of healing to the professional nurse. . . .[84]

Although I would strenuously dispute the last point, the fact that this statement was made by an authority in hospital management undoubtedly reflects a commonly held view. Most hospital administrators likely find that the nursing staff appreciates even minimal kindness and especially anything that reinforces and elevates their status; whereas dealing with physicians usually poses difficulties and problems. Physicians are less likely to be grateful than angry; in contrast, nurses are more likely to be thankful for recognition of their obvious skills and their rising status. In short, the physician–surgeon–plastic surgeon is no longer the cock of the walk. We physicians are witnessing our status and power within the hospital decrease while the opposite is happening to nurses, administrators, and skilled and even semiskilled workers [251].

When I first entered the hospital as a medical student (and it was *not* in the nineteenth century), nurses rose when the attending made his (it was always a "he") appearance. Now, as we know, the attitude is "get it yourself." There is more democracy and less rigid hierarchy. As plastic surgeons, we frequently have to fight for hospital beds, operating time, even a parking place. Although admittedly the patient has less control of his or her destiny in the hospital, the physician's perch, whatever his or her specialty, is less secure as well.

The Office

In the hospital, the plastic surgeon is but one of many, with little opportunity of putting his or her impress on the environment. This is not so in the office, where the physician has greater control. In fact, some plastic surgeons, especially those who exclusively do esthetic surgery, have transformed what may have been a large office into an imposing edifice. There the plastic surgeon reigns supreme, perhaps more so than in his or her own home, where the presence of a spouse forces compromise.

There are many types of offices, depending on the location as well as the occupant. For example, even the chief of a service is a temporary tenant in a hospital and cannot build an office according to only his or her liking; it must conform to the existing structure of the hospital and to its regulations and building codes. Hospitals, furthermore, are always short of space, for which many potentates compete.

In contrast is the office in a building owned by the plastic surgeon where the limitations are fewer and the possibilities greater to satisfy necessity as well as whim. Enough money can accomplish seeming miracles, at least structural ones.

For purposes of this book, I have chosen to focus on the private office, which is still the most common setting for the first elective interaction between a plastic surgeon and a patient. Nationwide, most plastic surgeons rent their offices.

During the time the patient is in our office, whether waiting for you or being with you, he or she consciously and unconsciously forms an impression of where you work, what you do, and what you are like. In reality, you are your office. The way you furnish, decorate, equip, and manage your office is an extension of yourself. For this reason, every physician is or should be aware of the image he or she projects or wishes to project.

A plastic surgeon who wants to do only esthetic surgery, for example, is more likely to have as reading materials *Vogue, Town and Country, Mirabella,* and perhaps a foreign magazine, such as *Réalités,* than *Popular Mechanics, Scientific American,* and *Baseball Digest.* The intended slant in the former instance is toward upper-class women who wish to maintain their beauty and not toward the factory worker with a hand injury or a basal cell carcinoma of the face. Whatever the reading material, keep it current. Patients resent out-of-date magazines that are crumpled and torn. Their displeasure is compounded if they note that the magazine is a discard from the doctor's home. No one likes being considered second best.

The way a doctor desires to be seen is frequently not the way others see him or her. Some patients in a lavish office may feel reassured and comfortable because the doctor seems to understand the rich and powerful and would also appear to be successful and wealthy. Other patients may regard fancy furnishings as a facade and as evidence of a doctor's penchant for expensive things obtained by charging excessive fees. That patient may believe that the doctor, through presumably competent, is a poseur and is on the make professionally.

Qualities that patients universally appreciate are those that we like or should like most in ourselves: honesty, competence, and concern, which should be reflected in the office [249]. In addition, most patients would prefer that the office be clean, orderly, and attractive.

2 The Initial Consultation

This is especially true in regard to plastic surgeons, who should know the importance of appearance. William Carlos Williams, a poet-obstetrician, was not that concerned about how his office looked:

> *Oh,* I suppose I should
> Wash the walls of my office
> Polish the rust from my instruments and keep them
> Definitely in order
> Build shelves in the laboratory
> Empty out the old stains
> Clean the bottles
> And refill them, buy
> Another lens, put
> My journals on edge instead of
> Letting them lie flat
> In heaps—then begin
> Ten years back and
> Gradually read them to date. . . .[279]

The sophisticated, urban patient seeking a facelift would have little sympathy with that attitude though it might have relaxed Williams' patients in Rutherford, New Jersey (population about 20,000).

Decor differs with geography. What may appear normal-modern in Beverly Hills might seem garish and distastefully slick in Boston.

These considerations about furnishings are not minor since they affect the relationship between patient and plastic surgeon, not simply because of appearance but because of the fact that how you may appear to the patient depends largely on how you think of yourself. Some plastic surgeons consider themselves plastic surgeons; some as general surgeons with special skills; some, simply as physicians; others as cosmetic technicians; still others, only a small minority now, as vendors. If the office and the demeanor of the doctor and staff resemble more closely a beauty parlor than a medical facility, the patient will conclude that no "real operations" with real risk are being done here. Any complication will then be hard for the patient to accept because the stage has been set for a hazard-free medical jaunt. The ambience of the office may actually produce a more vivid set of expectations in the patient than any informed consent with its detailed disclaimers.

The plastic surgeon whose image is that of a highly skilled cosmetician may be surprised that patients do not consider him or her a "real doctor." It is difficult to build and maintain two disparate images successfully.

One's personal style should be evident, not a decorator's fashion grafted onto the plastic surgeon like a poorly matched piece of skin—unless, of course, the style is somebody else's fashion. In the words of Yves Saint Laurent, "I like style—I don't like fashion. Fashion disappears. Style remains."

One recalls the statement of Buffon, the eighteenth century naturalist, who, in his discourse on the occasion of his admission to the French Academy, declared: "The style is the man himself." Of course, one has to add ". . . the woman herself."

One is what one is; despite seemingly endless variations, the basic theme remains. One cannot surmount one's personality; one can modify it and overcome certain unwanted characteristics. One may even be able to control one's behavior, to develop a new persona under specific conditions, but one can never totally transform the self into a new person.

ANATOMY AND PHYSIOLOGY OF THE INITIAL CONSULTATION

We will now consider the what and how of the first encounter between patient and plastic surgeon. Although the initial consultation may bring together two people who have never known each other, the scene, as has already been mentioned, has been set long ago [142]. Into that meeting, each carries an established personality with behavior patterns evolved from innumerable responses to countless previous social interactions and stimuli. The patient has likely had other illnesses and interactions with a physician. The doctor too has probably been a patient on more than one occasion. The patient and the doctor will likely behave in a way that each perceives as the proper role for being the doctor or being the patient—roles culturally defined and transmitted from one generation to another. Were Hippocrates able to witness a consultation in a Boston office in 1992, he would see a ritual familiar to him, although the dress and props would have changed.

In theory, the patient and the doctor could interact in infinite ways;

in reality, they do not [18, 19, 25]. What happens is remarkably circumscribed; perhaps there is unpredictable variation but always on a predictable theme. This does not mean, however, that correct judgment is not necessary for both the patient and the physician to take in order to find the wisest course for each.

The patient and the doctor are conscious to some degree, not totally, of the impression that each is creating; each is acting differently from how he or she would under other circumstances, for example, at a cocktail party or at lunch with a friend. The doctor-patient consultation could serve as an excellent illustration of what Goffman has called "the presentation of self in everyday life." He has written:

> When we allow that the individual projects a definition of the situation when he appears before others (a group or another person), we must also see that the others, however passive their role may seem to be, will themselves effectively project a definition of the situation by virtue of their response to the individual and by virtue of any lines of action they initiate to him. Ordinarily the definitions of the situation projected by the several different participants are sufficiently attuned to one another so that open contradiction will not occur. I do not mean that there will be the kind of consensus that arises when each individual present candidly expresses what he really feels and honestly agrees with the expressed feelings of the others present. This kind of harmony is an optimistic ideal and in any case not necessary for the smooth working of society. Rather, each participant is expected to suppress his immediate heartfelt feelings, conveying a view of the situation which he feels the others will be able to find at least temporarily acceptable. Maintenance of this surface of agreement, this veneer of consensus, is facilitated by each participant concealing his own wants behind statements which assert values to which everyone present feels obliged to give lip service . . . when an individual appears before others he will have many motives for trying to control the impression they receive of the situation [88].

This process of "impression management" and the awareness of self and role(s) that each of us is to play have evolved to prevent or lessen social breakdown [246]. Within any stable society, most people do what is expected—drive on the correct side of the road, give a gift when appropriate and receive a "thank you" in return, go to the restroom labeled *Men* or *Women,* and so forth. In any given situation, no person exhibits his or her full potential. We neither say everything we think nor do everything we could. Accordingly, we never or rarely know someone else's every thought. We see only some of that person's actions, and our vision is influenced by what someone wants us to see as well as what we are predisposed to see. Under most circumstances of everyday life, these limitations do not impede the successful outcome of our transaction. For example, consider the instance of my going into a department store to purchase a tie. At the counter, as I am making my selection, I am aware of the salesperson, who is a young, attractive woman (I have instantly noted her sex, race, age, and physical attributes, her face, in particular [204]). I may even deduce from her rings whether she is married. Unconsciously or consciously I have already observed how she is dressed and how she is interacting with other customers—well spoken, efficient, pleasant? And she has surveyed me but most likely not with the same thoughts as mine. She will know, of course, my sex, race, and approximate age. She may judge my appearance less in terms of physical attractiveness than in terms of potential for buying: He looks well dressed and prosperous. These observations become even more important if her salary is based on what she sells; however, chances are that her income is fixed. Perhaps it is 4:00 in the afternoon. She is tired and bedraggled, yearning to leave the store after just one more hour. Inwardly, she may groan when I appear. Yet, mustering a smile she will invariably say, "May I help you, sir?" From the many possible replies, I will most probably say, "Yes, please." I have noted that she called me "sir," and I have had a fleeting twinge of disappointment with that further evidence of my aging—I may also wince because she is about the age of my daughter. None of this, however, ever gets expressed and she will probably never know my thoughts. (For her part, she may think "He is my father's age.")

The litany of our relationship continues—predictably:

She: Cash or credit?
I: Do you take Visa?
She: Yes.

While she is processing the sale and as she puts the tie into a bag, she may think, "What a dull tie!" But she would never say it. To break the monotony, I may offer something like, "The store seems really busy today" (certainly not a Churchillian phrase to be treasured by posterity). Mechanically she will acknowledge it by mumbling, "Yes, it is." Or, to her surprise and mine, she might smile, look up, and say, "You should have seen it yesterday. I was really strung out then." Tie in hand, I leave the store. I have learned nothing about her background (unless she has a distinctive accent), her life's dreams, her pleasures, or her pains. Nothing intimate has been exchanged. Any attempt in this direction would have been justifiably interpreted as forward, inappropriate, perhaps bizarre. Yet, an hour and a half later, that same person will be relating in a much different fashion to the man or woman in her life. Under those conditions, her thoughts and actions will differ from what they were in the store, but they will follow a somewhat predictable pattern. Her boyfriend, who may pick her up at work (predictably at 5:15), gets a kiss (as soon as she gets into her seat she will lean to the left and he, to the right) perhaps a sign more of relief than of passion. Then she will settle back and light a cigarette, glad that the working day is finished. He or she will ask "How was your day?" And so on, each reacting with the other according to expectations and experience. Only in a mental hospital, perhaps not even there, could the following sequence occur:

He: How was your day?
She: Turnips are lousy to eat.
He: Cronin is running for mayor.
She: [No response—keeping silent for an hour.]

She will not pick her nose in front of him and he will not drive on the left side of a two-way street (even in Boston).

The vignettes of my purchasing a tie or the salesgirl with her boyfriend are mundane events in ordinary living; however, those happenings make up most of life. Let us now return to what might transpire at the time of the initial consultation.

The patient and the plastic surgeon will establish a relationship that has features common to any relationship between two human beings and between any patient and any doctor; yet it will also have aspects distinctive of the specialty of plastic surgery [266].

Recognition and communication characterize the process by which two people get to know each other [253]. An exchange of information and feelings takes place, largely through language and intonation, but what is not verbalized can be as important or more so than what is. The body also communicates—by facial expression, gesture, and posture, for example. Within the first few minutes or even seconds of the initial consultation, the patient and the physician have appraised each other. In a computer fashion, each receives and stores information about appearance (attractive, neat, well dressed, or not), about manner (concerned, likeable, friendly, honest, or not), and about intelligence (bright or not). The patient will quickly form an impression of whether he or she can trust that doctor with the diagnosis and treatment of the problem. The physician also rapidly judges the patient, not only in terms of the diagnosis and possible treatment, but also of the patient's capacity for cooperation. In what sequence and in what order of importance each evaluates the other is not generally known since it is complex and instantaneous; moreover, the assessment of the patient and physician will vary according to needs and values of the individuals involved.

Before meeting, the patient and the doctor usually know each other's gender. Undoubtedly, there are differences in the reactions of a doctor and patient according to the sex of the other. Though these dissimilarities in response may be subtle and momentary, they exist. Normally, the importance of the medical problem transcends or should transcend these considerations of sex. When there is ambiguity about gender, as with transsexuals, the physician, unaccustomed to these patients, may be visibly disturbed by not knowing how to classify them: whether to call them Ms. or Mr. or by what first name—and, in general, how to react to them.

Without venturing too far into the realm of psychoanalysis, one could safely postulate that the female patient will probably react to the physician who is male and older in some measure as she has related to other male authority figures: father, teacher, perhaps husband, and other doctors. Or she may sense the hostility of the male physician who has never liked women, perhaps because of an unsatisfying relationship with his mother, wife, or both. Depending on previous experiences as well as age differential, the male patient may view a doctor of the same sex as a grandfather, father, brother, son, or peer. I remember a male executive, about 10 years younger than I, immediately addressing me by my first name with the explanation that "I always called my father by his first name. I hope you won't mind."

Differences or similarities in race, religion, and socioeconomic status may also affect, at least initially, the interaction between patient and physician. In the United States, where we like to think that enlightened tolerance exists more than it really does, we avoid discussing these uncomfortable issues. Unfortunately ability and need are not the only criteria by which the patient and the doctor judge one another. Each unconsciously and consciously holds stereotypes. Although this process may allow valid conclusions, it may also permit harmful prejudices. The patient and the physician may disregard important individual variations in formulating comfortable categories—"comfortable" because the familiar gets imposed on the new; each is navigating unknown waters. The advantage is ease; the disadvantage may be error.

As has been emphasized before, the initial consultation does not arise de novo; the substrate has been present for a lifetime—two lifetimes.

Any action of a human being and any interaction with another can be broken down into component parts, small or large, and can be analyzed at different levels and from different perspectives: physiological, psychological (conscious or unconscious), personal, social, cultural, cross-cultural, religious, philosophical, cosmological.

Consider the geometric, stepwise description by the novelist Robbe-Grillet:

> Then, holding the letter in one hand A . . . closes the drawer, moves toward the little work table (near the second window, against the partition separating the bedroom from the hallway) and sits down in front of the writing-case from which she removed a sheet of pale blue paper—similar to the first but blank. She unscrews the cap of her pen, then, after a glance to the right (which does not include the middle of the window-frame behind her), bends her head toward the writing-case in order to begin writing [222].

Tedious, mechanistic, yet accurate. Another writer with a different purpose and style might have stated simply, "She took some paper from the desk and wrote."

Similarly, the tableau of patient and doctor can be presented with broad strokes or in *pointillism*. My purpose is to make the reader aware that more is occurring than one might previously have believed, and that the tableau is not static but changing. The patient and the doctor meet for a short time in the continuum and complexity of their lives.

If one could analyze the patient's first visit in a time-frame sequence, it would become obvious that hundreds and even thousands of events take place. These happenings, moreover, involve numerous decisions, unconscious and conscious. For example, is the patient required on arrival at your office to announce his or her name in front of the other patients? Where does your secretary (or nurse) tell the patient to wait, and where does he or she choose to sit? Is the waiting room for only your patients, or for those of doctors in the same specialty or in a different area of medicine? In this regard, one of my colleagues, who does esthetic as well as head and neck surgery (an unusual combination for these times), believes that those seeking cosmetic procedures will be repelled by the sight of patients who have had radical neck dissections, and therefore he sees each group on different days. Aside from the possible comfort of the cosmetic patients, he does not wish a prospective patient to wonder whether he who obviously does extensive ablation could also do or would even be interested in "delicate" esthetic operations.

A seemingly minor clerical procedure also involves complex decisions with various advantages, disadvantages, and consequences. Does one ask the occupation of the spouse? If so, who asks it, when, and why? Is it a means of reaching the family should an emergency arise? Is it to know the socioeconomic status of the patient in order to set the fee?

Other decisions concern how and by whom the past history and system review are obtained. Some doctors, like myself, view history taking as integral to the process of doctoring and they will use this occasion of securing information to help establish a relationship. Other physicians regard the history as a chore preferably done by someone else who, they feel, can do it as well, and thus they are unencumbered to see more patients, increasing efficiency and income as well as decreasing tedium. Another alternative is to have patients make out their own questionnaires. Some patients resent doing this because they feel it is the doctor's job and not even that of the secretary or nurse. Advantages of having the patient do it include efficient use of time, a greater chance of completeness, and the fact that nobody knows the patient's past better than the patient. Furthermore, any information that is lacking or erroneous would be a result of the patient's error and not that of the surgeon or of anyone in the office. This possibly could be an important benefit from a medicolegal standpoint. Even though the secretary or nurse or someone else in the office may have access to information in the record, a patient usually has a greater sense of privacy if he or she is not made to divulge personal facts to someone who is not a physician. A major benefit of having the doctor or a trained interviewer obtain the history rather than having the patient supply it is the greater likelihood of being certain that the patient has understood the questions. Also, one can pursue a point if the answer seems significant. This is particularly true with respect to ascertaining whether the patient takes drugs, e.g., cocaine, or imbibes too much alcohol. These points may be denied on the questionnaire, whereas an offhand inquiry, such as "Do you use coke for social or recreational purposes?" might evoke the information desired. Responses to a questionnaire also tend to be flat without clues to their possible importance for the patient. The purpose of this discussion about history taking is not to champion one way over another but to illustrate that whatever course is taken, others are excluded.

The variations in taking a history and in running an office reflect the differing styles and objectives of doctors. Specifically, some plastic surgeons think of themselves as furnishing a service—an operative procedure—and view their interaction with the patient as a necessary prologue to what transpires in the operating room. Consciously and unconsciously, they do not want their relationship with the patient to be more involved than what is needed to deliver their product. Perhaps they prefer distance in all their relationships. Other doctors, myself included, want more than a glancing encounter with a patient. I enjoy the depth and breadth of the more classic doctor-patient relationship. As a specialist, my surgical care is restricted to a relatively narrow-gauge track—but not my concern for that person and his or her life beyond the problem that has brought about our meeting.

In addition to varying with the personality of the doctor, the routine of the office differs also with the locale: Standard office procedure in Juneau, Alaska is not the same as in Manhattan. Moreover, the average type of doctor and patient in each of these cities is probably dissimilar, at least superficially in terms of life-styles, even though they may have the same ideals: peace, not war; kindness, not cruelty; longevity, not early death.

Since the patient has come to your office to get help, the reality is that the form and content of the initial consultation are determined more by your style and desires than those of the patient. Hopefully, your objectives will coincide with those of the patient, but frequently this is not true. The physician who is overly aloof and insular may not perceive, much less fulfill, the emotional needs of the person in his or her care. Under these conditions, if the relationship proceeds to an operation, events unfortunate for both can happen.

Face to Face

At some point you and the patient meet for the first time. After nearly two decades in practice and thousands of patients, I still find that moment exciting. Admittedly, I am less enthusiastic when I am tired, late, or both. Yet even then I am conscious that this moment could be the start of a medical adventure or misadventure.

Your encounter with the patient involves several choices and decisions, largely on your part. Do you see the patient in an examining room, relatively bare, where the emphasis is on the physical aspects of his or her problem—the diagnosis and treatment? Or do you routinely begin in your office, usually larger than an examining room and furnished in a style conducive to relaxation and to talking: rugs, pictures on the wall, mementos on the desk? In the former situation, your purpose is clear: No loitering allowed. You do not want to "waste time" with what you consider extraneous discussion or emotions. In the latter instance, you have provided more of a living room atmosphere and are trying to draw out the patient, to expand the boundaries of your mutual interaction.

How the patient arrives in the consultation area can also occur in more than one way. Is he or she led by the secretary or someone else who has called his or her name? Or does that person who is familiar with the patient from the preliminary paperwork preserve confidentiality in a crowded waiting room by a nod or a tap on the shoulder? Is the patient accompanied by someone, or is he or she too afraid to ask whether you would allow this? Does the secretary or receptionist, knowing your desires, encourage or discourage a friend or family member to be present?

Once the patient is with you, how does the initial consultation proceed? Do you rise to greet the patient, or are you already standing? Do you shake hands? Shaking hands establishes a physical contact, palpably bridging the gap.

Do you call the patient Mr., Ms., or Mrs., or by his or her first name? Do you call all children and most women by their first name? These matters involve more than manners. They are consequential acts for many patients. For example, some older persons resent being called by their first names; some women reason correctly that they are being treated like children. Others, however, do not consider this form of salutation an act of disrespect; rather, they feel relaxed by the doctor's friendliness.

I remember a 70-year-old Boston banker who, while pruning trees one weekend at his New Hampshire home, cut his hand and, still dressed in his workclothes, saw "a young surgeon locally. He said to me, 'How did you do it, Billie?' Well, nobody but my father ever called me 'Billie.' I thought that that was as good a time as any to part company and I walked right out of his office." While his reaction might be that of one's grandfather's generation, it is usually safer to be less informal initially and whenever in doubt.

Although the content and form of the initial consultation vary from doctor to doctor and according to the type and needs of patients, each doctor usually has a customary way of conducting the consultation [130, 273]. I am either standing or I rise when my secretary brings a patient in to see me—in my office (rugs, pictures, mementos). My secretary will say, "Mrs. Hodges, this is Dr. Goldwyn." I always shake hands and usually remark, "I am happy to see you." I then say, "Please sit down," and indicate a chair in front of my desk, behind which I then sit. A word about the seating arrangements: Next to the patient is another chair for a friend or family member. The desk, I recognize, is a barrier to communication. White [273] observed that when no desk intervened, about 55 percent of patients were "at ease," in contrast to 11 percent when there was a desk. I have consciously chosen to accept this impediment and to overcome it because I am more comfortable with structure that preserves distance while permitting friendliness. Right or wrong, I believe this is important, especially with female patients, who constitute about 75 percent of my practice.

I encourage all patients to bring in whoever may have accompanied them [97]. I will specifically ask the patient whether there is someone in the waiting room whom he or she would like to have present during this consultation. If there is, I sometimes ask either my secretary or the patient to go out to fetch that other person. Invariably, his or her presence will visibly relax the patient. By the time we are seated, I know whether or not the patient is somewhat relaxed or very anxious. What is the patient's affect and mood? Appropriate? Depressed? Manic? Hostile?

Instead of jumping immediately into a new patient's problem, I usually talk in general terms to relieve the apprehension as well as to establish a relationship. Though mundane, weather, geography (place of residence), or an occupation serve well to launch the interaction. "I see from the record that you are a schoolteacher, how did you get a day off during the week?" Or, "You are from New Hampshire. Has it started to snow there?" I might even ask the patient what he or she does or where he or she lives even though I have that information. Putting the patient at ease should be an early objective of the consultation. One should remember that a visit to the doctor is seldom a joyous occasion. Depending on the problem, the patient may fear that his or her condition is serious, or that his or her desire for surgery will be considered "vain" or that the treatment will involve considerable embarrassment (the patient must get undressed), perhaps even pain, maybe death, certainly expense, and always uncertainty.

You should never assume why the patient is in your office. I usually begin with a question, "How can I help you?" I am conscious of the word "can" rather than "may" because "can" implies an ability that

I would like to think I have as a result of training and skill. Other physicians might say "Why are you here?" or "What has brought you here?" or "What would you like to talk about?" If I know why the patient is here (from the record), I might say "I understand you are here because you are considering facial surgery" or "Your doctor called to tell me that you had a biopsy the other day, and I understand that it is a small skin cancer—the type that is usually easily curable" (if I know that the biopsy showed a basal carcinoma).

If possible, I refrain from telling the patient that I know that he or she is considering an esthetic operation. I do not wish to appear "too pushy." I am therefore aware of the impression I am creating by not appearing like a huckster with regard to esthetic surgery; however, in a noncosmetic situation, I may be more forward because the patient has been referred with a problem whose treatment expense is covered by insurance.

Never commit the grand gaffe of assuming the reason the patient has consulted you. I once said to a man who could have been the original Cyrano de Bergerac, "I guess you're here because you want something done about your nose," when, in reality, the patient was in the office because of a cyst on his back.

It is important to pay scrupulous attention to the precise words the patient uses in describing his or her problem. You will be able to learn the emotional reactions to it. For example, consider the difference in these statements of different patients:

> "I have this thing [a nevus] growing on my nose and I can't stand to look at it." [Patient's concern is primarily appearance.]
>
> "My wife is worried that this thing on my nose is growing. I had a sister who had a malignant freckle." [The patient's concern and that of his wife is melanoma. The patient has probably denied his fear for a while and lets you know that he has made this appointment at his wife's insistence.]
>
> "Dr. Smythe wants you to look at this on my nose. He thinks it's nothing, but he wants to be sure. If it does not have to come off, I would be delighted." [The patient's concern is malignancy; the message is not to do unnecessary surgery.]

The usual progression of the consultation is toward the present illness. How this process occurs varies with the patient and the physician. Henderson, the physical chemist, who depicted the doctor-patient relationship as a reciprocal social system, an analogy to the physical chemical processes and equations that he helped define, admonished:

> When you talk with the patient, you should listen, first, for what he wants to tell, secondly for what he does not want to tell, thirdly for what he cannot tell. He does not want to tell things the telling of which is shameful or painful. He cannot tell you his implicit assumptions that are unknown to him, such as the assumption that all action not perfectly good is bad, such as the assumption that everything that is not perfectly successful is a failure, such as the assumption that everything that is not perfectly safe is dangerous. We are all of us subject to errors of this kind, to the assumption that quantitative differences are qualitative. . . . When you listen for what the patient does not want to tell and for what he cannot tell you must take especial note of his omissions, for it is the things that he fails to say that correspond to what he does not want to say plus what he cannot say. . . [133].

In listening to the patient, in trying to elicit history, and in forming a judgment of the patient, here, as throughout your entire interaction with the patient, the focus can be narrow or broad. If, as I mentioned previously, you can see your role to be that of a vendor of a skilled service or technique, you will not let your patient stray from the business at hand (note the word *business*); you will want only the facts essential to determine fitness for operation.

In reading accounts of the doctor-patient interaction written by those who are not physicians, I am conscious of and frankly resent their blithe disregard of the reality of time, with which we in the medical field have to contend. Aside from the impact of the disease itself, we doctors must deal with the dictates of the clock. Even when the patient arranges the appointment, time is a factor. How much time has been allotted for the visit? In some offices, the patient is asked over the phone the nature of the problem. Although some might find this intrusive and annoying, it is necessary for the doctor's schedule as well as the patient's good. Generally, a patient with a small angioma of the cheek requires less time to see and evaluate than would a patient desiring a complete facelift or a breast reconstruction. Although some patients like the "in and out" approach, most do not. They have waited days, perhaps weeks, even months to see you, and, even if you consider their problem minor—it may be—they do not. In *The Thibaults,* by duGard [64], the chief of medicine remarked: "The only thing patients really want is—to be taken seriously." I believe that they want more, but the point is a good one.

A patient with a small lesion may have a large medical history. Most physicians are too clock conscious, having scheduled too much in their usual day. This awareness of time is frequently communicated to the patient, who senses the doctor's impatience and may even apologize: "I'm sorry to take up your time when I know that you are so busy."

I have heard many plastic surgeons say, almost as a boast: "I need to spend just ten minutes with a new patient." Although it may be possible to effect an exchange of information, it is usually impossible for anything more than the most tenuous connection with a patient if you give the impression that he or she does not really matter to you as a person but just as an object for an operative procedure. Admittedly, it is not only the quantity of time but the quality. Some physicians have the knack of being efficient without seeming pressed. Their manner is unhurried and the patient may feel that the time elapsed with the doctor has been at least half an hour when it has actually been only 15 minutes; however, there is for each patient an irreducible minimum below which he or she feels spurned and cast off. One of the most common complaints of patients is that "the doctor did not spend enough time with me." The patient usually does not mean that the doctor failed to diagnose properly or to recommend the correct treatment, but rather the doctor did not satisfy the patient's emotional needs. Patients generally want to talk not only about their specific problems but also their fears, values, and their lives—what two friends would normally discuss with each other. The patient has entered your office as a stranger but wants to leave as a friend. Is that unreasonable?

S. J. Aston [7], in describing his views and behavior during the usual preoperative consultation for esthetic surgery, offers a different perspective and has a different style.

> The first thing to understand is that the preoperative consultation is a business meeting during which you *may enter into a written and oral contract* [italics are in the original] with the patient—a legal contract which has all the ramifications thereof. In my preoperative consultation, I want to

obtain as much information as I need to decide if I want to perform the operation, and I want the patient to gain as much information as she needs to determine if she wants me to do it. I try to be honest, thorough, and, especially, *efficient*. Keep in mind it is not how long you spend with the patient—it's what you do with the time.

The patient arrives and is met in the reception area by two staff members. After filling out her own medical history form, the patient is given *a detailed information sheet on the facts about facelifts, eyelid and forehead surgery*. The patient is required to read this information before she sees anyone in my office. Prior to my personal consultation with the patient, a nurse has reviewed the medical history form, confirmed it with the patient and entered the pertinent medical history on the chart. The nurse also determines and records what bothers the patient and why she is seeking consultation. When I walk into the examining room, having the chart in front of me, I know every piece of relevant information about that patient—the first day she called my office, how long it took her to get an appointment, any previous surgery she has had, who referred her, what she wants changed, and so on.

The typical manner in which I would open the conversation might be something like, 'Miss Jones, I see you're healthy, happy—you're 41 years of age, and you're thinking about having your lower lids done,' or 'You're thinking about freshening up your face.' She will most likely answer a brief 'That's right.' She usually doesn't feel the need to repeat her history, because she sees that I am looking at the chart which she has already reviewed with my nurse. This allows me to *control the conversation* right from the beginning, which is what I want to do; that's the only way to be efficient. Then I say, 'Let me look at you. I'll tell you what I see, and then we'll talk about it together.'

My hand is on the patient most of the time. I touch the eyelids, I touch the neck, etcetera. I walk around the patient—always walking in front of her, not behind. The fact is, you don't really need to walk around the patient; you don't need to touch most patients to know exactly what it is you want to do for them. But this gives you an opportunity to perceive in the first two or three minutes, from that patient's reaction, if this is someone you have to be especially careful of psychologically. You can't always read them, but many times you can.

Then I'll hand the patient a mirror and say, 'Let's start at the neck and work our way up.' I go through each step, pointing out *what we can correct and what is (and is not) able to be improved*. At this stage, I will only talk about those appearance problems which she has already indicated are bothersome to her. I never try to suggest an operation to a patient, regardless of whether I feel she needs it, unless she herself has expressed an interest. Of course, I explain in detail about the surgery and the recovery. Finally, I ask if the patient has questions. It sometimes occurs that the patient wishes to focus on questions about possible complications (which were covered thoroughly in the informational materials she read previously); in this case, I am prepared to answer any questions directly and completely.

One of the last things I always say to the patient is, 'When you get home, you're going to have further questions. *Call me.* If I'm not available at the time of your call, I will call you back.' I probably call one out of ten preoperative facelifts at home, and, sometime between the initial consultation and the surgery, I see about 20 to 25 percent of them for a second consultation. I want my patients to know that I'm available for them, and I think this is important. I want them to arrive at the hospital feeling comfortable with me.

During the consultation, one of my nurses is writing down everything I say to the patient, positive and negative. We have a *coding system* on the chart, and the last thing I do in the consultation is turn to the nurse and go through the coding system starting with the forehead, the eyelids, the face and the neck. By the time I'm ready to walk out the door, the nurse has already written the fee on the chart which she hands to me. If it's a standard surgical fee, I glance at it; if it's not, I mark the change.

At this point, if the patient starts to ask questions about scheduling, finances, do's and don'ts before surgery, and that sort of thing, I introduce her to one of my staff members who is trained to discuss these matters. (By the way, it's always good to have more than one girl in your office who can do this, or any, job.) The whole process works out very satisfactorily for all concerned.

Aston's approach is obviously efficient, with the control palpably in the hands of the plastic surgeon. Randomness of behavior is not encouraged because the surgeon considers preoperative consultation a business meeting as well as an introduction to the patient; furthermore, the objective is to determine whether the patient is a suitable candidate for a specific operation. In addition, Aston has somebody else present—a nurse—writing down what he says to the patient. The fact that his approach is almost opposite from mine does not mean that either of us is wrong or right. It means that each of us has a different style, and adaptation is required by the patient. Some of my patients might prefer that I be less broad, that I focus more quickly on the problem, tell them as soon as possible what they need, whether I can do it, and, if so, what it will cost. These differences of approach may reflect not so much what the patient wishes to get out of the consultation but what the plastic surgeon desires from it. My needs and those of Aston are somewhat different; for whatever reasons, best left to the psychoanalysts, I want more reciprocity than does he. I need not add that his surgical results are outstanding and that he has a strong commitment to his patients. What I am trying to emphasize is that plastic surgeons vary in their consultations with their patients, perhaps as much or even more so than in their method of performing a specific operation.

The doctor, the plastic surgeon for our purposes, who is not attuned to the numerous times during the course of a day when he or she has emotionally short-changed his or her patients will remain oblivious to the rising well of dissatisfaction until something goes wrong; then an outpouring of hostility will come. A broader and deeper relationship with the patient is useful not only to avoid anger and unpleasantness but to give ongoing satisfaction to the patient and the plastic surgeon as well, if, indeed, he or she values the warmth of human interaction. Note the word "interaction" because, like Henderson [133], I believe that what happens when the patient meets the plastic surgeon sets off a reaction that is not linear or unidirected, but it is reciprocal, or, at least, should be. The surgeon can benefit as well as the patient. For this to occur, the physician-surgeon must not be overly preoccupied with diagnosis and treatment. The patient must be more active than he or she traditionally is and the physician less active than he or she is usually depicted (I am not referring to psychoanalysis). In short, there must be more reciprocity with regard to activity and passivity.

In addition to the plastic surgeon's values concerning his or her profession, the consultation with the patient depends also on the individual personalities of both. Because the patient has sought the plastic surgeon and has initiated the encounter (and goes to his or her office), not vice versa (unless there has been active advertising on the part of the plastic surgeon), the doctor's preferences for the content and form of the initial consultation usually prevail. The word is "prevail" not "obliterate." The more authoritarian the plastic surgeon is, the more structured the consultation and the treatment will be. Ideally, a doctor should listen as well as talk. The purpose in asking the patient questions is to obtain information. Why interrupt the patient who is furnishing that information at that particular time? The surgeon should not direct the consultation as if it were an operation, at least that is my opinion. Others might disagree. Letting it happen, I believe, may have important dividends. Questioning, of course, is crucial to elicit relevant data and to channel the consultation within the realities of time; however, queries should be gentle. One is a physician—a plastic surgeon—not a precinct captain or a tobacco auctioneer. If, for example, a patient who seeks an augmentation mammoplasty is asked too soon about breast cancer in the family, she may become extremely anxious and incapable of listening and remembering what you tell her about the operation and its possible benefits and hazards.

The primary objective of the consultation for the plastic surgeon, in my belief, is to know the patient medically and emotionally [160, 163]. If there is to be a surgical journey, it starts then. Rushing the patient, scribbling down information with one's head in papers, and paying more attention to form than to content will prevent you from attaining the perspective necessary for proper evaluation and treatment—the old "not seeing the forest for the trees" syndrome. The time one takes to sit back, observe, and listen will save much more time and may spare the plastic surgeon and the patient a serious error. The best occasion to know the patient is the initial visit. Someone once said in reference to psychotherapy: "All the major themes are present in the initial interview."

The consultation should glide and should not be a series of staccato acts. When it is time to "lay the hands" on the patient, it should not be done abruptly. If the patient's complaint concerns a usually unexposed part of the body, it would be best to take more time before examining him or her.

Who is Present at the Time of Examination

Some physicians always examine the patient alone. I prefer to have a female present (secretary or nurse) when examining a woman for an operation on the breasts, buttocks, thighs, or genital area. Some patients request that only you be present; these patients have usually come for an operation on their breast or chest. They are embarrassed by what they consider a deformity: small, large, or asymmetric breasts; or a pectus excavatum.

Frequently patients are accompanied by a family member or friend whom they want in the examining room. I do not consider this an infringement on my domain or that of the patient but rather as an opportunity to discuss the problem and possible treatment with an individual who is probably the most important in that patient's life [97]. That person, moreover, will be able to recall the information that you gave the patient who is often so anxious about being there that he or she forgets what you have said. Also, an observer who is more dispassionate than either you or the patient might ask an important question that had not occurred to either of you.

On occasion, however, it is necessary to see and examine the patient alone. This is particularly true with a teenager, for example, inquiring about rhinoplasty. You may need information that the adolescent would be afraid to communicate if the parent were present. Similarly, by separating husband and wife you may be able to find out more about their marriage in order to assess the impact of the procedure on each partner and on their relationship.

Since patients differ, as do their problems, it is unwise to force everyone into a set sequence. Your system and style should have the flexibility of accommodating individual differences. The patient will then sense that he or she counts with you as a human being, not just another patient to be processed in your office machinery.

The Quality of Examination

The type of physical examination depends on the patient's problem: nasal deformity, parotid mass, mammary hypoplasia. How you examine is as important as what you examine. By that, I mean not only your competence but your gentleness and considerateness.

As physicians, we are so accustomed to inspecting, palpating, and probing the human body that we forget what it is like to be a patient. Since most plastic surgeons are male and since many patients for reconstructive surgery and most for esthetic are female, we must be aware of their feelings. In 10 or 20 minutes after having first met the patient, I may have learned about a problem that none or only a few of her intimates know; I have listened to revelations about her personal life and her family history usually not discussed openly; and now, for example, I may be examining her breasts. What is routine for us physicians is certainly not for our patients. When I have my annual checkup, I am conscious of the embarrassment of standing undressed before the doctor even though he is a friend of the same sex [229]. Our society is still not unisexual in its attitudes and actions. Although most females accept the fact that most physicians are male, being nude or half dressed in front of them is usually awkward and discomforting. I can empathize with their situation and usually say, "I know that most of us do not enjoy going to a doctor and being examined. I don't like it myself, but I guess it's a reality that all of us have to put up with." When I take their pictures, especially if they are unclothed, I say, "I know, Mrs. Burns, that you don't usually pose for such photographs—at least on Tuesdays." The acknowledgement of their ordeal with perhaps a little humor makes this part of the consultation more bearable for the patient and consequently for myself.

I am never present when a patient of the opposite sex undresses since I believe that my being there will make her more ill at ease. Furthermore, how a patient disrobes is not relevant to the purposes of my examination, unlike that of a neurologist, who assesses the patient's ability to button and unbutton clothes.

The Patient Knows

A common error of many physicians is to underestimate the intelligence of patients. This "intelligence" includes not only factual knowledge but perception as well. Most patients usually recognize hostility, hypocrisy, arrogance, avarice, and lack of sympathy, even when the physician thinks that he or she has these traits well hidden. Someone, for example, who has been kept waiting inordinately will appreciate and recognize an apology that is sincere, not pro forma. If you are rushed, it is better to acknowledge that fact to the patient and perhaps suggest that he or she return (at no charge) for a proper, unhurried consultation. Most patients will see through the pretensions of the room game, whereby they are moved from one place to another to give them the illusion that they are actually getting somewhere and that something is being done for them. As they go from room number 4 to room number 1, the scene becomes reminiscent of an Arthur J. Rank production, with the gong expected to sound as the patient is finally brought into the presence of the great plastic surgeon.

As much as possible, try to picture yourself as the patient. By doing so, you will find it easier to understand his or her emotions. That awareness will improve your patient rapport and your self-understanding.

> *No man values the best medicine if administered by a physician whom he hates and despises.*
> Jonathan Swift

Behavior by the Physician or Staff that Negatively Affects the Patient
Despite variations in personalities among patients and doctors and differences in office routines, certain actions by any physician, including the plastic surgeon, will be detrimental to the doctor-patient relationship [166, 168, 169]. Some I have already mentioned, but I wish to discuss them and others more fully now and also later.

The pressures of a professional life can easily make us take the patient's visit for granted. We lose sight of the individuality of the patient; successive patients become a blurred parade. The physician may view the consultations as another chore; for the patient, this encounter with the surgeon is a singular occasion, a happening to be recounted to family and friends. Consider for a moment what the patient has gone through to arrive in your office. He or she has made an appointment, probably having made numerous inquiries concerning the "best" doctor able to take care of the problem. Most likely, the patient has had to wait a few days, weeks, or possibly months to see you and has had to arrange home and work schedules, probably also planning transportation and perhaps arranging for child care. A married patient's spouse may have had to take time from work in order to accompany him or her. Most female patients probably have thought carefully about what to wear for the consultation. I remember one woman who came for treatment of a basal carcinoma of her face and then happened to think of another lesion on her lower abdomen. When I offered to look at it, she initially consented and then looked horrified and said, "I really can't have you see my undergarments today. I hadn't thought that you would be looking at me there."

Most patients worry about not only what you will say about their condition, but what they will say, how they will respond, and what will be the course of their visit with you. If, indeed, their reason for being in your office concerns a major condition, such as an extensive neoplasm or a significant problem in esthetic surgery, they will be even more apprehensive. As physicians, we are so accustomed to dealing with patients who are anxious that we easily lose our sympathy; we forget what trepidation is unless that patient happens to be ourself or a loved one [197].

Under these circumstances, the worst behavior on the part of the physician is a cold and uncaring attitude [29]. The patient may make allowances for your being brusque and harried but will not excuse your lack of concern and sympathy. The patient does not want to feel like an intruder, just another patient, or a penitent. The most important patient is the one in front of you. Keeping someone waiting excessively (without apologizing sincerely), not listening, accepting telephone interruptions, signing or reading letters, forgetting the patient's name, and asking the patient the same question twice are examples of not only bad manners but of inconsiderateness. They reflect your lack of esteem for that human being.

Writing about a house call Osler once made, a neighbor recalled: "In a room full of discordant elements, he entered and saw only his patient and his patient's greatest need, and instantly the atmosphere was charged with kindly vitality. Everyone felt that the situation was under control. . . . The moment Sir William gave you was yours . . . becoming wholly and entirely a part of the fabric of your life . . . he was one of those who having great possessions, gave all that he had" [150].

In the office, the patient rightly views your staff as part of you. Passively or actively, a doctor thus condones the behavior of his or her helpers and associates. To patients, some secretaries are the major obstacles to overcome because they are rude, unfeeling, and hostile. To surmount these liabilities, the doctor must labor hard in order to restore lines of communication. Frequently the patient is already angry before meeting the plastic surgeon because of being handled so carelessly when arranging the appointment and on arriving in the office. Without realizing it, the doctor is already behind and must do more to get approval from that patient.

Detrimental to the patient–doctor relationship is lack of confidentiality. A patient whose name is called out in a crowded waiting room may feel embarrassed. Records carelessly left about so that names are easily visible may be noticed. Telephone conversations by the doctor or the secretaries may be audible. Some patients may hear friends being discussed in the office or at cocktail parties, and they correctly assume that they will suffer from the same lack of privacy.

Inefficiency of the physician and his or her office erodes the patient's confidence in the care that will be provided. The patient may surmise, correctly or incorrectly, that the doctor is not sufficiently interested in his or her problem to do what was promised. For example, the physician or secretary might have mislaid a letter from the referring physician; or the physician might forget to arrange laboratory tests, might not communicate the results to the patient, or may fail to write to the referring physician.

Another point of irritation relates to finances. Pecuniary arrangements between physician and patient are admittedly important, but they should not dominate the relationship. Patients should understand their financial responsibilities but should feel that the doctor considers their problem more important than their money. The surgeon who charges "excessively" in comparison to colleagues may be explicitly or implicitly saying to the patient: "I charge more but my results are better." If, indeed, the results are not so good as what the patient had anticipated, that doctor deserves the inevitable boomerang.

Obviously, improper diagnosis and treatment can shatter the bond between patient and surgeon; however, most patients can accept error if they have received kindness and truth.

It is regrettable that many physicians never learn the reactions of their patients to their behavior and to that of the office staff. Physicians, like all authority figures, become insulated from the truth; they develop protective scotomata. Too often their reality is what is fed them by those in their hire. Part of the reason that it is harder to learn as one gets older is that fewer people dare tell you your faults. Occasionally, truth bursts forth from an angry patient, but you may reject its validity since you are so busy defending yourself from the onslaught.

Appraising the Patient

> To this fact, that we are each a secret to the other, we have to reconcile ourselves. To know one another cannot mean to know everything about each other; it means to feel mutual affection and confidence, and to believe in one another.
>
> Albert Schweitzer
> Memoirs of Childhood and Youth

After the physical examination, your interaction with the patient usually will concern his or her specific problem and your recommendations for treatment. In a later section, I will discuss types of patients and types of operations; however, a word here would be relevant about what you have been doing thus far during the initial consultation. You have been assessing the patient in terms of a condition or problem and that person's emotional and physical suitability for treatment, particularly an operation. After approximately half an hour, you and the patient will make a decision. In most instances, the judgment is correct although it is reached on the basis of incomplete evidence. No individual, even the physician with the greatest angle of vision, can see all facets of the patient. "A human life is always broader than we realize," observed Antoine, a physician in duGard's *The Thibaults* [64]. Besides imperfect perception by one human being of another, there is only partial comprehension of motivations. Blurred vision and faulty understanding are the givens of the human condition; yet despite these deficiencies, most of us adopt courses of action without fatal mishap.

Another point to remember is that the plastic surgeon in terms of the patient is still a plastic surgeon; the nature of the relationship—that of a patient to a surgical specialist—automatically has boundaries that prevent each of them from venturing too far. Although one may get a hint of marital discord, perhaps of sexual disharmony, you, as a plastic surgeon, are not the one to treat it or even to obtain detailed information about it. Similarly, if the patient has anxiety not only because of the condition that has brought him or her to you but, let us say, because of financial problems apart from your fee, you are not a financial advisor. The roles of being the patient and of being the physician–plastic surgeon carry with them "No Trespassing" signs. Perceiving just how far to go is the mark of a skilled physician, whatever his or her specialty, if any.

Another issue for consideration is that even the most talented of us are biased by our very skills. We are prisoners of our own strengths as well as weaknesses. No matter how exalted we may sit, we are trapped on our perch. How different our species has appeared to Socrates, Voltaire, Marx, Freud, and Camus! Sometimes we physicians, in a supposedly rational occupation, forget that the patient in front of us still eludes the philosopher, theologian, political scientist, biologist, psychotherapist, novelist, economist, and sociologist. We must also realize that we are connecting with that patient only briefly and at only one aspect of his or her being. The "care of the whole patient" is not only trite as an expression but is pretentious as an ideal, as mentioned earlier. If such a holistic view goads us to be more understanding, competent, and compassionate, then it is worthwhile; but if it leads us to believe that we can truly fathom the entire patient and fulfill all his or her needs, then the concept nurtures arrogance.

The best that we doctors can hope for is to comprehend the patient well and long enough to help him or her, physically and emotionally [22, 65].

Similarly, the patient will make a decision, perhaps more on the basis of trust than of knowledge. Ultimately, in every human interaction, the outcome is not guaranteed—marriage is an outstanding example. The patient, in reality, may know our reputation, may know patients or even family members whom we have treated, but can never be certain that our behavior toward him or her will be the same.

Today, when the atmosphere surrounding the patient and the doctor breeds suspicion, the patient may wonder whether the plastic surgeon in front of him or her will actually be doing the surgery, in spite of the reassurances that he or she may have received. Perhaps the plastic surgeon, the patient wonders, is an "impaired physician." Maybe he or she is on drugs or alcohol or is the type of person who will become irritable and definitely unavailable if needed. The uncertainty in life certainly does not end with a medical experience and the interaction between physician and patient; in fact, the uncertainty persists despite the attempts of both the physician and the patient to leave little to uncertainty.

A perfect relationship between a patient and a physician would bring an ideal doctor and an ideal patient together in harmony: a competent, caring, honest surgeon placing the patient's needs above his or her own, always being there for the patient, and charging well within the patient's ability to pay; and a patient with a significant problem for which a relatively simple solution exists, a trusting patient who will follow instructions with few complaints and few questions, someone who is grateful and will happily pay the bill.

Unfortunately, the world has few faultless people and consequently few faultless patients and surgeons; *perfect* therapeutic dyads are regrettably less common than desired. This does not mean, however, that most patients and most doctors will not have a satisfying interaction. The likelihood is that they will.

In this society to date, most patients are not assigned to a specific plastic surgeon, and most plastic surgeons need not accept each patient. In general, the more urgent the medical situation, the less important become the personality characteristics of the surgeon and the patient in their choice of each other. Whether a patient whose thumb needs replantation is hostile and neurotic will not influence the surgeon's decision to operate; however, if that same patient were there for an elective procedure, such as a musculocutaneous flap for osteomyelitis, the surgeon would do well to consider that patient's aggression before consenting to operate. Hostility in the individual who is in the office for a rhinoplasty would be or should be a reason to refuse that person's surgery. In contrast to several decades ago when there were few plastic surgeons in the world, today's patient has more choice, as does the plastic surgeon, who need not feel guilty for refusing to operate if he or she believes the patient is a poor risk emotionally if not medically or perhaps even both. When and how to say "no" under what conditions will be discussed later.

3

Plastic Surgery: Reconstructive and Esthetic Surgery

Unlike Gaul, plastic surgery is divided into just two parts: reconstructive and esthetic. A further dissimilarity is that these parts overlap.

To the public, despite the significant advances in reconstructive surgery, the "plastic surgeon" is the one who does esthetic surgery. This distortion of image is not totally the fault of the laity since individual plastic surgeons as well as their organized societies have expended money and effort to make a prospective patient think of a "plastic surgeon" (board certified by the American Board of Plastic Surgery) whenever he or she contemplates a cosmetic procedure. No matter how frequent or sensational the stories in the media are concerning replantation of limbs or reconstruction after burns, the reflex image evoked in the public's mind to the title "plastic surgeon" is that of someone who changes a nose or erases the signs of aging, and now, suctions fat.

Many plastic surgeons who do both esthetic and reconstructive procedures would feel demeaned if someone at a party said to them, "I suppose you don't bother with noses since you are doing much more important work." The usual reply to that type of question is a defensive denial. It is as if plastic surgeons have become enamored of the image that they have helped to create but are somewhat ashamed of having.

The current definitions for both cosmetic surgery and reconstructive surgery that the American Society of Plastic and Reconstructive Surgeons is using, and which the American Medical Association House of Delegates approved in July, 1989 are as follows:

> Cosmetic surgery is performed to reshape normal structures of the body in order to improve the patient's appearance and self-esteem. Reconstructive surgery is performed on abnormal structures of the body, caused by congenital defects, developmental abnormalities, trauma, infection, tumors or disease. It is generally performed to improve function, but may also be done to approximate a normal appearance [230].

Most plastic surgeons (certified by the American Board of Plastic Surgeons or eligible) do both esthetic and reconstructive surgery. A survey published in 1988 indicated that the "typical practice profile is 58% reconstructive and 42% esthetic which is only a slight variation from 1984, when the ratio was 60/40." [5]

The fact that the majority of plastic surgeons do esthetic as well as reconstructive surgery regularly does not mean that we can precisely fit a procedure into either category. For example, if one accepts as part of the definition of cosmetic surgery the statement that it "is performed to reshape normal structures," how do we classify a 17-year-old girl who has severe breast asymmetry with a nubbin of a breast on one side and a massive pendulous breast on the other? Are we reconstructing the smaller breast (probably so) and performing esthetic surgery on the other? Yet, the hypertrophied breast is not really a "normal" structure, but an abnormally exaggerated one. Operations for cleft lip are usually covered by insurance since they are deemed reconstructive, but who would argue that a major factor in prompting secondary, tertiary, and even more procedures on the lip-nose is the strong factor of appearance.

In attempting to make the decision regarding coverage of a procedure, insurance companies try valiantly, sometimes even honestly, to determine whether the operation is cosmetic (esthetic) or reconstructive. Frequently they will invoke the criterion of "being necessary for the health or survival of the patient." Although that may appear to be a logical index, most insurance companies will not consider an endangered psyche as a cause for operation and therefore coverage. I recall a patient, a 16-year-old girl, with a truly enormous nose, who was severely depressed and wanted a rhinoplasty. Unfortunately, she had normal breathing, and one could not invoke a deviated septum with compromised airway as a reason for operating. The insurance company stated that they could not defray the cost of the operation, but they would be willing to pay the expenses of a psychiatrist as an alternative!

In other words, esthetic surgery is not covered for psychological reasons since the plastic surgeon is not a mental health worker. Perhaps the insurance companies are correct in general; otherwise, they would have to underwrite almost all esthetic operations since the objective in most instances is to improve self-esteem.

Because reconstructive surgery is performed to undo the effects of trauma, infection, tumors, or disease, the patient may not have recently been in good health as a result of having sustained those medical problems. In contrast, the esthetic patient is usually in good health. Furthermore, much reconstructive surgery is done as an emergency, especially that undertaken in association with trauma, for example, a flap to cover an exposed wound with a comminuted open fracture of the ankle.

The patient for reconstructive surgery, though obviously not enviable, does have the advantage of society's support: He or she has been a victim, and society, both the individual and its institutions, is there to urge the treatment, to provide it, and to pay for it. This is in sharp contrast to the patient for esthetic surgery.

SPECIAL FEATURES OF ESTHETIC SURGERY: CONFUSION ABOUT NAME AND DEFINITION

The first singular characteristic of esthetic surgery is the confusion about its name and definition as well as its spelling. Many plastic surgeons prefer the word "esthetic" over the word "cosmetic," wishing to avoid the connotations of makeup and a beauty parlor. The "a" that precedes "esthetic" in most communications from official organizations of surgeons doing this type of operation also serves to upgrade the image by conferring on it a classic lineage. Since esthetic surgery is still fighting for rightful respect from the medical profession, even from many plastic surgeons who do mostly reconstructive work, another common practice is to use more impressive names for operations commonly called facelift (rhytidectomy, rhytidoplasty), meloplasty, or eyelidplasty (blepharoplasty), nose job or nasal surgery (rhinoplasty). The evocation of Greek roots is indicative of insecurity, frequently unconscious, among many cosmetic surgeons. In my presence, the head of a prestigious plastic service chastised a resident who listed the procedure as a facelift instead of a rhytidectomy, which the chief said would "look better to our colleagues."

Some surgeons favor calling cosmetic or (a)esthetic surgery the surgery of appearance or body-image surgery to imply more than the effecting of merely superficial changes. Gertrude Stein's comments are pertinent: "A difference to be a difference must make a difference," and "A rose is a rose is a rose is a rose." The schoolteacher's maxim that "You don't know it unless you can define it" is not always valid when it comes to distinguishing between esthetic and reconstructive surgery. Furthermore, good reconstructive surgery almost always has an esthetic objective [159, 226].

Visibility

Although the range of operations in both esthetic and reconstructive surgery is extensive, and although the results of many reconstructive operations are visible, all esthetic surgical procedures are directed to areas where the human eye can reach under certain conditions [129]. The face is usually in view [171, 172]; the breasts, only occasionally and then only to special observers. Although one might not readily be able to see evidence of a previous esthetic operation, detailed scrutiny usually reveals telltale surface scars. The fact that the results of esthetic surgery are generally apparent means that they can be judged in terms of appearance (favorable or not) by patients, friends, or others. This is certainly not the situation with the outcome after a cholecystectomy.

Enhancement

An important feature of esthetic surgery is that the patient considers the result of the operation, if all goes well, to be an enhancement [40, 86], not a loss as is usual after other types of surgery, such as a hysterectomy. These benefits are objective as well as subjective. Because of an improved appearance, the patient becomes more socially desirable to others and to herself or himself [92]. Walster and colleagues [264] found that physical attractiveness was the most important personal characteristic influencing how much one is liked in a man-woman dating situation. Especially for the woman, good looks are the passport to popularity and upward mobility. The confluence of beauty, wealth, and power is a universal phenomenon. Literally, it pays to be beautiful. Kalick [148] conducted an experiment in which subjects viewed preoperative and postoperative photographs. Individuals pictured postoperatively were judged to have more desirable personalities, to be better potential marriage partners, and to have happier lives than the same persons photographed before surgery. Since all the impressions were from photographs, actual personality was not a factor in his study. His findings and those of other researchers suggest that esthetic surgery may have a stronger social impact on patients' lives than had previously been assumed. The "enhancement" of appearance from the operative procedure is not only in the mind of the patient, but also in the minds of those around him or her [92]. The improved social reception reinforces the patient's sense of well-being; glowing in these reverberations, the patient may become even more outgoing, possibly even charming.

Numerous studies have shown that after a successful esthetic operation, the patient's self-consciousness about a displeasing feature decreases as do anxiety and depression. At the same time, self-esteem rises as does the patient's perception of herself or himself as more attractive sexually. For males there is an enhanced masculinity; for females, an increased femininity. In a study of 40 female cosmetic surgery patients, Burk, Zelen, and Terino [35] found that their average patient was "a normal woman in terms of self-esteem when attempting to remediate a consciously felt inconsistency between general and specific body-part esteem. Cosmetic surgery seems to reduce this inconsistency."

Behavior patterns, sometimes complex, designed to camouflage an unpleasant body part and concomitant feelings of poor self-esteem and inferiority disappear. New nonverbal as well as verbal behavior comes to the fore, and the patient becomes less socially withdrawn [181].

Cash and Horton [39] found that in the patients they studied, cosmetic surgery was undertaken to improve looks (87%), to improve feelings about self (80%), to receive compliments (67%), and to decrease self-consciousness (64%).

At first thought, it may seem perplexing that so many women today are seeking esthetic surgery during the burgeoning of the feminist movement, many of whose leaders are opposed to such operations; however, the "Be what you are" message is not as important to some women as the other message "Be all you can be"—actualize your potential [186].

A recent patient, a woman in her early 50s, coming for a facelift said, "I have been a good mother, a supportive wife, and now I want to do something for myself." This was the expression of someone who was seeking *equal* entitlement—equal to what she thought her husband and her children had received from her.

The beneficial effects of esthetic surgery extend even to the patient's life at work, where advancement may be partially the result of an improved and younger look [170]. In fact, some executives have credited their rise to a cosmetic procedure [162]. The point here is that it is not only how that person looks, but how that person feels he or she looks.

As plastic surgeons, we tend to be wary of the patient who wants an esthetic operation for a massive change in his or her life or, more specifically, for a better job. Our hesitancy is due to our fears that such patients will expect too much from the procedure, and that if they fail to achieve their professional or personal objective, they will be disappointed and even hostile. What we might consider unrealistic about that patient's expectations may actually be realistic. The ripple effect of an anticipated outcome from esthetic surgery is hard to judge. Commonly, the plastic surgeon hears from patients or their family that "the operation changed my [her or his] life." The more modest among us may believe that such a statement is hyperbole when, in fact, it may not be.

The plastic surgeon should not tell the patient that if he or she has the procedure, it will change his or her life. Such promises may be fatuous and misleading. It is better to recognize the benefits of the procedure after the operation rather than predicting their occurrence when, in fact, they may never come to pass.

Unequivocally I would state that no patient in my experience has ever undertaken an esthetic procedure without expecting a positive change somewhere to something (perhaps only the anatomic part) on his or her body and in his or her life. In short, every cosmetic patient expects an enhancement of some sort from undergoing the ordeal—or for some, the opportunity—of esthetic surgery.

Elective Nature
Unlike almost every other surgical situation, operating for esthetic reasons is completely elective, more so even than in other areas of plastic surgery, as mentioned in regard to reconstructive surgery. For the esthetic operative patient, survival in terms of life is rarely the issue. An esthetic patient is almost always in good health, which he or she is willing to risk in order to achieve a better self-image and an enhanced degree of self-esteem. The plastic surgeon is in the odd position under these circumstances of making well patients ill in order to make them feel better about themselves.

In esthetic surgery, the patient who is least sick physically is in fact the best candidate. That individual least fulfills the classic sick role: The expected prognosis in terms of morbidity and mortality is excellent; anticipated pain is minimal; complicated ancillary procedures and prolonged nursing care are not needed. In contrast, the sicker the patient, the greater the likelihood that the operation is reconstructive, and the more the plastic surgeon, rather than the patient, becomes the judge of the result.

The fact that esthetic surgery is elective allows the patient and the surgeon time to decide. The patient can obtain additional consultations and frequently does.

Brief Physical Examination

The initial examination of the esthetic surgical patient is regional and does not ordinarily encompass the entire body. A 40-year-old woman seeking a rhinoplasty, for example, would consider a breast or pelvic examination inappropriate if performed by the plastic surgeon, yet she would expect those examinations in the office of her internist, family doctor, general surgeon, or gynecologist, and if they had failed to do them, she would consider them delinquent.

In most instances, evaluation of esthetic surgical patients involves simply looking; of course, we examine with our fingers by palpating, but we do not usually do complex physical or diagnostic examinations. In a sense, we are assessing the patient as he or she assesses himself or herself: by looking, most usually in the mirror.

Thorough physical examinations in other areas of medicine are usually done to establish a diagnosis as well as to evaluate the general health of the patient. Much of this has already been done for us by the patient through his or her history. The diagnosis we may seek is more in the nature of what is causing the external anatomic condition about which a patient complains. For example, is the pendulous and ptotic breast the result of stretched, redundant skin or of excess breast tissue? Is the sagging of the tissue in the neck due to skin only or to the platysma as well?

In short, patients seeking esthetic surgery expect an operation, usually are healthy, and require minimal diagnostic acumen to determine the nature of their problem. Therefore, the jump to structuring the consultation in terms of treatment occurs with more rapidity under these circumstances than it would most likely with complex reconstructive problems in plastic surgery or ordinary problems within other surgical specialties, such as orthopedics and neurosurgery.

Guilt and Embarrassment

Esthetic surgical patients often feel guilty about wanting an operation that they, their family, or their friends consider "frivolous" or "vain." They are ashamed above having an operation when they are not truly sick.

Although the popularity of esthetic surgery is increasing, the acceptance within the ethos of our Judeo-Christian heritage is still lagging. The Old and New Testaments speak against vanity, and many patients coming for cosmetic surgery worry about being vain. Many, in fact, openly express that their vanity, which has led them to your office, might be punishable later by some complication because they did not "leave well enough alone." They are conscious of perhaps desiring more than fate or God has given them and fear their impetus for physical improvement may turn out to be a mistaken venture, maybe even a disaster. This fear of celestial reprisal is evidence of their guilt. Jacques Joseph (1865–1934), the father of modern cosmetic rhinoplasty and a founder of reconstructive surgery as well, declared that "it is inhuman to ascribe to vanity the driving motive for these patients, seeking correction, as is often done. One may speak of vanity . . . only in those cases in which a person desires to be more beautiful than the average human being. Those who want only to be freed from disfigurement, whose aim is only to achieve average looks and, therefore, to become inconspicuous, should not be labeled with that odious word *vanity*." [145] He called it *antidysplasia*—"the feeling of being disfigured and the aversion to such disfigurement and its emotional and material consequences."

In the United States, we admire more the people who gain their money through work (achieved) than through inheritance (ascribed) [149]. In both instances, however, when people have either beauty from birth or wealth from their own work, the implication is also that fate and God have favored them.

Esthetic surgical patients are not the only ones embarrassed about their problem and their need for help [246]. Consider the person with a venereal disease or an emotional illness. In the former situation, society, while providing treatment, still is judgmental: "He should have known better." In the latter case, the often expressed message is that with enough will (ego strength), patients should be able to overcome their mental difficulties.

The patient for cosmetic surgery, especially if older, may receive little or no emotional buttressing from loved ones, unlike those persons with life-threatening disease or reconstructive surgical problems who are cajoled and sometimes even carried to the doctor. Many esthetic surgical patients think that even the family doctor opposes the surgery they want, and, in many instances, they are correct. The fact that the patient does something of which friends and family disapprove increases guilt as well as anxiety.

Rapid Recovery and Little Regression
Since most esthetic operations can be done under local anesthesia (usually with intravenous supplementation), patients do not lose consciousness but are awake or drowsy. They maintain contact with the environment. Patients for cosmetic surgery not only want to resume their normal activities as soon as possible but are able to do so sooner than those undergoing more major procedures requiring reconstruction. The cosmetic patient has little incentive for secondary gain by prolonging recovery. Less regression thus occurs; the esthetic patient does not break stride for long. Serious strains in the patient-doctor relationship may arise, in fact, if a complication delays the anticipated early return to normalcy.

One of the major reasons that patients wish a rapid recovery and regress minimally is that they do not want others to know that they have had the procedure. In soon, out soon, back to work soon— become the ideal sequence of an esthetic operation.

George Bernard Shaw would not have wanted esthetic surgery for at least one reason: "I envy convalescence. It is the part that makes illness worthwhile." Moreover, cosmetic patients do not think of themselves as ill.

Minimizing Surgical Reality
In the relationship between the surgeon and the esthetic patient, features and pressures lead each to minimize the surgical reality [59, 99, 245, 250]. The surgeon may tell the patient about risks but not in such a way that the patient is put off; the patient may screen out the information because he or she very much wants the operation. If the patient truly expected, for example, an ectropion, infection, or blindness from an eyelidplasty, he or she would never have it done. The surgeon, by doing the procedure under local anesthesia

on an ambulatory basis (especially if it is in the office) wittingly or unwittingly perpetuates the notion that this is not "real surgery," which usually involves general anesthesia and at least one or two days in the hospital, with the implication of a greater likelihood of serious complications and a longer recuperation. If, indeed, the surgeon believed that the patient would develop a complication, such as ectropion or blindness after an eyelidplasty, he or she would never undertake the procedure. Both the patient and the surgeon are hoping that chance-probability will favor them, while realizing that chance cannot favor everybody.

Our culture in general fosters unrealistically high hopes about many, if not most, of its activities. An apparent paradox in our society is the mixture of myth and science, of rationality and irrationality. Technological prowess has led us to expect that "all is possible." We are primed to anticipate more than we are likely to receive. It is hard not to become a victim of false hopes in a land where cigarette smokers are depicted as winning a pliant beauty, not a fatal cancer; where cosmetics, clothes, dyes, and esthetic surgery hide the natural state; where perfumes, sprays, and deodorants mask normal body odors; where the media stroke the fantasy zones; where the citizenry are told that they are "created equal" to have and become what they wish, as if mere desire could transform somebody ordinary into a Giotto, a Garbo, or a Getty; where people believe that with more money we will soon conquer cancer, heart disease, and aging, enabling us to live "happily ever after"; where politicians thrive by avoiding unpleasant truths and by promising the undeliverable. For a populace spurred to grasp the golden carrot in this world, it is not surprising that frustration, disappointment, and anger are likely to be high if medical treatment does not meet expectations. These expectations are further elevated by unrealistic presentations in the media.

Even if the patient has fairly read and carefully signed a proper informed consent, when a complication occurs, he or she is likely to blame something or someone [10, 12]. As a member of a technologically advanced society, he or she is not likely to accept the explanation that "fate," "the spirits," or "bad luck" did it. The attorney thus becomes the ombudsman, offering those who have unrealistic expectations an enormous self-entitlement. Even the concept that everyone has the right to sue and to anticipate recompense is not realistic, since obviously not all plaintiffs win, but, nevertheless, the malpractice march keeps going on.

The surgeon, as mentioned, not just the patient, may have fanciful expectations, and these are not simply about complications or the lack of them. It is always the next patient who may be the recipient of his or her first perfect operation. Perhaps the surgeon's practical sense has been muddled by the articles in professional journals and presentations at meetings that show only flawless outcomes. Ideally the surgeon will be more objective than the patient, but both are interacting as members of the same society.

Pain

Every incision can cause pain in almost every patient. Excessive pain is unusual in esthetic surgery and even in reconstructive surgery. When it occurs, it likely indicates or heralds a complication such as bleeding, infection, nerve injury, or irritation. However, great is the variation among our patients and ourselves in tolerating pain. We should keep in mind Samuel Johnson's remark about pain: "Those who do not feel it, Sir, seldom think that it is felt."

Happiness as an Objective

Esthetic surgery involves the elusive objective of "happiness," which is implied in the enhancement patients expect after a cosmetic operation. The results of psychotherapy are judged also in terms of that hard-to-define (and acquire) mental state, whereas in most of medicine, the efficacy of therapy is usually measured in terms of decreased pain or increased motion or function (e.g., ability to defecate or urinate or grasp normally). It would be unusual to ask a patient after a colectomy whether or not he or she is "happy" with the result. Being "alive and well" and "free of disease" are the common indices of success. The term *patient satisfaction* is rife in esthetic surgery but rare in neurosurgery or general surgery, for example.

Preponderance of Females

Another distinctive feature of esthetic surgery is that at least 85 to 90 percent of patients are females. The reasons are not anatomical, as in gynecology, but cultural and personal. Our culture places a higher value on the attractive appearance of the woman than on that of the man; and the woman, deprived of the many sources of gratification available to the man in terms of achievement, has undoubtedly learned to use and value her body, consciously and unconsciously, to please herself and others [113]. This behavior is rewarded, perpetuated, and reinforced throughout her life by such acts as using makeup, adopting hair and clothing styles, and keeping "young and trim." In *Beauty Bound*, Freedman [80] has written:

> Beauty counts for everyone, but more so for women. From the moment of birth, beauty is sought, perceived, and projected onto girls. When parents were asked within twenty-four hours after delivery to rate their first-born infants on a variety of characteristics, daughters were described as beautiful, soft, pretty, cute, delicate and little. Sons were rated as firm, strong, large-featured, well-coordinated, and hardy. The baby boys and girls in this study had been carefully matched for equivalent length, weight and level of responsiveness. Despite the physical similarities of these infants, their parents nevertheless brought home 'beautiful' daughters and 'strong' sons. A baby dressed in blue was described in another study as bouncing, strong, active; the same baby dressed in pink was called sweet and lovely. Studies confirmed that throughout childhood girls receive more attention for their appearance than do boys.

To emphasize the point, Freedman quotes the poet Tagore: "O woman, you're not really the handiwork of God, but also of men; these are ever endowing you with beauty from their own hearts. You are one-half woman and one-half dream."

Inculcated with the desideratum of attractiveness and bombarded by measures and stratagems for acquiring it, many women feel obligated to change or maintain their bodies to promote pleasure for themselves and others [81]. Aiding them in the battle for beauty is the plastic surgeon who is generally a man (95% of certified plastic surgeons in the United States are male) and does not think it is unusual for a woman to enhance her appearance through surgery [245].

Finances
For the cosmetic patient, going it alone as a *modus operandi* applies also to financial aspects. Insurance plans generally do not cover so-called luxury surgery, and they will not defray the expenses of treating its complications. Prepayment is customary for esthetic operations, unlike other areas of medicine except, perhaps, orthodontia. Prepayment will be discussed later (see pp. 100–101).

PATIENT SELECTION FOR ESTHETIC SURGERY: THE IMPORTANCE OF CAUTION

Some patients should not have cosmetic surgery; their soma or psyche makes them unsuitable [9, 16, 89, 91–94, 103, 216–218]. As plastic surgeons, we justifiably place great reliance on technique; but contrary to the message in most surgical atlases and sex manuals, technique is not everything. A well-executed procedure does not necessarily produce a happy patient. When one considers the vagaries of surgery and wound healing, as well as the complexities of human nature, it is surprising that so many patients seem satisfied with their results. The unhappy few, however, loom large in the surgical landscape. In my experience, one dissatisfied patient can dominate days and even weeks of one's professional life. Let us now consider identifying those who might prove to be poor selections for esthetic surgery. I emphasize that these categories represent *potential* patients to avoid and not absolute indications for rejections; however, as André Gide once remarked: "It has been said before but because no one listens, it must be said again." In frankness, I believe that we do listen, perhaps not enough to remember, when we talk to each other about patients whose quest for self-improvement through surgery we wish we had not attempted to facilitate.

The Patient Who Writes an Excessively Long Letter to Arrange the Initial Consultation
The patient who approaches you with a tedious communication is not simply providing information in a less than readable fashion, but is pleading his or her case. Generally, such letters contain an obsessively described saga of repeated dissatisfaction following multiple

treatments of a condition that may be objectively less major than the patient believes. This compulsive quality in recounting the excruciating litany of medical misfortunes is pathognomonic of a neurotic, rigid person who tries to relieve anxiety by attempting to control every item in life. Such individuals tend to be so perfectionistic that no result would ever please them.

Alternatively, the patient may truly have had a series of maldirected medical acts that now has produced a problem warranting detailed description; however, in my experience, such is not usually the problem. You have become the patient's last resort because of your "great reputation." The letter is thus not only an outpouring of grief but also a means of manipulation—to get you to don the armor of the knight errant for the patient's next surgical crusade. Almost always the patient will strongly criticize another plastic surgeon for lack of skill and sympathy. A common expression is "Now he won't see me or even return my call." Indeed, that might be so. Although this patient might appear pathetic and wronged, tread warily before deciding to operate, since you may well end up not as the knight errant but as the erring knight. Obtain all possible information from the patient, the family physician, and the other plastic surgeon(s). Most likely there has been more than one procedure by more than one surgeon.

The Rude or Demanding Patient

Some patients refuse to accept the next open appointment but insult or try to bypass the secretary to have you see them earlier. Frequently, a beleaguered referring doctor will apologetically call to have you see the patient as soon as you can just as a "personal favor." This type of patient wants to be treated as an exception because he or she (and it is usually a woman) feels exceptional. That person has a high titer of self-entitlement that he or she will maintain until the last good-bye, which perhaps should be soon after the first hello. The sense of entitlement is astronomical and, in the words of one of my residents, represents "malignant entitlement." The patient will want the earliest possible date for surgery, a private room, and will insist on being first on your operating schedule. Later the demanding patient may not accept your instructions and may become hostile should even the slightest thing go awry. These patients are usually well-to-do and may be accustomed to having all obstacles wither before their financial clout. As physicians, we should not discriminate against patients because of their economic status—poor or rich. It might be helpful to recall the interchange between Ernest Hemingway and F. Scott Fitzgerald, who observed: "The very rich are different from you and me." Hemingway replied, "Yes. They have more money."

A patient with excessive entitlement may never realize that he or she is part of the human race, a minor figure on the globe, subject to the "uncontrollable whims of fate and circumstances." Illness, death, and the surgical act are levellers; the laws of chance sometimes overcome those of skill and expectation.

The Unkempt Patient
The unkempt patient is not out of place in an emergency room but is unusual in the setting for cosmetic surgery. Although some patients with a pervasive deformity such as overly large breasts may let themselves become obese or slovenly, that kind of appearance may indicate a severely disturbed personality. Not every patient can afford a Ralph Lauren dress, but all can purchase or acquire a bar of soap. With this type of patient, it is important to obtain an extensive medical history, including possible previous or current psychotherapy. One should ask specifically about drug and alcohol abuse.

The Patient Who Makes Your Office Her (or His) Home
Occasionally, you may find in your consultation room a patient who has taken over; looked through your papers and at the pictures on your desk, and removed books from the shelves. In my experience, these patients who aggressively rummage around your office are women. They wish to be in control by establishing an immediate intimacy. Some may ask whether they may be on a first-name basis with you. Their behavior may indicate underlying anxiety about dependency and perhaps they try to allay their disquiet by dominating every situation. This type of patient is trying to direct her own care. If you plan to operate on her, you must establish early that you are in charge. To your surprise, they usually acquiesce quite easily, almost thankful that you now carry the responsibility for them.

The Patient Who Praises You Excessively and Denigrates Your Colleagues

Some patients have discovered an eternal truth: Few doctors can resist flattery. By plumping your ego, this kind of individual may get you to perform an operation whose results he or she will never like. You will soon join your colleagues on the hate list.

The usual dialogue is like this:

She: I am glad you could see me. I've waited many weeks to come here. I'm thankful to be here. I've learned a lot about you. You certainly have some reputation!

You: [Shifting uncomfortably in your chair] Thank you, what can I do for you?

She: I am here to get your opinion and your help about my nose, which, I dislike saying, has been butchered. I am sure you have heard of Dr. _____; he is supposed to be good, but twice he operated on me, and my nose is worse now than it ever was before. My husband and friends don't know how I ever went through all I did—the pain and expense, and for what? A ruined nose? If he really thought he couldn't help me, the least he could have done was to tell me and refer me to someone like you.

And so it goes. The web is being spun.

The Patient Who Gives a False History

You may suspect an occasional patient of lying. Although apparently alert and intelligent, he or she may give contradictory information or appear surprisingly vague; dates may not jibe; the social and occupational history have an unconvincing, fictional quality.

I have had several patients who have denied previous cosmetic surgery but had the stigmata of a rhinoplasty and the scars of a facelift. The patient may say that you are the first plastic surgeon she has seen, but her questions and reactions to your queries belie her. One woman on whose lids I noted scars confessed when I questioned her, "I didn't want to tell you I had my eyes done a year ago. I wanted to see if you thought I needed surgery. If you didn't, I would have known that he did a good job." In that instance, fortunately, he had done "a good job."

Other patients have an abnormal affect, as if they are sedated or tranquilized. Indeed, some are on psychotropic medication. They will try to hide their emotional illness, perhaps fearing that you might reject them for operation. In this regard, they are not unrealistic.

If you believe that the patient has not been truthful, you should try to determine why—usually by gently confronting the patient with the inconsistencies of the history or physical findings or both. You need not be a district attorney in your manner, but you should present a realistic appraisal of them and the story they furnish. In general, with patients who dissimulate, you are unlikely to establish a mutually satisfying relationship. Once the golden moment for trust is past, it is seldom regained.

The Indecisive or Vague Patient

Sometimes a patient may be unable to tell you what bothers him or her. A woman may say that she is unhappy with her nose—her whole face—but, "What do you think, Doctor? Look me over and tell me."

Although it is possible that this woman is placing herself under the scrutiny of the "expert" (and she may even state that "since you are the expert, I will leave it to you"), it is my experience that this attitude characterizes a patient with poor self-esteem. Although that is not a reason to reject the patient and, in fact, it is one of the reasons we do operate, it can mean that the patient has a generalized lack of self-esteem with only a murky focus on her physical features in the desperate hope that changing one of them or even more may make her more confident about life. It is important with these patients not to venture a harsh appraisal of all their physical defects; this would increase that person's dissatisfaction and expand the area of his or her poor self-image and surgical concern. The indecisive patient may schedule and reschedule surgery, to the exasperation of your secretary. Such vacillation is an indication of a lack of preparedness to undergo the operation and possibly even indecision as to what body feature really disturbs that individual. If you make the decision for the patient, he or she can blame you for later dissatisfaction, saying that you talked him or her into an operation—and, indeed, possibly you did.

A few years ago, a fellow surgeon consulted me for an eyelidplasty. On three occasions, he made arrangements and then canceled. Finally, I wrote him a letter (marked "personal"), in which I pointed out that his behavior suggested a conflict about having the operation or, at least, having me do it. I proposed that he seek another plastic surgeon. It was a hard letter to write because he was a doctor, but I fought against the temptation of treating him differently from any other patient. Later, he did have an eyelidplasty but was not pleased with the results, which to me looked satisfactory when I saw him on another occasion.

The Patient with Minimal Deformity

The worst combination for a satisfactory surgical result is the patient with maximum concern about a minimal deformity [67]. Since surgery is potentially hazardous, the objective of the procedure should be of sufficient significance to warrant the risks. A patient whose emotional energies are directed toward a minute bump on the nose had better first see a psychiatrist. If, indeed, a rhinoplasty were performed, the focus of that person's dissatisfaction would then be on either the postoperative result or another part of the body as well as you, the plastic surgeon.

I do not believe in tightrope surgery, in which you place the patient and yourself at hazard—one little mistake results in a catastrophe. If the operation is successful with respect to a deformity that is almost imperceptible, what really have you done? If you fail, you have given the patient an unfavorable result, which ultimately leads to another operation whose result may still be deficient and unsatisfying.

The Patient Who Refuses to Undress for Proper Examination or Refuses to be Photographed

Understandably, few people like to disrobe before a doctor or nurse, particularly if he or she is of the opposite sex; however, if a patient absolutely refuses to submit to a proper examination, then you cannot recommend proper treatment.

Many patients fear that their photographs will be used in a publication without their consent. They need specific reassurance about this.

Unwillingness on the part of the patient to be photographed may also prevent you from having an adequate record for planning. Furthermore, should medicolegal problems arise, your defense would be much weakened. The problem here is more than shyness. You should emphasize to the patient that you cannot proceed to help unless you can visually document the problem and thereby properly plan surgical treatment. Photographs to plastic surgeons are like an electrocardiogram to a cardiologist, and, in fact, you may offer the patient this comparison. Help the patient to understand that your office routine has evolved from the care of many others with similar problems.

The Perfectionistic Patient

The perfectionistic patient is the individual who wants everything in life, including surgical results, to be "perfect"—every wrinkle gone or "the nose just so." It is usually impossible to satisfy that person because surgery and wound healing are beyond absolute precision and control. The skin is not marble. Perfectionistic patients are hard on themselves and on others: The restaurant never prepares their meal properly the first time; their seamstress or tailor never listens to instructions; the weather is either too hot or too cold. They may obsessively pursue health, constantly dieting, always exercising [11].

We plastic surgeons who tend to be perfectionistic may sympathize with anyone seeking a faultless outcome; however, the combination of a perfectionistic plastic surgeon and a perfectionistic patient is frequently imperfection, so far as that patient's appreciation of the result is concerned.

The perfectionistic patient frequently becomes the shopper.

The Shopper

> There are many very good people who are not what I call good patients. I was once requested to call on a lady suffering from nervous and other symptoms. It came out in the preliminary conversational skirmish, half medical, half social, that I was the twenty-sixth member of the faculty into whose arms, professionally speaking, she had successfully thrown

herself. Not being a believer in such a rapid rotation of scientific crops, I gently deposited the burden, commending it to the care of number twenty-seven, and, him, whoever he might be, to the care of Heaven.

Oliver Wendell Holmes
The Young Practitioner, in *Medical Essays*

The surgical shopper usually does not look for the lowest fee but for the surgeon who will guarantee the result. By going only to "the best plastic surgeon" (how that can be determined, I am not sure), that type of patient will feel more secure; however, like any shopper, this person thinks of surgery as a commodity—something to purchase and to return if defective or if the buyer is dissatisfied [143]. Unfortunately, most surgical results are not totally reversible. Do not be flattered that this patient has selected you from the six others already seen. They are by far the luckier.

The Plasti-Surgiholic

The plasti-surgiholic, usually a woman, is the seeker and bearer of multiple operations. She may proudly recite a list of famous plastic surgeons who have operated on her. Though relatively young, she may have already had her nose and eyelids done, her breasts augmented, and her abdomen tightened. She may want repeats or something new. That she has needed to submit her body to surgery and its attendant pain indicates a masochism and low self-esteem [283]. This patient needs a psychiatrist [258], not a plastic surgeon, but characteristically, she will refuse your referral and will continue her search for a willing surgeon, whom she is very likely to find, especially if she can easily pay for the procedure.

It is easy to get trapped into operating on such a person to correct a deformity, such as unsightly scars, resulting from her previous surgical escapades. You may delude yourself by thinking that you are not doing an operation but a "revision" or a "touch-up." Your remedial procedure still counts as an operation—it is still surgery—and it will be just one more notch on her belt.

In this era, however, when so many people begin at a young age to have plastic surgical procedures, it is possible to have a woman in her 50s who, though not the classic psychoneurotic described by Freud, has had a rhinoplasty and breast augmentation and now contemplates a facelift. To have a body that looks perfect, to maintain weight and life in control, and to be a high achiever are the characteristics of many younger women and men of today. Their overemphasis on exercise, weight, and diet—even caliber of their stools—constitutes a syndrome of our era: the compulsive pursuit of perfection in the hope for happiness, the latter becoming more elusive as the chase becomes fiercer. Some of these women have a history of eating disorders: anorexia or bulimia, or both.

In assessing a patient who has had multiple procedures, it is important to know over what interval. If a 63-year-old woman reports three or four previous esthetic operations, it may be of less concern than if a 35-year-old gives the same history. Sometimes the person who seems addicted to plastic surgery is either an individual with poor self-esteem or someone with enormous narcissism; the latter usually more satisfied with the result than the former, who might have expected that an operation would magically transform his or her life and noticeably improve his or her self-image and self-esteem.

Knorr, Edgerton, and Hoopes [153] found that the personality characteristics of those addicted to cosmetic surgery were similar to those with other addictions: low self-esteem and feelings of inadequacy in personal and sexual relationships and at work.

The plastic surgeon, not the patient, has the responsibility to prevent further unnecessary surgery whose end point is not finite or anatomical but psychological and infinite.

The Acquiescing Patient

Sometimes a patient wants an operation to please someone else, often to save a failing marriage. It is a form of masochism in which no surgeon should get involved. Someone willing to risk harm, to undergo pain, and to pay the expense of an operation—all in the name of patching up a relationship—is doomed to failure. It becomes a *folie à trois* when the surgeon joins that person in holding still another individual within a relationship. Psychotherapy is what that patient should have and not esthetic surgery, at least at this point.

The woman or man who has a deteriorating marriage and on whom you operate is frequently dissatisfied with the results of the procedure because the expected result is not anatomical but interpersonal, between spouses or intimates. Later you may be surprised to see the husband and wife, as an example, lovingly unite to blame you if the operation has not produced what was secretly desired. There is always a wrinkle to find, always a scar to criticize, always the possibility of having done "too much" or "too little."

A 55-year-old man, accompanied by his wife, came to see me because he wanted his nose made smaller and his chin larger. Significant in this history was a serious myocardial infarction two months before. In listening to his desires and seeing the marital interplay, it was obvious that his wife was the instigator. Her commitment to the surgery was strong and did not waver when I pointed out to her the risk of operating on someone so soon after a heart attack, especially for an elective procedure. I refused to do the operation at that time and referred them both to their family physician, who at first seemed surprised that I doubted that this couple had a happy marriage. Later he called to say that after having talked with them further, he found out that the husband was impotent and his wife "could not stand him because of his big nose and small chin." Subsequently, they went for marital therapy for problems that, I am sure, were of greater importance than the size of his chin and nose. I have not since heard from them or about them.

Another common instance of an abnormally compliant patient is the adolescent who accedes to rhinoplasty to placate an overbearing parent (see p. 114).

The Paranoid or Depressed Patient

Elective surgery, especially if esthetic, is best not performed on individuals who are paranoid or depressed. With psychotherapy, and with the use of proper medication, perhaps that person may be prepared for operation, but its timing must be carefully chosen. The plastic surgeon must communicate with the psychiatrist, whose clinical judgment hopefully will be sound. Occasionally, because of an impasse in therapy, a psychiatrist might refer a patient for plastic surgery—as a means of surmounting the obstacle. Whatever the opinion of the psychiatrist, I would not perform the operation if I had strong doubts. The patient may go into a reactive depression, and you will have to bear the brunt of his or her dissatisfaction and anger.

Depression is not always obvious. Many seek plastic surgery after a loss, such as a divorce, a breakup with a lover, or the death of a loved one. Usually the patient is middle-aged and a woman. The operation is desired to attain a younger appearance, almost as if the patient were trying to be born again—to start life anew, to be more attractive, more saleable. Often such patients could benefit anatomically from esthetic surgery, but it must be correctly timed to avoid further depression. Sometimes a consultation with a psychiatrist is helpful to be sure that the patient has experienced a proper grief reaction.

With so many marriages failing, it is almost impossible to have a full day at the office without seeing a middle-aged person who is either separated or divorced or may be considering either. It is important to inquire when that patient became concerned with an unwanted feature. She (the majority of these patients are women) may say: "I never liked my nose and when I was a teenager I wanted it done but my parents wouldn't let me. Then I got married and I sort of forgot about it although I admit that I never liked having photographs taken, especially from the side. But now when I am no longer married and have gone back to work and would like to go out more, I think of the nose more and more and I like it less and less." This may be a realistic response from a patient who is not depressed and who is an excellent candidate for the operation, but, should she, on questioning, admit that she cannot fall asleep and then wants to stay in bed most of the day, has crying spells but no appetite, and does not seem to enjoy life any more, she probably has a clinical depression and should have treatment, which takes precedence over rhinoplasty. Perhaps at a later time, when she is no longer depressed, the operation will give her a result that is satisfying both anatomically and psychologically.

The loss in a person's life with its subsequent depression need not always involve a person. The cause may be a change in financial status (down usually but up occasionally), or the loss of a body part, as after a mastectomy or hysterectomy.

A 43-year-old single woman sought a facelift four months after having had a hysterectomy and bilateral oophorectomy for enlarging fibroids. She was still angry at the gynecologist whom "I just can't talk to; he says I am babying myself." She thought that she had aged dramatically since her operation, although, in fact, she had only the most minimal signs of aging—nothing sufficient to warrant a facelift. Listening to her, I noted that she was obviously depressed by what she considered her loss of femininity, fertility, and youth. She said that recently her spirits were better than when she had called for an appointment. At the end of the consultation, she seemed relieved to hear that many women under similar conditions have a depression and seek a facelift or other cosmetic surgery, from which they (herself included) would benefit very little. She also admitted that even though she never planned to get married, the presence of her uterus, now gone, had given the fantasy and the hope that some day she might be able to have a child.

Although some surgeons have reported success from esthetic surgery in patients with severe emotional problems [140], including depression and paranoia, these happy outcomes should be considered feats and exceptions but not routine outcomes. The surgical blade is not a psychic knife.

The Patient in Psychotherapy

The fact that a patient is in psychotherapy is not by itself a contraindication to esthetic surgery; it may actually be an advantage. It does mean, however, that you must ascertain the nature and degree of the emotional problem that led him or her to seek therapy. In addition to making observations, you must rely on the therapist for information about the patient [211]. You must communicate with that therapist to be certain that what the patient seeks surgically is appropriate and realistic in relation to the ongoing psychotherapy, as well as to other aspects of the patient's life. It is surprising how often a patient who has been seeing a therapist for many months, even years, has not discussed arranging a consultation with you for a problem that she has willingly discussed with you but never with her therapist. In these circumstances, as with any patient in psychotherapy, you should offer to call or write the therapist. I find a letter preferable because my thoughts are then on record; also, it may elicit a letter in return, which will be part of the patient's file. Customarily, I dictate the letter in the presence of the patient or send the patient a copy, or both, indicating to the therapist that the patient has either heard or will read my opinion. This openness helps to eliminate ambiguity and the patient's feeling that if surgery is refused, it was because of a collusion between you and the therapist. Frequently the patient will ask you to defer writing until he or she has discussed the consultation with the therapist. I then insist that the patient call me in a couple of weeks to let me know whether he or she did talk to the therapist about the problem.

For many patients, the undertaking of esthetic surgery represents progress toward resolving emotional problems and improving their life. Sometimes, it may be a hopeful shortcut around an obstacle in therapy as mentioned. One must be very wary of that situation, since the procedure, even if done well, might not alleviate the patient's emotional problem. An exception to this might be if the therapy is now centering on a physical feature that is grossly displeasing to the patient and would be so to most observers, e.g., a very large nose or an underdeveloped chin.

When a patient states that he or she is "in therapy," it can mean many things. A patient may be midstream or may be ready to terminate by agreement with the therapist or may be impulsively ending the therapy without the therapist's approval.

Who the therapist is also makes a great difference [271]. The task of treating emotional disease has been undertaken by many who are poorly trained and who are not psychiatrists, social workers, or clinical psychologists. Even within those groups are persons of varying judgment and experience. You may find yourself in the disquieting position of disagreeing with the therapist—almost always being more dubious than the therapist about the patient's ability to benefit psychologically from the operation. You may be forced to request an additional consultation, even to the point of suggesting someone else whose experience and judgment you trust.

Sometimes a psychiatrist may refuse to give an opinion about the patient's suitability for surgery, perhaps responding to your request for guidance with the comment, "The decision is the patient's." Although not making decisions for the patient—at least openly—is a standard stance of many therapists and ultimately may be beneficial to the patient, it may be exasperating to you. One should resist the impulse, so common to surgeons, to resolve the ambiguity by action—by operating. Since the patient's condition is not urgent, you also can be and perhaps should be noncommittal. To the therapist and the patient, you may suggest postponing a decision and reviewing the matter in a few months.

I would never operate on a patient whose therapist is opposed to the surgery. Frequently, I refuse even when the therapist is in favor if I sense trouble ahead. One should remember the plastic surgeon still has a primary responsibility for the patient should he or she be dissatisfied after the operation. Just as the psychotherapist can be wrong, so can you. I am sure that some patients whose operation I would not do have gone to someone else and have had a satisfactory outcome, anatomically and emotionally. Yet, being safe is always better than being sorry. Calvin Coolidge once remarked: "You don't have to take back what you don't say." It is far worse in terms of a surgical procedure that never can be erased once it has occurred.

The Patient Whose Spouse Says "No"
Although theoretically and legally an adult can decide on an operation, if competent mentally, it does not mean that you, as plastic surgeon, must do it. The reluctant spouse is more likely to be a husband who strongly disapproves of his wife's desire to alter her nose or, more likely, to reduce her breasts. Although that is her privilege and although we live in an era of feminism, I am still fearful to initiate an elective operation to which a spouse is unalterably opposed—even after, let us say, I have spoken to the spouse in person in an attempt to determine his or her objections and anxieties. Often I have observed that a displeasing feature to the wife may be important in the power relationships within the marriage, e.g., the woman has poor self-esteem, a fact that the husband exploits consciously or unconsciously.

I do not want to enter the marital fray as the surgeon. I once had the experience of the husband and wife then combining against me, perhaps as a way of resolving their marital problems. If the patient has a significant complaint, for example, with massive breasts, and I believe the operation should be done because it would benefit her, I suggest marital counseling first. If they are unwilling to do this—

not just the wife going alone—then I will not consent to be the surgeon. They may go elsewhere. It is their right to do so, but it is also my right to refuse to operate.

The "Special" Patient (VIP)
The danger with the "special" patient is that surgical judgment may defer to status. The patient may want you to treat him or her differently from others because he or she is "important." Without your being asked, you may be making medical decisions unconsciously for that individual that you would not make for others. Departing from your routine increases the chance for error. Realistically, no doctor treats everybody the same since we must take into account a patient's personality, intelligence, and background; however, you should be treating primarily the patient's problem, not his or her socioeconomic position. Throughout our residency training, most of us saw errors of management that would not have arisen had the patient been poor and from the clinic rather than rich and from a Cadillac. Fame or wealth does not change basic anatomy, physiology, and biochemistry.

The Patient Whom You Dislike
Fortunately, the disagreeable patient is infrequent. He or she is the type of person who, if presented with a dozen roses, would note only the thorns. Their bitterness about life, their insatiability, and their hostility will focus on you and the postoperative result, no matter how technically acceptable it may be.

In an emergency situation or for a condition that threatens the patient's life, we must accept the difficult individual; however, for elective surgery, particularly esthetic, there is no virtue in baring your neck to the guillotine. For taking care of that patient, you will receive not a medal but more likely a subpoena.

In general, never do an esthetic procedure on a patient who is hostile to you at the time of your initial meeting. Seldom will you be able to avoid becoming the target of more aggressive feelings. Furthermore, if the patient has diffuse aggression or if it is centered on some other surgeon, you will most likely become the next target.

Unlike psychiatrists whose work is to deal with many unpleasant emotions such as anger, we, as plastic surgeons, do not need and should not wish to become therapists. We may have to manage the patient's aggression during the course of treatment, but to embark on a surgical enterprise with an already angry individual calls for more masochism or megalomania than I possess or wish to acquire. A few of us may want to be an Osler or a Freud, but one should remember that they did not operate on such patients either. Realize that at best a surgical procedure may only temporarily calm or defuse a hostile patient, but, more often, it may be another stimulus to his or her punitive sentiments.

As mentioned, the situation is very different when the patient becomes hostile during the course of your treatment—postoperatively. Your responsibility then is to find the cause and hopefully to resolve the problem (see p. 246).

Another circumstance in which you confront an aggressive patient with whom you must deal responsibly is when someone hospitalized has become unhappy and angry (hostile in the hostel) because of failure in management or simply because of the length of confinement. The medical problem and the patient's reactions are identifiable and understandable—frustration, fear of never getting well, and loss of power. Weiss [267] has written,

> A sick patient feels he no longer has control of his own destiny, for his role as an independent doer has suddenly been reversed and has become one of relative or complete dependence. Not only must he depend upon his physician, but upon those who previously depended upon him, his family. It is not surprising, therefore, to find the patient is equally hostile to family members as he is to the physician himself, demonstrating the global nature of this loss. He has figuratively become "impotent," and he sees the physician, his sole treater, as omnipotent. This precipitates with him new sources of hostility—the first is a function of the newly-developed dependence and the second is a secondary manifestation of his rage at the physician when he discovers that his intense, immediate narcissistic needs cannot always be gratified.

The patient in the hospital or even one who has been discharged and for whom things are not going along smoothly is much different from the physically well patient seeking a facelift, for example, but who has a palpable anger toward life and you.

For some surgeons, the issue is not so much the patient they dislike but the operation they detest. The ill-fated patient then becomes by association the recipient of the surgeon's irritability and displeasure. One plastic surgeon told me frankly that he found facelifts "boring," and he did them only because they were an easy way to make money.

Other surgeons do not like the kind of patient who might wish a certain operation. A colleague confessed that he thought "rich women" who sought cosmetic surgery were "vain, childish, and self-indulgent." His attitude was reminiscent of a line in one of John Cheever's short stories, "God preserve me from women who dress like *toreros* to go to the supermarket." [45] Fortunately, this surgeon had enough insight, if not to change his feelings, at least to avoid operating on these patients.

Rarely can one do well what one does not like doing. Without enthusiasm, success is difficult.

The Patient from Afar

The out-of-town patient may present a problem not only in relation to cosmetic surgery, but reconstructive as well. Furthermore, distance is a matter of degree and the patient's and doctor's conception of it. For example, I have patients for whom a 40-mile drive into Boston is a fearsome ordeal, much worse than for other patients who may come from much greater distances. To some doctors with an international practice, nothing is "afar." Yet, some general points deserve mentioning about the patient who is not from your backyard.

As a physician's reputation grows, so will the radius of referrals. Most surgeons may actually feel a glow when patients come great distances to get their opinion and to use their skills. Despite the obvious advantages, there are, however, certain potential problems [2].

The first is that both the patient and the surgeon are under pressure of the moment to decide on a course of treatment. Frequently, a patient may actually be scheduled before he or she has seen you, a situation that is not ideal but occasionally unavoidable. If that same patient had lived nearby and could have returned for a second visit, it is possible that the decision would have been not to operate.

Another problem with the patient from afar is that communication with the referring physician or other consultants is not so facile and direct. Proper discussion with family members, such as parents or spouse, may have to be sacrificed to the exigencies of scheduling.

The fact that the patient has made the trip to your office alone and has decided to have the operation at a great distance from home may lead you as a surgeon to overestimate that person's self-sufficiency and to underestimate his or her anxiety, fear, and loneliness. The patient then goes through the operation outside his or her customary orbit and ordinarily without the usual support systems. These realities become especially important should a complication occur, when the patient may then become increasingly anxious about separation from home and family. An unfavorable result will necessitate contending with mounting expenses, since their stay may have to be lengthened or additional treatment may have to be undertaken. The patient may even be discharged and forced to return for another hospitalization. The fact that the patient's family may have disapproved of the operation in the first place or of his or her having had it far from home will engender more guilt. In the event of a postoperative problem, it is essential that the family, the referring doctor, and anyone else close to the patient be kept informed about what went wrong and your present plans for its management.

Every patient from afar who has had an operation must remain nearby long enough for proper observation and care. In addition to the physical realities of an operation, the patient needs emotional support to deal with the inevitable stress. For example, after a facelift the patient commonly will become depressed and will require periodic reassurance. The doctor must be there to answer questions, which are not so much to elicit information as to renew the patient's confidence. When the patient goes home, it is helpful to have him or her write or call regularly.

The postoperative patient returning home may also have difficulty obtaining proper follow-up should it be necessary. She or he may have seen a plastic surgeon locally and then decided to go to you for the operation. It will be embarrassing for that individual to return to the home surgeon, who might also resent being asked to do the cleanup work. Even the patient who has not consulted another plastic surgeon may correctly dread his or her displeasure at being passed over for the operation and now being called on in an emergency. It is axiomatic that the patient should not have to arrange for follow-up care; you should do this in a telephone call or letter, preferably both, to smooth the way. Hopefully your colleague will not be hostile because the patient exercised his or her right of choice in medical care.

Some patients want to have their surgery done out of town to avoid the embarrassment of having people know that they have had it; this is particularly true for facial surgery. Although that attitude is understandable, it sometimes makes things difficult when a complication ensues.

Other patients, however, come to you because they do not realize they could obtain excellent treatment where they live. For them, the appropriate advice is to have their operation at home. Their physical and emotional resources and perhaps fiscal as well would be needlessly depleted by having you as their surgeon, particularly if staged procedures were necessary.

With the patient from a distance, as with every patient, the surgeon's decision should be in the interest of the patient and not simply for personal gain or ego boosting.

The Patient Who Is Dissatisfied with What Is an Objectively Good Result of Another Plastic Surgeon's Operation

I have always been interested in the phenomenon of a patient who, having had a successful procedure by another plastic surgeon, has come to me. When I have asked these patients why they did this, a few have even questioned my questioning them. One woman, obviously angry, retorted: "That is my right—to see anyone I want." Deruffling the feathers was the next task with her. Other patients, however, may say that they did not think that the first plastic surgeon did this procedure although they had never asked; still others may say that they decided to switch plastic surgeons because one of their friends had come to me and had liked me and the result; my question surprises others whose response discloses their total lack of allegiance to the first surgeon. A typical answer is: "I never thought of going back to him. He did a good job and I suppose I should have thought of it—but it never occurred to me."

However, the patient to be wary of is the one who says, "I have had plastic surgery before and the result was really not good, in fact, it was terrible. That's why I'm here to see you because I don't want the same thing happening again." He or she seeks not to rectify the outcome of that operation but to have another esthetic procedure. You must determine what that operation was, the reason for dissatisfaction, what the patient did about it—simply complain, consult another plastic surgeon, or hire an attorney. Perhaps a litigation was justified, but frequently the outcome, when you evaluate it, is not by any means as grossly inferior as the patient believes and would have you believe.

I am writing about this kind of potential problem patient having just encountered one in my own practice: a woman who came to me for a facelift but complained of the result from her reduction mammoplasty done elsewhere. I examined her breasts—she had asked me to do so—and I thought that the outcome, though not magnificent, was good. I told her this but blithely proceeded to undertake her rhytidectomy. I was surprised, though I should not have been, that she did not like the result. The clue was present if I had heeded my intuition and advice, but I did not. I was foolish or arrogant to think that I could satisfy her expectations in another part of her body when someone competent had failed to do so elsewhere.

When, Why, and How to Say "No"

For most physicians who have been trained to say "yes" to tasks and responsibility, it is sometimes difficult to say "no." Yet saying that two-letter word may occasionally be a brilliant and sanity-saving decision. Under some circumstances, refusing to operate is relatively easy if the patient requires no operation: someone who has come for a facelift that has only very minimal signs of aging, for instance—or a patient whose problem is best managed by another specialty, such as dermatology. In the latter situation, the patient comprehends and appreciates your unwillingness to operate. Incidentally, I do not charge a patient who, for example, came for surgical excision of numerous seborrheic keratoses but whom I immediately refer to a dermatologist for simple management with liquid nitrogen. I even send a letter to that doctor. If the family physician originally made the referral, I generally suggest that he or she be consulted for the name of a dermatologist; thereby, I do not preempt that physician's prerogative.

Gorney [120] has identified another type of patient to avoid, whom he calls "the truly ugly patient." He has written:

> The patient whose deformity borders on the monstrous usually has great mental or deep ineradicable psychiatric problems. Except for the brilliant cranialfacial techniques, those persons are rarely candidates for traditional esthetic surgery. If the 'challenge' becomes too much of a temptation, the surgeon may wind up converting the merely grotesque into the simply ridiculous.

That individual should be referred, in my opinion, to someone specializing in cranialfacial surgery.

There is another kind of patient for whom one probably can do very little although one would like to do very much: the plain or unattractive woman, such as the person I recently saw in my office, a 50-year-old unmarried typist who wanted to know whether I could do anything to improve her looks. Her features were coarse: her skin thick, her eyes almost slits and deep-set, her nose was large more because of the skin than because of the bone. I thought that her appearance was beyond my surgical talents; I would not know where to start, what to do, or where to end. I referred her to another colleague for possibly a different opinion. Although I felt sorry for her, I would not want to compound her problems by a useless surgical effort that would not only cost her money but inflict scars, pain as well, and perhaps even disappointment over the result.

Another situation in which saying no should be unambiguous is one to which I have referred and that is when you do not feel competent to do the operation required by the patient's problem. None of us should be reluctant to admit that someone else may be better qualified in a specific situation. It would be unwise and unethical to attempt an operation that you do poorly or have done so rarely that the patient would be in jeopardy. In most areas of the country, plastic surgeons are nearby who probably have the needed skills. Remember the guideline: Treat the patient as you would want yourself or a member of your family to be treated. In fact, admitting your limitations will ultimately increase your stature in the estimation of the patient, his or her friends, and the referring doctor. The longer one is in practice, the greater appears the wisdom of the saying "You make your living by operating and your reputation by not."

In some situations, I actually point out to the patient that it is in my financial interest to operate, but it is in her best interest for me not to.

Another reason, obviously important, for refusing to be the surgeon is that the patient's health will not permit it. This judgment is made for elective procedures, usually esthetic, and is reached in conjunction with the patient's family doctor or internist. The patient will understandably be disappointed, and you must emphasize that your decision has not been made for your convenience but for his or her welfare. One should spend more time with these patients so that they will not feel coldly rejected.

A more difficult situation is one in which the patient could benefit anatomically from surgery, but because of his or her personality, you do not want to undertake it.

To the "perfectionist" patients (see p. 70), I usually say that "I am afraid that my skills are not such that I can predictably give you what you want. I doubt whether anyone will guarantee that kind of result. Unfortunately, the state of plastic surgery now is not at the point where you can be sure of getting specifically what you want. Perhaps some other plastic surgeon might be able to do better for you." [7, 9] That technique allows you to withdraw without offending the patient, who has the option of going to someone else.

Much more difficult is refusing the patient whom you dislike (see pp. 78–79). As gently as possible, I usually say: "For some reason, you and I do not have the same personality. I sense the friction. If I operated on you, I really believe that we would be on different sides of the street. You would be better off with someone else."

It would be unwise for you, the surgeon, and unfair to the patient to proceed when you have many negative feelings. The patient will perceive your hostility and will react aggressively. Far better for both to disengage at the outset.

For a doctor, how *not* to say no is illustrated by what Oscar De La Renta allegedly replied to an obese woman who asked him why he did not make dresses for people built like her. He said, "I am a designer, not an upholsterer."

Where to Start and Where to Stop
This cryptic heading refers to a common clinical situation: A 45-year-old woman wants only a bilateral upper eyelidplasty, but her lower lids could also benefit from a blepharoplasty. I am usually reluctant to widen the scope of surgery, particularly for a condition that consciously, at least, does not bother the patient. She must understand that the lower lids, if left alone, will probably look worse by comparison once the upper lids have been improved. The risk, however, is that the patient may think that you are talking her into more of an operation and, should there be a complication, she will be angry at what she now interprets as your insistence and at her capitulation.

The issue here is not simply a matter of esthetics or finances but of philosophy as well—yours and the patient's. In general, the concept of "while you are there" or "while I am here" can be dangerous. My advice would be to stick surgically to what truly annoys the patient. You should not assume the obligation of refashioning that individual. Admittedly, the face is a totality, but it does not necessarily follow that operating on one aging feature inevitably necessitates including another.

We all know plastic surgeons of the "soft sell" and the "hard sell" variety: the former may have in his or her waiting room a "show book" of past triumphs; naturally no complications are shown [104, 106]. More subtle but, in my mind, equally crass is the small sign in the waiting room: "Anyone wishing to see a book of photographs illustrating the kinds of procedures that Dr. _____ commonly does should speak to the secretary."

Elsewhere I have described a "marketing stratagem," abhorrent in practice as it is in thought, of having the secretary, who knows why the patient is there for the visit, pretend to be mistaken [104]. "Oh, Mrs. Jones, so you are here to speak to the doctor about your nose." Mrs. Jones, in fact, has come for a breast reduction but now, in horror, has added something more to her list of "the ten most unwanted features."

This kind of game playing, while amusing perhaps from a distance, is not what medicine and plastic surgery should be about.

"Have You Ever Done This Operation Before, Doctor?"
This query, which may come from the patient or from family or friends, is easy to answer if you can honestly reply in the affirmative. If the contemplated procedure is relatively rare, then an answer of "no" will not diminish you; however, if you have not done the procedure, but others in your community do it regularly, you may feel reluctant and embarrassed to admit that this would be your maiden voyage. (It would also be your patient's.) Obviously, you should reply frankly and refer the patient if it is best for him or her. Some patients are more subtle about asking a doctor whether he or she performs an operation frequently. When I was younger, patients would frequently say, slyly, "You certainly are young to have had all this experience." I was never sure whether they expected me to say that I was really twice my age or so brilliant that everyone sought me out for that particular procedure.

Some patients will actually ask what you did last week in the operating room. I tell them, and if it happens not to include their operation, I might add that I did perform that procedure a few weeks ago (if it is true) or will soon be doing it (again if it is true). I need not point out that if a surgeon has lied when a patient asks whether he or she has done a procedure, that fact could later be used very effectively in court by the plaintiff's attorney.

When it is a question of an esthetic procedure, some patients think they are being very clever by saying: "I am sure that you do so much serious surgery [they mean reconstructive] that you would not spend much time doing this type of work." The plastic surgeon doing cosmetic procedures will then have to protest, without, I hope, carrying it to the extreme of saying that "to me a facelift is as important to health as is an emergency heart operation." Far better to tell the truth, which might sound like the following: "I do both reconstructive and esthetic operations and I try to do each operation in both of those categories as carefully as possible. I frankly like a variety in my practice; others may not."

INFORMED CONSENT

For thirteen years, I taught my tongue not to tell a lie; for the next thirteen years I taught it to tell the truth.
The Korester Rabbi

Although the subject of informed consent itself deserves a book, certain general points need mentioning here; other aspects and specific examples will be discussed in association with individual operations (see Chap. 4).

Properly informing the patient about contemplated treatment is not only logical but essential, both medically and legally. In the latter context, with respect to malpractice, doctors are accused usually either of negligence or of failure to inform adequately (or both). Not only must the plastic surgeon inform fully and correctly, but he or she must be able to document it.

There are obviously various ways of informing a patient [10]. The main principle is that the plastic surgeon truly wishes to inform the patient and should put himself or herself in the patient's position about what he or she would like to know about the operation: how generally it is done; what likely result can be obtained; what complications frequently occur and what can then be done about them. Aside from death, there are complications whose treatment is problematic, at best. An example of that would be severance of the mandibular branch of the facial nerve, observed late. It is the plastic surgeon's duty to communicate reality to the patient. This is possible only if the surgeon knows and acknowledges the reality [105].

It is possible to inform without imparting information. An example, spectacular, I admit, is that of billboard advertising for cigarettes. The hard sell is in massive letters; the part about "hazardous to health" can be read only by an eagle. In regard to a patient, it is much easier to recite a litany of possible complications without highlighting the most important. The monotony of their presentation will obtund the patient's critical faculty, which should not be the objective of the disclosure. So that the patient will not slip away, the surgeon, consciously or unconsciously, is following the letter of the law but certainly not the spirit of either the law or medicine.

Written Information

For almost 20 years, I resisted giving patients reading material concerning a contemplated procedure. Although I recognized that such information would be helpful in decreasing ignorance, ambiguity, and anxiety, I was reluctant because I feared that unconsciously I would rely more and more on the handout to answer questions to allay fears while trying less hard in the initial consultation and subsequent interaction with the patient to accomplish the same thing. I also dislike the fact that such booklets tend to be impersonal and lack the warmth that I believe is essential to the relationship between a physician and a patient. And leading the patient from the cold to the hearth is one of my primary professional aims.

However, I realized that patients began to expect such information and wondered whether I was either out of date or out of the mainstream by not giving them pertinent reading material. Therefore, I now routinely give patients something to read after we have met and discussed the problem and possible treatment. Others would prefer to give this information even prior to the initial consultation by having the patient receive it in the mail or in the waiting room after he or she arrives in the office.

I have yet to overcome my feeling that printed sheets are the quintessence of what someone once called "retailing information." Yet, on the balance, I believe that printed information educates the patient, particularly by making him or her remember some of the points discussed during the consultation. In addition, the patient can talk about these things with important people in his or her life.

Another reality and a major benefit of a tastefully done handout is that patients forget, either consciously or unconsciously, most of what is told them by the physician, be he or she a plastic surgeon or a family doctor. Yet, one should not expect that printed information will solve the problem because many patients do not even read what you have so consciously prepared yourself or purchased in order that the patient comprehend his or her operation.

It is not surprising that patients are least likely to forget what they perceive to be the most important, especially if these things are mentioned first. Any minister, teacher, or politician would recognize the truth of that observation. The attention span of patients, like everybody else, wanes, and one should take advantage of the initial few minutes to present the most important material.

Having the patient take home something to read is helpful in the event that you have inadvertently omitted a topic. A thoughtful patient will use the written word as another opportunity to ponder the proposed procedure and ask questions if he or she wishes clarification.

Still another advantage of written material is that the surgeon can record having given the patient such material. Patients, however, differ in their ability to read and retain.

That this printed matter may find its way into beauty parlors where it may have been left by one of my patients makes me uneasy, since I am aware that some plastic surgeons of "overweaning ambition" have resorted to this ploy.

Audiovisual aids, such as films about the operation (preferably with you as the surgeon dubbed in) help reinforce the message. The plastic surgeon must be careful, however, that not just the best results are depicted. Otherwise, one can be accused of implied guarantee, as would occur if you had shown a patient the slides of your most favorable outcomes. It is also important to be sure that if you are spliced in to be the surgeon that you agree with the technique depicted.

Availing oneself of a blackboard is also a good way to demonstrate what you want the patient to remember, but I would advise doing so only if you can draw well; if not, the patient will conclude that you are as poor a surgeon as you are an artist.

Further information about esthetic surgery is available free to patients in the form of telephone messages sponsored by Blue Cross and Blue Shield in some states and various medical societies throughout the country. These recordings can be dialed by the patient from his or her home or even from your office. Obviously, before recommending these tapes, one should listen to them to be sure that they reinforce what one is trying to tell the patient. Although you can have the patient sign a statement that he or she has heard them, just as with written and verbal information, there is no guaranteeing that the patient has either understood or will remember. One should be wary of the patient who repeatedly asks the same question that you think you have already answered satisfactorily. That patient may be in conflict about having the procedure or may have an abnormal affect whose cause you should probe.

Consent Forms
Consent forms usually are remarkable for their complexity and obliquity [126]. Most patients regard them more as a means to protect the doctor legally than to inform them medically [42, 168]. In the Appendix are a few examples of what I use for various procedures. Other plastic surgeons have different preferences. The objective, however, should be the same: clarity and honesty in letting the patient know the treatment proposed, the possible complications, and having the patient legally document that he or she has understood the objectives but also the limitations and the complications of the procedure.

In giving this information, one must be wary of overwhelming the patient with facts and jargon. Some colleagues make the patient sign the bottom of an information sheet and each paragraph of a consent form in the space next to which is printed, "I have read this carefully. I understand this. I have no questions about this."

However, in the courtroom, a plaintiff attorney can point out to a jury who might be in total agreement that in the pressure of seeing the doctor in the office or even in contemplating the procedure at home, the anxiety about a future operation prevented the patient from really understanding what would be done to him or her and what could possibly go wrong. After all, the patient is not a physician—I can hear the attorney and even fantasize him or her making this point with great emotion to the jury.

I do not believe one should spare the patient the reality of a possible catastrophe. With every eyelidplasty, I discuss the probability of blindness and death. Hearing about these disasters rarely causes the patient to decide against the operation—at least in my experience. The human being adapts by believing such misfortune happens only to somebody else.

The logical question is, when should the patient sign the consent form? Although it is more practical if it is done at the conclusion of the consultation in the presence of a witness—someone in your office or the patient's friend or family member—the patient may want more time to read it through and think about it. Taking a copy of the form home and discussing it with family is better for many patients who are not calm or in their usual state of mind following the consultation because of the excitement and anxiety that it may have provoked. In my experience, many patients who go home with a consent form return it improperly witnessed, for example, having a child who is a minor sign it. Despite this possibility, even if it is stipulated on the form that a minor should not sign it, it is better to have a signed form than not to have given the patient a form or to have the patient sign it in the office and then plead that he or she was "pressured into something I did not really understand or want."

Like Sisyphus, condemned to push a heavy stone up the hill only to let it roll down and then to begin the process again, the physician, with every patient, must inform honestly and clearly, a point that has been repeatedly made here. If the patient gives up the idea of the operation or goes to another plastic surgeon, you have lost very little. In fact, you may have spared yourself much trouble. If you are not operating on that patient, you will probably still be doing surgery but on someone else, or a few hours of free time is not the worst onus.

Even with verbal and written information, calls and questions continue. As one patient confessed, "You probably have mentioned it somewhere on what you gave me but I guess I'm calling more for psychological support." Her statement confirms the observation that when someone asks a question, the primary objective is not always to get information; it may be for reassurance.

Finally we should remember that the patient, no matter how well informed, and the surgeon, no matter how skilled, must be content with a certain amount of irreducible ambiguity; something may go wrong, and over a period of time and as the number of operations mounts, something will go wrong. Fortunately, the unwanted event happens only infrequently. Yet, when it occurs, the fact that it is an uncommon circumstance or that the patient was informed about it and that the surgeon realized it could happen—all this does little to console either the patient or the surgeon.

Being Understood Is No Disadvantage

> *In the presence of the patient, Latin is the language.*
> Medieval Maxim

The matter of informed consent emphasizes the need for adequate communication between every doctor and every patient. Communication between two people who have the ability to speak and to hear a common language theoretically should not be a problem. Unfortunately, the reality is different. Witness the many books and seminars on ways to improve communication. Consider also the innumerable psychotherapists working with clients on bettering their capacity to say what they mean to people important in their lives.

The first requisite to verbal understanding between two human beings is a mutual desire to communicate and to be understood—a comparatively recent development in doctor-patient relationships. For centuries, physicians controlled the process and may have even exploited the mystique of the metier; they kept a veil between the patient and their diagnosis and even their treatment [28]. The rationale, conscious or unconscious, was that the ignorance of the patient worked to the benefit of the doctor. They never needed to explain, for example, the presumed mechanism of the medications they prescribed. In retrospect, had doctors been forced to do so, some of the outlandish treatments of past centuries would never have come to pass.

Perhaps there is a law of medical dynamics: Respect for the doctor increases in proportion to the ignorance of the patient. The shaman knows the value in not telling all, even today; however, unlike the physician in modern Western society, the shaman has few scientifically proven measures at his command.

Not until the fifteenth century did a medical text appear in the vernacular rather than in Greek or Latin, the language of the educated minority. Traditionally also the prescription was written in Latin or illegibly, or both, accomplishing the same objective of bypassing the patient's comprehension. As a resident, I remember the momentous change in the hospital when the decision was made to label the patient's medications on discharge. Society and medicine had finally reached the point that allowed the patient to know. It seems obvious to us today, but it was not so obvious then that patients do own their bodies and have a right to understand what is being done to them.

At times, however, failure in communication is due to the patient's not wishing to understand. These situations, although few, mostly occur in association with a terminal illness, particularly cancer, or with some other grim disease, but they may also happen with patients seeking esthetic surgery who may deny to themselves the possibility of postoperative complications (see pp. 60–61).

Johnson [144] has commented on another aspect of "doctor talk." "The doctor's 'we,' by the way, is of special interest. Medical pronouns are used in special ways that ensure that the doctor is never out alone on any limb. The referents are clearly vague. The statement 'we see a lot of that' designates him as a member of a knowledgeable elite, 'we doctors.' " The use or overuse of *we* occurs less often in an office than in a hospital, where the very complexity and the many support systems provide ready refuge and a tempting labyrinth for the badgered physician. Furthermore, the patient perceives that the doctor in the hospital is only one of many. Johnson [144] is correct that often the physician does not wish to be "alone on any limb." Doctors should remember that the patients also do not want to be alone and, of course, being or becoming ill—having an operation— tends to isolate them.

Talleyrand said, "Language was given man to hide the truth." Although we might disagree with his cynicism and his explanation of the origin of the spoken word, the message is irrefutable: People lie. This fact is responsible for much of the chaos in personal lives [27] and on an international scale—wars. Human beings have yet to evolve to the norm of saying what they mean and meaning what they say [30]. For example, I had once heard that the National Park Service was going to kill a large number of wild donkeys in the Grand Canyon—for conservation purposes. To avoid public outcry they termed their plan "direct reduction." Although not a lie, this lack of forthrightness has its similes in many other euphemisms that the government invents to do what it wants without public knowledge. In that instance, the government is acting apart from the people who supposedly elect it.

Those outside government take refuge in euphemisms that give either an exaggerated or understated meaning when reality would be too harsh. For example, we call garbage collectors "sanitary engineers," salespersons "marketing representatives," and, in the lingo of retailers, *shrinkage* means stolen goods.

It should not be surprising that doctors and patients may also talk near or around something unpleasant or bury it with words. The dreaded cancer is not labeled; at rounds *cellular proliferation* takes its place, as an example.

If carried too far, this lack of clarity and this refuge into ambiguity augur poorly for what should be a collaborative effort between the patient and his or her physician–plastic surgeon. This matter is not just a moral issue to be addressed at a symposium of doctors and theologians; it has practical relevance, particularly in the matter of informed consent.

FEES

> *I got the bill for my surgery. Now I know what those doctors were wearing masks for.*
> James H. Boren

> *A hospital should also have a recovery room adjoining the cashier's office.*
> Francis O'Walsh

Every relationship between the patient and the physician must involve a consideration of some kind of payment to the doctor and possibly the hospital. This is true even if the payment is waived.

With few exceptions, most physicians that I know do not enjoy the process of securing recompense for their services. Perhaps this is a result of their having in their core the image of the unselfish, "dedicated" physician. I admit that this type of image may have been more prevalent when I went to medical school and where I trained in general surgery—at a university hospital in Boston (Brigham and Women's Hospital, then the Peter Bent Brigham). The process of how the physician was paid was not discussed or learned. Only during my plastic surgical residency in Pittsburgh was I allowed to see how an office functioned and how the matter of fees was handled. I observed then that plastic surgeons of great competence and compassion actually got paid, and that they did not reek of the marketplace. Someone once commented that it is fortunate that money exists. What else would we use for payment of services [33]? Think of how many chickens a patient having a facelift would have to bring to the office!

Until recently with the appearance of what is now called the Hsaio report, there was little discussion about what determines physicians' fees [138]. Despite this complex and thoughtful relative value system [138], with data sufficient to choke a computer, many inconsistencies, inequities, and absurdities remain.

Before getting lost in specific enigmas, let us first try to recognize a few guiding generalities [99]. Physicians are paid according to the service performed without regard to outcome. A radical mastectomy, for example, has an associated monetary value, irrespective of morbidity, mortality, or cure. Perhaps the genesis of this *modus operandi* was the justifiable reluctance of the earliest physicians, and of us even today, to guarantee health and survival, which are not completely within the control of any human being. With or without a skilled doctor, disease and death eventually supervene.

Another feature often forgotten is that a third-party medical payment does not depend on the skill with which the service is performed. A careless colectomy will bring the surgeon the same fee (although the patient does not get the same result) as one done with finesse—in fact, perhaps more if the surgeon has to operate again because of complications.

Physicians are paid differently for their time and treatment. A total gastrectomy garners a larger fee than a herniorrhaphy. Such variations are allegedly related to differences in the complexity of the procedure, the skill required, and the potential hazards. Less understandable are the fee discrepancies among disciplines. Is a cataract operation twice as difficult as a cholecystectomy? Then why does an ophthalmologist get far more for that procedure than does the general surgeon for taking out the gall bladder? Is an hour of the surgeon's time intrinsically more valuable than that of a psychiatrist, pediatrician, or internist? These considerations are obviously at the heart of the Hsaio report, but even there they are not completely resolved. Why is the diagnosis of mitral valve prolapse worth the same as that of the common cold? Is it all based on time or how the time was spent or who spends the time?

Differences in monetary recompense among surgical specialties are not due solely to the realities of supply and demand. Less tangible factors are important [98]. Therapies requiring manual dexterity earn more than cerebration alone. A doctor performing a coronary bypass generally gets more for his or her efforts than does a colleague managing a patient with a coronary occlusion. Yet, in both instances, the physician is supposedly directing his or her efforts toward the same objective: restoring the health of the patient. Is the monetary hierarchy in medicine related to a hierarchy of the body? Are the brain and heart king and queen and the large intestine and liver merely the knaves? It becomes a "mediphysical" riddle.

What about the fees charged by plastic surgeons for operations for appearance, such as rhinoplasty or facelift? Since these procedures are elective and are an enhancement rather than a necessity, the argument is that the usual standards for fees for nonelective procedures do not apply.

Although for many of these patients, "cosmetic" surgery is rehabilitative, some might question whether the cost should be more than that of a lifesaving operation. Few surgical acts are more lifesaving than a tracheostomy or drainage of an abscess. Should those command a higher fee than an eyelidplasty or a carpal tunnel release?

The practice of medicine, like other activities of human beings, lacks apparent consistency. Paradoxes abound. Cultures vary in their values. A ballet dancer in Russia, for example, engenders the great excitement and top money that a professional football player does in the United States. And here, a rock 'n' roll singer makes far more money than any elected or appointed official, including the president. Pecuniary reward, of course, is not the only measure of society's esteem. A Supreme Court justice gains a different kind of respect than does a speed car racer, but he or she has much less take-home pay.

Setting the Fee
When I began practice about 30 years ago, I had available a fee survey prepared by the Massachusetts Society of Plastic Surgery to give its

members an idea of prevailing charges, their range, and their average. Because of the Federal Trade Commission's view that such documents were contrary to the best interests of the consumer and are therefore illegal, this fee schedule and others throughout the country have been abandoned; however, the young practitioner must still decide what to charge. The present method is to ask other physicians, generally those who are older.

There are three alternatives: to charge less than the usual, the same as the usual, or more than the usual. The first might have the advantage of attracting more patients who believe that they will save money. It also has the disadvantage of convincing some that you are offering less. Charging the same as others has the benefit of allowing the young surgeon to blend with peers. Charging more has the advantage of making more money, if the flow of patients continues, and perhaps convincing some patients that the higher charges reflect better skills.

Ultimately, the decision as to what to charge is determined by the attitudes and values of the physician and the local community as well as the means of the patient. From my observations it seems that the younger plastic surgeons, just beginning in practice, are likely to charge more than the average older plastic surgeon because the younger plastic surgeon enters practice possibly knowing what his or her mentors were receiving for their fees. Since many have had their residency with premier plastic surgeons, they may have learned the high scale of fees.

With regard to reconstructive surgery, what one charges might be totally irrelevant if the plastic surgeon is bound to accept the payment allowed and not permitted to bill the patient in addition. With regard to esthetic surgery, the situation is completely different. There is no third-party regulation; theoretically, the plastic surgeon can charge as much as the patient can bear and even more.

Some plastic surgeons charge so much that they are the pariahs of the medical profession and of our specialty. They have paradoxically earned a bad reputation for which they would have willingly paid considerable money to a public relations firm to untarnish. They would have been wiser to curb their materialism, if they could, for the sake of a better name among their colleagues. Yet, patients go to them since they think that they are the best. Sometimes it is true; more often it is not.

With plastic surgeons who are notorious for their excessive fees, I have observed an inexorable cycle. The more their colleagues resent them, frequently because of envy, the more these surgeons charge, perhaps getting satisfaction in making more than anybody else. They then get caught in the "the more you make, the more you spend" trap. They become unhappy with less and require more and more. Their life-style becomes more demanding: They work harder, charge more, make more, but do they enjoy it more? Perhaps not as many of us would like to think.

How another person conducts his or her life is not the issue here. But how a physician wishes to live and to charge to live does affect his or her relationship with patients.

Another aspect of fees deserves mention: the practice of some to charge excessively as a deterrent to the patient. I have heard colleagues say, for example, that they "dislike doing facelifts." Therefore, they set their fees so high that patients wishing that operation will be discouraged. The obvious question is why these plastic surgeons do not tell patients that they prefer not to perform a specific procedure. The reason is that an admission of a deficit in their repertoire would seem a weakness, and such a confession, as they would interpret it, might damage their image. They would like the patient to feel that he or she is inadequate financially, but not that they are inadequate surgically. The irony is that patients undeterred by the high fee will be paying a premium for the procedure at which the surgeon is least proficient.

Since very few physicians enjoy discussing fees with patients, many resolve the conflict by delegating that matter to someone else in the office. This tactic undoubtedly increases their income since patients are less likely to persuade someone other than the doctor to reduce the fee; in fact, they are less likely to ask the secretary to lower the fee than they would the plastic surgeon because the secretary lacks the ultimate power to do so. I admit that I still do not enjoy the process of discussing fees with my patients but I do it. Sometimes I believe that lowering the fee is justified, and it would not likely happen unless I was part of the discussion.

Prepayment

Most plastic surgeons and most patients desiring esthetic surgery expect prepayment. Since insurance does not usually cover cosmetic procedures, the patient must pay his or her own way beforehand. But this practice arose because of other factors besides the lack of third-party payment.

Empirically, collecting the money before esthetic surgery, rather than after, is easier. If patients postoperatively fail to honor the bill, the surgeon has only two alternatives: to forget it and be consoled that he or she has helped someone and probably also has learned something; or to engage in unpleasant encounters with the patient and the court system.

You cannot take back a performed eyelidplasty as you could a refrigerator that is unpaid for. Many surgeons believe patients are happier with the result if they have already purchased it. They complain less about scars, swelling, or residual wrinkles.

Basic, however, to the issue of prepayment is the fact that many cosmetic procedures fail to give the patient what he or she had expected. This may be particularly true with regard to facelifts. A year or even six months later, a few patients look as if they could use still more facial rejuvenation. Furthermore, not everyone comes out as well as those shown in slides at meetings and in photographs in journals and books. And even if the plastic surgeon should achieve a surgical nirvana for the patient, a few will still be dissatisfied. In retrospect, because of their unrealistic hopes, they should have been weeded out during the initial consultation.

Aside from the patient and surgeon, prepayment has affected the emotions of our non–plastic surgical colleagues. Many are envious and angry since they perceive this practice as evidence of the easy materialism of our specialty. Explaining the reasons for this financial arrangement sometimes increases our colleagues' understanding but seldom eliminates their negative feelings.

For perspective regarding prepayment, it is interesting to realize that in the time of Hippocrates, physicians were accustomed to being paid before they rendered their care. When a doctor took on a patient, a certain fee was agreed on for the entire treatment. The physician was not paid for every service. Hippocrates and his disciples, however, advised the doctor not to be "too greedy" and "to take the economic status of his patient into consideration, even to be prepared to give free services occasionally, either because he has some obligation toward an individual or for the sake of his reputation. This is especially desirable in the case of some poor foreigner who has fallen ill far away from home, without the possibility of obtaining the funds necessary for treatment." The doctor was urged not to raise the question of fees in the beginning with patients suffering from acute diseases, since worrying about finances would worsen their health. Like many other precepts of Hippocrates, this still has validity, although it may not be current practice.

Professional Courtesy
The term "professional courtesy" refers to the traditional reduction in charges to certain people, primarily physicians and their family; however, other patients commonly receive this special consideration, such as nurses, medical students, residents, and clergy. Great is the variation, both among doctors and geographically, in the interpretation of professional courtesy. In my practice, for noncosmetic surgery, I accept third-party coverage as complete payment even if I had the opportunity to bill the balance of my charges. If the patient has no insurance and I believe that he or she should have professional courtesy, I generally do not bill for consultation and in unusual instances even for the operation itself. For cosmetic procedures, I do not charge doctors at my hospital with whom I have had a close relationship, and it is a problematic matter of what to do with their family. I have never charged residents and medical students or their spouses for cosmetic surgery. With nurses, clergy, and with doctors whom I do not know, I reduce my fee. For dentists and veterinarians, I charge the usual. I realize that in stating all this I am perhaps out of date, but I am a product of my upbringing professionally just as is everyone else and every reader of this book.

The financial aspects of professional courtesy sometimes are not so important as other, more subtle considerations. For example, a colleague, who is a friend, may bring his wife to me not only because he may like me and trust my work but because he knows that I will not charge him the full fee or I will markedly reduce it. His wife might be embarrassed by going to me because I know her and her family. Later, should a complication occur, she will probably not directly express her anger for fear of creating a disagreeable scene in front of me, a family friend, or for fear of seeming ungrateful after I have performed her operation for nothing.

The treatment of fellow physicians and their families takes place in the hazardous zone along with any other VIPs, who are imperiled by considerations of who they are as well as what they have medically. All of us recall with anguish instances when we changed the rules and the routine to oblige a colleague or friend—with unfortunate consequences for everyone concerned. Professional courtesy, then, may still be for some a gracious act; an exception that affects the ledger and not the therapy. That this ideal is not always possible to achieve is another reason to abandon this practice, which financially squeezes the doctor, whoever he or she is and especially the one who may have many colleagues and their families as patients. My impression is that professional courtesy has become an anachronism [13], yet I am still struggling with it. Rees [219] had a tastefully printed card given to those patients who might expect professional courtesy. It read as follows:

> During the many years that I have been in the practice of Plastic Surgery, I have extended courtesy fees to close friends and doctors as a matter of principle. As the years pass, I have been fortunate in accumulating more friends and enjoyed the professional confidence of families, to the extent that almost one-half of my time these days is consumed performing such surgery. With the increasing costs of overhead in the practice of surgery today, not the least of which is our excessive and growing insurance premium for malpractice insurance, it is not longer possible for me to fully extend such courtesies. Needless to say, it is embarrassing and distasteful for me to have to charge my usual fees to close friends and colleagues; however, the practicality of the matter dictates that I do so. I hope you will understand and forgive me, since all I have to offer is whatever experience I may have developed and my time.

Financing Schemes
Recently plastic surgeons have received information about plans that make loans available to patients seeking esthetic surgery. That this phenomenon would come to plastic surgery was not hard to predict; it seemed an inevitability of marketing. The rationale for financing

plans is that it does little good to attract patients if they cannot pay for operations. My reaction is that the plastic surgeon is not a financier and should not be a money lender or even a middle agent to bring about such a transaction. If a person tells me that he or she cannot afford the procedure, I would advise the patient not to go into financial jeopardy. In my experience, the majority of patients refuse the alternative of becoming a "resident's case."

Occasionally a patient will request that you perform the operation and then let him or her pay if off in installments with interest. My response is that I am not a loan shark, a money lender, or a banker. I advise them to consult others in those areas for possible help, although it gives me an uncomfortable feeling to know that a patient may have economic stress as a result of an elective procedure. Furthermore, it is always possible that he or she could sue, alleging that the result was unsatisfactory, when, in reality, the reason is to recoup the money by threatening a court action. Plastic surgery is hazardous enough for me anyway without adding the burden of becoming a mini (really micro) J. P. Morgan. Today, it seems, with the collapse of the savings and loan institutions, banking may be more perilous than plastic surgery!

SCHEDULING FOR SURGERY: WHEN AND WHERE

Numerous ways exist for scheduling patients for operation. In some offices it is done while the patient is there, immediately after consultation. Other surgeons communicate later with the patient. For some patients, calling or writing at a future time is more convenient because they do not have their appointment books with them and they usually have to arrange for time off or for a babysitter or other types of support. Some surgeons prefer that the patient call at a future time in order to give that person and his or her family a sufficient interval to ponder the procedure as well as the cost of having it.

Whatever the plastic surgeon's personal preference, he or she must deal with the reality of available beds and operating room time. Most patients want their procedure as soon as possible after they have decided on it. Under some circumstances, either because of the patient's schedule or that of the surgeon, the date may be months away. The long interval between consultation and operation can cause uneasiness for the patient. I have found it helpful to encourage that person who wishes another visit to return a month or so before the operation. Aside from reassurance for the patient, this occasion allows one a second look, to rethink plans, and to better understand that person's personality and expectations. One is surprised and even disheartened by questions that were in fact answered in detail before. One realizes the wisdom of the Baptist preacher who emphasized that repetition improves retention.

Some surgeons will never schedule an esthetic operation without seeing the patient again. Although that may be an ideal arrangement, I have found it too cumbersome. I simply do not have the time to see patients again unless the patient requests it. Some would argue that one error in patient selection is so costly in terms of time, effort, not to mention possible legation, that prevention through "a second look" is by far wiser.

One should remember that for us in an office, scheduling is a routine matter; for the patient, however, it is a singular event, ambivalently contemplated: the pleasant hope of improvement, whether through reconstruction or cosmesis, coupled with the disquieting fear of failure.

Several doctors and a few patients have told me that it is inadvisable suddenly to fit someone into the operating schedule with the explanation that "someone canceled," even if it is true. The patient may then imagine that one is not good enough to hold the other patient and that he or she got away, off to someone better. The patient may then follow that example, real or imagined. I have been surprised by the frequency of patients who leave the office while begging for an earlier operating date—then when it is suddenly presented to them, say that they cannot accept it.

Frequently two patients will have consultations on the same day. They may have arrived in tandem. They will ask to be scheduled for operation also on the same day. Generally these patients are a mother and a daughter for rhinoplasty or two women friends for facelift. They may even request the same room. Their plan seems reasonable and easy, but one should be careful because of the possibility that one of the patients will do better than the other in terms of pain, ecchymosis, swelling, and final result, including scars. Even if both results are objectively very good, one patient, in the instance of friends, is likely to envy the other as she probably did prior to operation, and since she cannot rationally direct her hostility toward her friend, the plastic surgeon may be the easier target. Practically also, who is scheduled first on that same day? The one who is having the later operation will predictably feel slighted.

I require every patient on whom I do an operation to sign appropriate forms (see Appendix). I cannot claim that mine are superior to others, but they do have the guarded blessings of several attorneys specializing in medicolegal matters. In truth, these forms have been written as much to protect me, perhaps even more so, than to protect the patient. One of the forms stipulates that the patient is financially responsible for any hospital costs arising from the necessity of a secondary procedure to improve the initial result, such as might be necessary in patients having augmentation mammoplasty. Furthermore, that form makes it clear that in the event of a complication, which is not likely to be covered by insurance if it is a cosmetic operation, the patient assumes complete financial responsibility with reference to hospital payments.

Because I do not perform surgery in my office, I discuss scheduling with regard to a hospital setting. Like any institution, hospitals are cumbersome to deal with. For the esthetic surgical patient, especially as an inpatient, care in the hospital is more expensive and less efficient than it would be in an office operating room with a facility, such as a motel or hotel, nearby for overnight stay. The other advantage of one's own surgical facility is that it saves time for yourself and the patient. In addition, in your own surgical unit it is easier for you, not a hospital secretary, to decide when you may operate. The patient preserves anonymity; uniform, presumably higher grade, medical care is easier to give, and it is done according to your preferences and not the fiats or whims of distant, unidentifiable bureaucrats. In one's own operating arena, the patient as well as the plastic surgeon and his or her staff can enjoy a relaxed atmosphere because it is within the control of those responsible for the patient's treatment.

Pertinent, however, is the fact that a hospital does have the advantage of providing better backup of personnel and facilities in the event of an emergency, cardiorespiratory or otherwise. As the proprietor of an office surgical facility, one's legal responsibility is greater, especially if the plastic surgeon does not have a board-certified anesthesiologist in attendance [207, 234]. Another aspect to consider but not to belabor here is the progressive isolation of those who do office surgery from their colleagues and trainees not in plastic surgery. I am assuming that plastic surgical residents would be rotating through the plastic surgeon's office, although not every full-time chief sees the wisdom for this kind of exposure. As the office-based, office-operating plastic surgeon becomes further separated from the main channels of medical care, the potential good that plastic surgery can do for other fields in medicine and surgery and for those patients diminishes in his or her horizon. Likewise, the opportunities available to the plastic surgeon to use his or her skills for this type of sharing with colleagues and their problems decrease. I express these thoughts not to oppose office surgery, which I think has been a great advance [234], but it has to be performed according to the highest standards of patient care—and in the safest possible facilities that hopefully have been inspected and accredited recently and regularly.

Another disadvantage of being a patient staying in a hospital and one to which I have alluded is the possible confusion and mismanagement that can occur because of the large size of the institution, its inherent complexity, and the presence of so many people participating directly or indirectly in a single individual's treatment. Unless nurses and residents are accustomed to dealing with an esthetic patient, the patient may be the target of hostility. The attitude may be: "With all we have to do, why do we have to look after someone like her who is healthy and vain," or "I really can't stand people who have nothing to do but to get their face lifted." Envy may also be the basis of the aggression: The nurse may wish that she could have the same procedure, complete with a private room. There is a low threshold to considering a facelift patient as "demanding," and, in fact, many are. One nurse reacted in this fashion when a patient, following eyelidplasty, asked the nurse to help her get a glass of water; the patient could not see because of the ointment in her eyes and the ice dressings.

The plastic surgeon who has hospitalized patients must be a fence mender, taking the time to listen to complaints, minor to major, justified or not. While maintaining allegiance to his or her patient, the plastic surgeon must hear both sides and not reflexively champion the person who is paying for the services. Most unpleasant incidents in the hospital readily resolve themselves with the realization that they probably arose because the patient was anxious and the staff overworked. As the patient's physician and as someone known to those who run the hospital, the plastic surgeon should be the constancy amidst the flux. His or her availability and concern will reassure the patient and the participants in the treatment. For example, if one does not make rounds on a Sunday, calling the patient and nurse to inquire about progress or problems can be very satisfying to all concerned. Most hospital rooms now have phones; certainly each nursing station does. Speaking with the patient requires a willingness and only a three-minute effort on your part; the patient and the staff will greatly appreciate it.

In another context, after outpatient surgery, there is truth to what AT&T claims about the phone—that it is "the next best thing to being there." For a patient who has had a somewhat extensive procedure on an ambulatory basis, such as an augmentation mammoplasty or facelift, hearing from the plastic surgeon or one of his or her staff the following day can be gratifying and helpful. Even with instruction sheets, questions arise. The patient, however, will value your caring (if you truly care) even more than the information.

Of course, doing these things requires the plastic surgeon to be available. One must avoid the "will-o'-the-wisp" behavior—now you see the plastic surgeon, now you don't. Unlike the average physician of 75 years ago, today's doctors are not homebodies. The automobile and the airplane as well as the second home have made quick getaways a routine life-style for many. Leaving for a weekend or junketing to meetings is commonplace. But where does that leave the patient? Behind, and often angry, and maybe even in trouble. Although you may have provided competent coverage, your surrogate is not the same as yourself. If possible, you should introduce the doctor covering for you to the patient if they do not already know each other. This is not simply good manners but good medicine; it cements your colleague's responsibility and lessens your patient's anxiety (also yours) over being placed under the care of someone else.

Previously I noted that a possible problem patient could be the one from afar; a possible problem plastic surgeon can be the one who also is far away. A bad reputation results from being in the operating room to do the procedure and being in the office to see the patient initially but being scarce at all other times. I have found it particularly advisable after every esthetic operation to be in town for a few days to handle possible urgent complications and not to be unavailable or away too long in order to manage other problems such as transient depression that may later occur. One's presence may mean even more than one's words. If you have to go away on a trip and you know about it well in advance, you should inform the patient who is having that procedure that you will be away. You should not continue to operate up to the moment that the cab arrives at the door. Unfortunately, the economic realities as well as the demands of patients may make this advice sometimes impractical. The patient who has been warned that you will be away will be much more understanding should an emergency result than if he or she had never been told. Some patients will choose to postpone the operation until you are there for the postoperative care.

Admittedly, doctors like anyone else need a respite. Some patients, however, require your availability as much as you do your vacation. They do not want to feel deserted. Proper patient selection and scheduling can usually accommodate both of you satisfactorily.

WHO SHOULD KNOW?

Sometimes it is difficult to decide whether to discuss the patient's problem and visit with anybody else: a family member, another physician, or a friend of the patient.

Take the least ambiguous instance first: Any plastic surgeon would consider it mandatory to reveal the content of a consultation with a parent(s) or guardian if the patient is a 14-year-old girl who had been seen alone for nasal surgery and may have been accompanied only by a schoolmate. Because of her age, it is legally required in most states to obtain (parental) consent for operation (we are not talking here about abortions).

But what about an 18-year-old girl who wishes a breast reduction but does not want the family to know about it since "they would only worry and they would be against it anyway?" Under these circumstances, I try to convince the patient that communication with her parents would seem logical and fair. With proper understanding and knowledge, I venture, the parents may even support her plan. I usually tell the patient that if she is still opposed to speaking with her parents, then I feel ill at ease at "being in the middle," especially if something went wrong. If a complication arose, she would then have to tell them but under more stressful conditions. Almost always the patient consents—but not always. I must then decide whether I am willing to proceed with that extra burden. The enormous geographical mobility of our population has fragmented the family; children and parents often lead separate lives, and sometimes we are asking a patient to communicate when lines have long been down. I usually never operate on such patients without having informed the parents. Yet, when such a patient tells me that she has told her parents and has not done so, I can do little to validate her story, and I do not feel that I should, but I do make her statement part of the record.

The fervor, success, and validity of the feminist movement have made women less dependent on their husbands' approval in deciding about an operation, a point made earlier. Although the law does not require a spouse to be informed, it also does not require that under those circumstances I have to perform a procedure.

The Referring Doctor
Like most plastic surgeons, the initial form that the patient fills out has a space for "Who, if anyone, referred you?" My custom is to send a letter to the referring doctor after I have seen the patient. I always inform the patient of my intention, since some occasionally will object, because, she (almost always a female) will say, "I asked him at a party if he knew of a good plastic surgeon, but I didn't tell

him what it was for." Some patients even use the ploy, not too difficult to see through, that "I asked him about a plastic surgeon because a friend of mine wanted one."

In this situation, the patient has usually come for a breast augmentation, an eyelidplasty, or a facelift. Frequently the referring doctor is a neighbor from whom the patient obliquely extracted your name. The patient would not want him, and particularly his wife, to know that she has had esthetic surgery.

In addition to writing to the referring doctor, it is advisable also to send a copy of the letter to the patient's internist or family physician. Sometimes that doctor, if not informed, may feel hurt, even angry, and may retaliate by telling the patient that he or she was foolish to have undergone an elective operation.

In addition, by writing to a family doctor one can learn a lot about the patient, about his or her health and reactions to previous operations. I always request in the letter "any advice that you may wish to give me to make the patient's care optimal." Occasionally, this relatively minimal effort will prevent considerable difficulties. I recall an instance in which I wrote such a letter to the family doctor, who had not referred the patient, but he called me and told me that "Mrs. _____ is a very difficult patient. In fact, she tried to sue me on two occasions—once because I did not return her call that evening for a relatively minor complaint, and the other because I prescribed a medicine that made her nauseous." I should emphasize the fact that the doctor did not impart this information by letter. I asked the patient to return for another consultation and was able to recognize her hostility, which I had not detected previously. We parted: she perhaps disappointed but I definitely relieved.

THE END OF THE CONSULTATION

As with the beginning, there is an art to ending the initial consultation. It should be terminated naturally, or apparently so, not abruptly by you while you are unexpectedly standing up and saying, "Well, I think we've covered everything." The use of "we" is offensive and may not be warranted since the patient may still have some questions and concerns. One who is even moderately perceptive will sense when the skein has run out: when the patient and you truly have nothing more to ask or say. I then accompany the patient to the door, open it, and usually remark, "I enjoyed meeting you [if I did enjoy it] and I look forward to helping you [if that is true]." Often, before scheduling the operation, I prefer to let the patient think more about the contemplated procedure and to discuss it with family and friends, as mentioned, now that the patient presumably has more information than prior to the consultation. He or she may ask, "How do I schedule surgery if I decide on it?" My reply is, "Just call my office and speak with my secretary," and I indicate to her which secretary and may even introduce the patient if they have not previously met. I also say again that I would be pleased to answer more questions that might arise. If a spouse or some other important figure in his or her life is present, I state again my willingness to communicate with him or her, either in person or by phone.

If the patient is an adolescent, I encourage him or her to call me directly. I will say to them, "After all, you are the patient, not your mother"; however, the reality is that the parent will frequently call, and I tell the parent that I would be pleased to hear from him or her. I then say that "If I'm not in, I will get back to you."

On a few occasions, when I have spent a long time with a patient who has unending lists of questions, I have had to say, "Please forgive me, Mr. or Mrs. _____ [it is usually a woman], but I am afraid that I am keeping others waiting. If you think you would like another consultation, we can arrange it." Rarely is my suggestion accepted. Some physicians charge for a repeat consultation; I do not and tell the patient that I would not.

Occasionally a patient's final query will be, "Could I speak to someone who has had this operation [generally a breast reduction or reconstruction]?" I try to discourage this practice, primarily because I believe that the patient ends up talking to someone who is pleased with the operation—hardly an unbiased sample. Only someone who is happy with a surgical result would offer to converse with a prospective patient. I point this out, but if that individual persists, I will then tell her that my secretary will try to arrange it, since we have a list of those who have expressed a willingness to serve as "informants." In order to preserve confidentiality, only first names are used.

The patient is told to call at a certain time (set by the former patient) and to ask for "Mary," who has been informed that a "Janice," for example, will be telephoning.

Just as I like to show a patient a range of photographic results, for example, with breast reconstruction, I wish I could make the patient speak to someone who considered the outcome unsatisfactory; however, it is impractical because neither the patient nor I would relish further communication; it is difficult to ask a favor from a dissatisfied patient and to grant one to a doctor from whom you feel estranged.

By the end of the initial consultation, you as the plastic surgeon should have an accurate idea of whether that patient will be suitable for the operation, from the anatomical and emotional points of view. The patient should also come to a conclusion concerning whether he or she wants you to be the plastic surgeon. Although your competence may be hard to judge, it is hoped that your empathy and commitment should be evident.

4

Types of Operations and Types of Patients

In this chapter, which is a discussion of specific procedures, I have resisted the temptation to include more operations than I regularly perform. Although the book would gain in completeness, it would be offset by a loss in authenticity. All surgeons, myself included, have a basic defect, perhaps congenital, but certainly developmental, that predisposes them to believe that they have performed a greater number and a greater variety of procedures than the facts allow. Whether we like it or not, this is the era of the "incomplete" surgeon.

First I will characterize cosmetic operations and the kinds of patients who seek them. Subsequently I discuss reconstructive procedures along with patients. To generalize about patients and even operations is admittedly hazardous, but it is necessary. We live and even survive by casting someone or something new in the context of our previous experience. Undoubtedly inaccuracies arise, but it is a useful crutch in our daily life.

In a 1987 survey, the number (estimated) of cosmetic surgical procedures performed by members of the American Society of Plastic and Reconstructive Surgeons, in descending order of frequency, were liposuction (about 100,000), eyelid surgery (about 78,000), rhinoplasty and breast augmentation (each about 70,000), abdominoplasty and facelift (each about 50,000), and breast reduction (about 35,000) [4].

RHINOPLASTY

Rhinoplasty is a popular procedure among plastic surgeons and patients for the improvement it gives anatomically and psychologically [225]. It is also an operation that many who are not plastic surgeons do. Because cosmetic rhinoplasty is not a hazardous operation and can be done quickly and because it is not covered by insurance, it has a high income-to-time ratio, a fact that has not escaped the observation of others. Notwithstanding this, rhinoplasty is not an easy technique if judged in terms of results. And the ultimate outcome is how the procedure must be evaluated. That is why watching others perform a rhinoplasty may be less helpful than in the instance of other procedures where the result is more apparent at the conclusion of the operation, as, for example, in a breast reconstruction.

Rhinoplasty is the procedure the public expects most plastic surgeons do, but, in fact, not all plastic surgeons, even board certified, do it well or enthusiastically, and some may not even do it at all. Just as surgeons vary in their technique and in their results, a variety exists among patients. One must attempt to select the patient who will be satisfied with an objectively good surgical outcome.

The Adolescent Girl
In my practice, a large segment of patients are adolescent girls. Generally, the patient has initiated the idea of modifying the shape of her nose, but occasionally the mother, much less often the father, is the instigator. The mother might have had the procedure or might have wanted it but did not perhaps because of financial reasons, parental unwillingness, or her own anxiety about the result. Sometimes the mother, who has an attractive nose by nature, will observe

that her daughter has her father's nose. The mother then might subtly or not so subtly encourage the daughter to have a rhinoplasty.

Most girls do not say that they want a beautiful nose; rather, they wish to get rid of an "ugly" nose. They want to blend with their peers and not stand out because of an unattractive feature. The father may be the last person to agree with this child's wishes since he may see nothing wrong with the nose and, in fact, with his daughter in general.

How one teenager coped with her father's disapproval of a rhinoplasty is worth citing. She wrote him this letter:

> Dear Dad,
>
> I'd like to get your approval before I get a nose job, so please try to see my point of view.
>
> Getting my nose fixed is very important to me. I try to improve myself by going to school, reading, playing the piano . . . this is just another way that I can better myself. I think it's important that you allow me to change what it is I don't like about myself, because it would make me a much happier person.
>
> I'm asking you to be totally unselfish and approve of something I want for the sake of my ego. I'm asking you to cater to my wishes and allow me to improve my appearance—which means so much to me. You've always been receptive to my needs, though, so I don't think I'm asking for too much.
>
> Please think about this carefully, and try to understand how important it is to me.
>
> Thanks.
>
> Love, Ann

It would take a strong father not to be persuaded by that letter. Ann's father replied, and I think the points he made are worth our pondering also.

> Dearest Ann,
>
> The measure of a person is composed of many things. These include the character of an individual, how one responds to internal and external events—the maturity one has, the intelligence, the accomplishments, how interesting one is. In all of these ways you are tops and Mother and I are very proud of you because of this. You are very intelligent, you are an excellent pianist, you read and learn so that you are very interesting. Your mind is always active and seeking to do other things such as gardening, weaving, etc. And on top of all this, you are energetic and physically attractive. It is because of these characteristics and your marvelous personality that you are so very popular and sought after by all.
>
> You are also very pretty and have an excellent figure. This is fortunate

because physical attractiveness is important to anyone's ego. But beauty of this type is very much an individual matter which has as much to do with fantasy as with anything else. Consequently, this physical beauty is very much a secondary characteristic that is totally unrelated to and very unimportant when compared to matters of character and achievements such as those you possess. Beauty is *not* an accomplishment.

This is difficult to understand when you are in your teens, an age when so much emphasis is placed on physical perfection. But it is important to try to understand so that now and, in the future, you become comfortable with yourself. Such comfort derives from the realization that each person looks different from another. Not only are noses different but hands, feet, other aspects of the face differ. It is just this variation that makes life so interesting. If you do not fully appreciate this and become comfortable with it, then restructuring your nose will be of no consequence—in fact, it will make your discomfort about other physical matters worse. If you do understand this, then restructuring your nose or any other part of your body would be unnecessary.

If your nose were so grotesque or so misshapen as to be obviously abnormal, I would not hesitate to agree with you. Fortunately, such is not even close to this situation. Never for one minute have I ever taken notice of your nose or thought that it looked unusual. I would suggest that you think about the matter for some time. If after a few years you still feel that it should be done, then perhaps this will be a correct choice.

Ann, I love you very much and I want to give you everything that I can and to feel that it is justified. One of those things is any guidance and insight that I might possess. I hope you believe and understand that.

Love, Dad

What is obvious from these letters are the love and respect each has for the other. The father was correct about his daughter: She was attractive and accomplished; however, her nose was not beautiful, although her character was, and her face was very pretty. Ann was still unhappy with the nose, a fact that her father was somewhat slow or reluctant to realize. Ultimately, he did not insist that she wait "a few years," but after more discussion and a visit with me, he approved of the operation and was warmly supportive.

History

The plastic surgeon should be sure of one basic piece of information: the patient's age. In general, I prefer to wait until the patient is at least 14, although there are exceptions, depending on the physical development such as age of menarche and degree of breast enlargement. Also, some 12- and 13-year-olds have such a disfiguring nose that psychological adjustment at school may be impossible because of the taunting they receive. As a result, their school work in addition to their psyche may suffer, and a rhinoplasty might have to be undertaken earlier.

Sometimes harried parents will call to ask what to tell their 12- or 13-year-old daughter who is pestering them for a rhinoplasty. In that situation, I advise them to have the patient be seen; she will likely follow a doctor's advice about waiting, whereas she will not heed it if it comes from her parents.

During the initial consultation, it is necessary to establish whether the patient herself or himself desires the rhinoplasty. This is a very important part of the history. As mentioned, parental prodding can lead an adolescent into your office. A good opportunity for ascertaining the extent of pressure from parents is during the physical examination, which logically allows you the opportunity of being alone with the patient.

Some patients exhibit what Linn [167] has termed the "rhinoplasty syndrome":

> It is not meant as a joke to say that these patients did all they could to preserve a low profile. In public settings they tried to avoid side views of the nose. They dressed plainly. They avoided the use of jewelry. Hair styles and hats were selected to achieve inconspicuousness and anonymity. Because they were chronically and painfully aware of the nose in profile, they adopted various mannerisms with the hands calculated to cover the nose. They were often awkward in their manner and distracted in their thought so that they functioned at a distinct disadvantage in social settings.

Occasionally, you will see the patient actually cover her nose with her hand. Sometimes patients wear their hair in bangs, almost as a frustrated attempt to cover their nose. In fact, such a hair style, by concealing the upper face, makes the nose and the lower face more prominent and might even accentuate an underdeveloped chin if present.

The Adolescent Male

In my experience the adolescent male, in contrast to the much older male, who seeks a cosmetic rhinoplasty is generally satisfied with the result if he has initiated the consultation and very much wants the operation. With teenage boys, it is not unusual for trauma to have initiated the desire for a change in the appearance of the nose, whose shape may not be due as much to the accident as to genes.

In addition to a thorough past history and systems review, one must inquire of every patient about breathing difficulties. Respiratory obstruction is not always easy to establish because occasionally the parents may have schooled their child to mention a "deviated septum" or "troubled breathing" in order to obtain insurance coverage. The physical examination should later clarify the situation. It is fairly common for parents to attribute mistakenly, but honestly, their child's nasal deformity, such as a dorsal hump, to an injury rather than to heredity. Since children may bang their nose from time to time, parents can easily recall an instance of trauma. This kind of thinking by the parents absolves them of guilt from transmitting to their offspring a displeasing physical feature, and it also makes the operation "necessary" for functional reasons, not for vanity.

One must be certain to question the patient or the parents, if the patient is a minor, about allergies, especially to medications and antibiotics, and bleeding tendencies, personal and familial. Does the patient, if a teenager or older, sniff cocaine [244]? That question should be asked obviously away from the parents if they have accompanied their child. Before focusing on the nose, one should first try, as with every patient, to think more broadly. Find out about self-esteem, relationships with family and peers, adjustment or maladjustment at school, favorite subjects, summer plans, extracurricular activities, and future directions in life, college or whatever. One should get a sense of what the patient thinks the operation will do for him or her at this particular time of life, both emotionally and socially. For the plastic surgeon who enjoys young people, and is not too harried, these questions come naturally; others may have to work harder to remember asking the young patient about himself or herself.

Adolescents generally have not learned to dissimulate their emotions as well as their elders, even though they may be crafty in their conversation. A direct question usually provokes a direct verbal response, and when it does not, the discomfort and reluctance on their face is obvious and gives the answer.

I have mentioned that bleeding tendencies should be thoroughly investigated. The reason for my repeating it here is that I recall with anguish a patient who had spectacular bleeding about a week after operation as a result of von Willebrand's disease. Although he gave no history of this condition, a maternal aunt did have "life-threatening bleeding at the time of a gall bladder operation," as the mother related when I questioned her—sadly after the fact.

One should keep in mind that adolescents, females more than males, are usually preoccupied with their physical appearance [212–214]. Offer, Ostrow, and Howard [195] found that about 60 percent of females and 30 percent of males desired some change in their appearance. In a medical survey of body image, Cash and colleagues concluded that adolescence for females was the time of greatest dissatisfaction. Yet, objective deformity—with regard to the nose or any other part of the body—was not necessarily consonant with what the adolescent thought about himself or herself [154]. The "inside view" may be very different from the "outside view" (what others think), but the ultimate reality, at least at the time one is seeing the patient, is what he or she considers the self-image to be. That is why Cash and his colleagues [41] warned that the plastic surgeon should never impose his or her esthetic standards on the patient's own desires, desired appearance, and self-image.

Physical Examination
On physical examination, it is important to ask the patient how he or she would like the nose changed. Occasionally what the patient wants is anatomically impossible. It is better to establish that situation before the operation than afterward. I often give the patient a mirror and ask what he or she would want done to the nose.

Although initially one should exam any patient alone, it is helpful to call in the mother, father (or both), spouse, or friend if the patient wishes. Parents particularly, I believe, should be invited to hear what you plan to do in terms of their child's expectations and desires. Sometimes one can easily detect that the child would be an easy patient if it were not for the parents.

Williams [276] has emphasized the value of being gentle during examination. The patient is usually apprehensive and, as Williams has observed, may worry that you will find something "dirty" in the nose, such as normal mucus or crusts. If the surgeon forcibly grasps the nose, the patient may justifiably deduce that the surgical hand at operation will be just as heavy and clumsy.

One should carefully inspect the complete extent of the nasal passages with an otoscope, nasopharyngoscope, or a speculum and headlight; one should note the presence or absence of septal or turbinate obstruction [56]. One should also look for damage to the nasal mucosa and for a perforation, which might be due to cocaine sniffing. In that regard, questioning the patient about cocaine in the presence of the parent will predictably fail to yield an answer. When the patient and you are alone in the examination room, it is fairly simple to ask the patient whether he or she uses cocaine "for social purposes."

As one examines the patient's nose, one must view it in relation to the entire face: forehead, midface, lips, occlusion, and chin [152]. Be attentive to any thoughts the patient may have about those features or any dissatisfaction from previous plastic or maxillofacial surgical or nonsurgical treatment [76].

Informing the Patient
As mentioned, the patient and the family must understand your surgical objectives. This is possible only if you understand them. Examine now and think later is a poor *modus operandi* Although I refrain from showing pictures of other patients who have had a rhinoplasty, I believe a patient is entitled to know your operating plans since he or she must display your handiwork for the rest of his or her life. It is helpful to take a Polaroid picture, which then allows you to discuss immediately the shape of the nose as it is now and in terms of your contemplated modifications. A thorough discussion during the initial consultation usually obviates seeing the patient and the family for another preoperative consultation. A second visit, however, might be necessary if you, the patient, and family wish it, usually because of lingering uncertainty about your surgical objectives and their expectations. This additional visit is advisable for those for whom you can do less than what they wish, as in the instance of the patient with a bulbous, thick-skinned nose without a dorsal hump but with a history of acne. If one plans external

incisions (along the rim, at the alar base, or in the approach to an open rhinoplasty), one must inform the patient and the family about the expected scars although they may be almost imperceptible.

I emphasize to the patient and to whoever has accompanied him or her that rhinoplasty is not like sculpting marble. Human flesh is different and healing is unpredictable. Furthermore, one cannot throw away a nose as you would a piece of wood or stone if the result is unsatisfactory. Because the operation involves changing the foundation of the nose, its bone and cartilage, you and the patient must rely on the soft tissues to contract to produce the final result. At the time of the operation, it is almost impossible to know precisely how the nose will ultimately mold and heal. Adding to the problem of knowing the final shape of the nose is the swelling from the local anesthesia and surgical trauma as well as individual variations in the shape of the cartilage, thickness of skin, and intrinsic ability of the patient to heal.

I outline the sequence and details of the procedure and the hospitalization. I do not generally do this operation on an outpatient basis, except for revisions or tip rhinoplasties. I discuss the pain that the patient may expect (usually little); the type of anesthesia (local with intravenous medication, or general, if the patient insists and has obvious anxiety about being even partially awake); the length of the operation; the nasal packs that may be necessary; the nasal splint worn for a week after the operation; the expected time for discharge (usually the day after); and the fact that the initial swelling and ecchymosis will largely disappear in two weeks, but many months will have to elapse before the nose assumes its ultimate configuration. The patient must be warned to avoid sports and other strenuous activities for at least three weeks after the operation and contact sports for three months unless they wear a nose protector.

Complications
The patient and the family must clearly understand that complications might arise. I state openly that it is possible to die from the operation, but that it would be a rare event, and, at least at this writing, I have not had a fatality from a rhinoplasty. Infection is uncommon. Unexpected nasal bleeding does occur, but it may be in only one percent

or less of patients [114] and is almost always controllable. I do tell the patient and the family that in approximately five percent of operations, it is necessary to do a minor revision, such as a minimal rasping of the dorsum or taking a little bit more from the junction of the upper and lower alar cartilage, in order to achieve the wanted result. If one is contemplating septal work, the patient should know about the possibility of a perforation.

Many patients have misconceptions about rhinoplasty and the postoperative regimen. For example, a common myth is that they cannot ever or for a long time expose their nose to sunlight. The objective is to avoid ultraviolet and thermal injury on the healing nasal skin. This is not the same as to forbid sun for several years, although it might be a good idea in terms of sparing all sun-exposed skin from premature aging.

A worse misconception of some patients is that they believe you can produce the type of nose they wish according to the picture they might bring to you [46]. They must understand that the reality is often different. I have refused many patients because either they or a strategic family member, usually the mother, expected a precise anatomic result and was so perfectionistic that the daughter or son would ultimately be dissatisfied with the nose even if the outcome were satisfactory. Most parents and most older patients will express the desire that they "don't want too much done." Like myself, they dislike intensely the artificial nose, the surgical creation that may look better at a distance in a picture or on television screen than it does in person. The telltale signs of a rhinoplasty are those with which we are all too familiar: the scooped out dorsum and the excessively shortened, pinched tip.

Although adolescent males want a nose that is straight and generally smaller than the one they had (without a dorsal hump), they do not want a girl's nose—at least those males that have heterosexual identification.

During the Operation
Since most nasal operations in this country are done under local anesthesia with intravenous medication without the patient asleep, it is axiomatic that the patient should not hear unnecessary noise and

careless talk: for example, "Whoops!"; "Even if the nose comes out fine, do you think it will help her look better because she is overweight?"; "The nose still doesn't look straight." These remarks and others that are similar or worse cause the patient anxiety that may be reflected in an increased heart rate and blood pressure along with more bleeding [131]. Sometimes the patient may act as if he or she had not heard an unwise remark or an uncalled-for witticism, but when the result is not what was expected, the patient may give back to you word for word the sentiment that you had let fly in an unguarded moment.

Even under general anesthesia, when the patient is apparently asleep, there is some evidence that hearing and memory may not be totally impaired. Many unsettling and as yet inexplicable reports in the anesthesia literature document more patient awareness than is usually assumed.

Another precaution is to send to the pathologist all tissue that is removed. This is wise not only to conform with the usual hospital rules but also to provide evidence to an insurance company who may allege that the operation was totally "cosmetic" when, in fact, it was also reconstructive in the sense that its objective was to restore normal breathing.

A colleague and I reported a patient on whom we were doing a secondary rhinoplasty for a deformity partly caused by an unsuspected adenoid cystic carcinoma, diagnosed for the first time from the tissue that we had sent at our operation [119].

Should the patient experience inordinate pain or have excessive bleeding, one should remember that it is not his or her fault. Too often I have seen surgeons becoming angry at the patient in the operating room instead of directing their energies to rectifying the situation.

After the Operation
Since rhinoplasty is the first of the operations to be discussed in detail in this book, I will emphasize something here that I need not repeat but is mandatory for every operation: As soon as the patient is in the recovery room, you, not your secretary or resident, should communicate with the key family member or friend. The apogee of

callousness is for a surgeon to dictate the operative notes, gab, have coffee, and then go to lunch. One should immediately call or see to inform an anxious spouse or parent, for example, about the patient's condition, the findings at operation, what you did, and what you think the result will be. It is also imperative to tell a spouse or parent if the patient is a minor about any complications that may have occurred intraoperatively. It is better to have their support now rather than anger later because you "hid" something important from them.

A surgeon who believes that he or she is too important or too busy to perform the relatively minor act of communicating with the patient's loved ones reveals a character fault and is also making a serious tactical error. Should anything go wrong, the family might remember an uncaring attitude and might attach to that more emotional significance than the complication itself.

With regard to rhinoplasty, it is fortunate that almost every adolescent girl will be happy with the result of at least a good rhinoplasty. This kind of patient ignores flaws that might bother her family and even her surgeon. Sometimes I feel guilty because the patient is ecstatic with a result that is far from faultless. I should add that I resist the temptation to point out the shortcomings. An occasional patient might have a fairly good result—not an excellent one—and the parents will harp on its deficiencies to the point that they make the patient displeased with the result and, more important, displeased with herself or himself. In their zeal to be "perfect parents," they are more destructive than they realize. If the parents, relative, or friend of great importance to the patient does not provide emotional support, crucially needed immediately after the operation, what would seem to others to be an objectively good or even excellent result might seem a mediocre outcome [220]. In a closely knit family where every event, even minor, gets top billing in their emotional life, it is not surprising that an operation, its process and its result, should hold a meaningful place in that family's life.

The Older Woman
The older woman patient has usually debated more than half her life, probably since puberty, about having the shape of her nose changed. Although she has been somewhat accustomed to seeing her nose,

she may still resent possessing it and may not wish to die with it. Like most patients, she probably wants a nose to fit her face, but she does not want it changed significantly. In this regard she is being wise because after several decades of living with her body and having a specific image of herself, she will not be able to accept a dramatic change with aplomb as can most teenagers.

The older woman does not usually want her friends to know she has had a rhinoplasty, at least this is what she says before the operation [254]. On her hidden agenda might be a desire for a greater change than she had articulated to you or admitted to herself [132]. She might even surprise the plastic surgeon by saying that he or she did too little because nobody had noticed.

In my experience, many older women have come for a cosmetic rhinoplasty after the death of their husband. Frequently they will say that their parents did not allow them to have a rhinoplasty and their husband was also opposed to it. Now they will say that they are free to do it.

The older patient should understand that her tissues are less firm, and tip definition is harder to achieve. More than in someone younger, subsequent drooping of the tip is likely unless one takes precautions against this eventuality at operation. Often a middle-aged woman will consult a plastic surgeon for her aging face and eyelids and, in passing, ask about a rhinoplasty—with the comment that she has "always hated" her nose. She may settle on the eyelidplasty or facelift but not on the rhinoplasty. It is as if she is exerting her prerogative of being able to have a rhinoplasty without necessarily going through with it. The older woman may have become resigned to her nose but not to the effects of aging. Some patients who have inquired about rhinoplasty have done so with the prefatory statement that "at my age, having a rhinoplasty seems a little ridiculous"; however, they usually have little difficulty in accepting the *idea* of facial surgery, such as rhytidectomy, because many of their friends have had it. A facelift is as common at their age as rhinoplasty was when they were in their teens.

Since these patients are older, a careful medical evaluation by an internist is necessary, especially to rule out hypertension or any other cardiovascular abnormality. The plastic surgeon, of course, should be able to take the blood pressure, which should be done to determine the presence of hypertension.

In older patients, as Kaye [151] has noted, a partial rhinoplasty may accomplish a good deal, e.g., rasping the dorsum or refining the tip, which can be performed either solely or with a forehead lift if the patient is having one.

Napoleon and Lewis [189] have counseled, based on their work and that of others, that in elderly patients over 65, a good predictor of a successful emotional response to cosmetic surgery is when the patient feels younger than his or her chronological age [188]. These individuals usually have more optimism, more energy, and less depression than their peers who may think of themselves as old or older than their true age. An interesting aside is that we tend to feel ourselves younger if our fathers also did when they became older.

The Male Patient

Although more males are seeking cosmetic surgery, the majority of patients for esthetic surgery, about 85 percent, are still female. From their findings, Jacobson and colleagues [140] concluded that male patients are more likely to be "psychologically ill" than their female counterpart. Frequently they have a "conscious desire to dissociate themselves from the undesirable traits of their fathers, and an unconscious desire to dissociate themselves from the primitive rage at the mother from whom the father failed to rescue them and toward whom they have ambivalent feelings." These men are particularly sensitive to "any perceived threats to male effectiveness. The cosmetic complaint is a symbolic representation of an alternative to more direct ways of dealing with these conflicts."

With cosmetic surgery becoming more popular among men, those having it now are more likely to be emotionally stable than were male esthetic patients two decades ago. Some investigators have not been able to document the importance of family relationships, especially that with the father, in the motivation of males wanting rhinoplasty. Even in a long initial consultation, the plastic surgeon will likely be unable to dissect the profound motivations that account for that patient being in your office; however, one must still be very wary of older males who want a cosmetic rhinoplasty in the absence of trauma or respiratory obstruction. In my experience, they are likely to have more psychological problems and postoperative dissatisfaction than those for facelift, eyelidplasty, hair transplantation, otoplasty, dermabrasion, abdominoplasty, liposuction, scar revision, or correctional gynecomastia. I agree with others who have noted the basic problem of sexual identity in men who desire rhinoplasty. They are apt to be in their late 20s or 30s, single, and inwardly confused about how masculine or feminine they want themselves and their nose to be. I well remember one man who sought more surgery after he had already had five operations by three other plastic surgeons. The nose that he desired was that of a youthful French actress (he had brought me her photograph). I told him frankly that he should avoid another operation but should definitely see a psychiatrist. I doubt that this patient ended his quest for a change in the appearance of his nose. Sheen and Sheen [239] have written:

> The male rhinoplasty patient represents a silent minority. Although the percentage of male patients is increasing, men in my practice [J. Sheen] now make up only 25 percent. But the problems they pose are not proportionate to their number . . . my experience corroborates studies that have shown that the male patients have a higher rate of psychological disturbance than their female counterparts . . . frequently the postsurgical course for a man is both troubled and troublesome. There is more demon ecchymosis. There is a higher incidence of epistaxis and infection. Men ignore postoperative instructions: they blow out their nasal packing and braise themselves in hot sun. Their dressings fall off. They are intolerant of discomfort, and syncope is far more common than with women. Men need extra reassurance and patience . . . whether it is because the man comes in with a greater level of disturbance or because of a basic difference in response, the adult male patient (not the adolescent) more frequently experiences a stormy period of adjustment postoperatively. He may be preoccupied with small irregularities and impatient for resolution of postoperative artifacts. Many male patients describe going through an extreme 'identity crisis.' In fact, most male secondary rhinoplasty patients (who represent a higher percentage of secondary cases) request a reconstruction that closely resembles their original nose. . . . Most complaints of male secondary rhinoplasty patients are based on undesirable feminine qualities, such as being too low, too narrow, too short, or having too much ertrousse. Bigger and stronger

are qualities associated with masculinity and which many patients want to preserve.

As mentioned earlier, my experience has shown a conflict in what they say they want and what I think they want. Although one might debate the psychodynamics, few would dispute the ordeal that older male cosmetic rhinoplasty patients pose for the plastic surgeon and also for themselves.

In the man, the nose is the only projecting midline structure other than the penis, and through displacement, it may be the focus of sexual inadequacy. The nose contains erectile tissue similar to that of the genitalia, and in both males and females it responds to sexual excitement. In many cultures and at different times in history, the size of the nose was equated with the size of the penis, hence virility. A common punishment for adultery in India 3,000 years ago and in Germany in the Middle Ages was amputation of the nose—another displacement, cultural rather than personal.

These psychoanalytic considerations aside, the important decision for the plastic surgeon is whether or not to operate on these patients [53]. If the plastic surgeon chooses the surgical route, he or she must be prepared to deal with the sequence of operation → dissatisfaction → re-operation → possibly another plastic surgeon for another operation.

Since the patient may be undecided about what characteristics he wants for his nose, for example, how long or short it should be, whatever the surgeon does to the nose, the essential psychological problem and conflict persist. This situation may account for the postoperative dissatisfaction of these patients, who easily become hostile and litigious, and, if paranoid, may even become homicidal [228]. Being murdered is not the postoperative result that most plastic surgeons would want.

From her own experience and a review of other studies of rhinoplasty patients, Wright [286] has concluded that the rhinoplasty patient, especially the male, is more psychologically disturbed than "other surgery patients; and that psychological disturbances are usually long-term and tend to reflect 'an identity conflict or a somatic conversion of a conflict.' " She goes on to say that the degree of deformity cannot be equated with postoperative satisfaction and that the surgeon often becomes the recipient of the patient's repressed hostility [285].

Acquired Immunodeficiency Syndrome
Any surgeon who treats any patient today but particularly males should be concerned about acquired immunodeficiency syndrome (AIDS). Despite the fact that a plastic surgeon's risk of getting AIDS is minimal, no surgeon, male or female should be cavalier about contracting a disease for which there is no cure. At the moment, there are only three known ways of contracting AIDS: direct sexual contact with a carrier, parenterally usually through a contaminated needle or direct infection from blood transfusion, or congenital transmission from mother to child. As Gorney [120] has pointed out, in addition to the fear of getting AIDS, "what . . . makes our colleagues most nervous is the frustrating, if not impossible, legal situation imposed by many local state statutes." He then gives a few examples: If a patient seeks a consultation for just an esthetic procedure and is in every other way a good candidate, but you suspect that he may be a high risk for AIDS, can you refuse treatment? At this stage in which no established doctor-patient relationship exists, the law in no way obligates you to treat anyone you do not wish to; you can refuse treatment for any reason. This is particularly justifiable in a situation where no health considerations are involved; however, in asking patients to submit to a voluntary human immunodeficiency virus (HIV) test as a condition of treatment, one could conceivably require this if there are no local or state anti-AIDS discrimination regulations; however, one could be in danger of being sued because you are treating that patient differently from other patients, and you would be acting "contrary to the American Medical Association's strong ethical statement on the issue." Gorney [120] has stressed that "under no circumstances should patients be tested [HIV testing] without their full knowledge and written consent. Pragmatically, it would be of no value anyway. You could not utilize the information without revealing how you got it—which would be enough to create considerable trouble for you." Gorney then gives another situation that requires a different kind of action: A man with a unilateral breast mass presumed to be gynecomastia has an axillary node that you

biopsied. The node proved to be malignant, but, in addition, you discover that the patient also has AIDS-related complex. In this instance, as Gorney [120] has stated, one has a "firmly established doctor-patient relationship. Failure to follow through with your commitment to surgery could be, first, breach of the AMA's [American Medical Association] policy statement, and then an invitation to a lawsuit on the basis of discrimination and abandonment. The crucial point here is that now you *are* dealing with matters affecting the health and even a life-or-death situation." This is a far different situation from a male patient who wants an elective cosmetic rhinoplasty.

Do you operate or not operate in this elective situation? If so, one takes the obvious precautions: double gloves, eye and face shield, assiduous disposable needles, linen, and so forth. If you do not operate, what do you tell the patient? The hard truth is probably something that most of us would not want to say, namely: "I am afraid that if I operate on you and stick myself, I might get AIDS even though the chance of contracting it is minimal. I do not want to die because of your nose."

More likely strategems would be to say something such as, "I would like to operate, but I get the feeling that you (the patient) won't like the result." Or, "You may have difficulty in healing with a good chance of getting a serious and overwhelming infection" (no evidence for this in someone who is HIV positive and asymptomatic or, in fact, in those with AIDS). Or, do you create a situation in which the patient or any reasonable human being would have to say "no," e.g., triple the usual fee or be so abrupt and discourteous that the patient will flee the office, or do you say "yes" and then schedule the patient two years down the line, hoping that he will go elsewhere? I admit that I have not been in this situation myself, but I would probably tell the patient the truth, realizing that I might have to answer to it in court. I certainly would not tell it harshly but would probably say that from an anatomic point of view, he probably could be improved by operation, but that many male patients are dissatisfied with the results (a point that I make to all male patients). I would then say that I am fearful of contracting AIDS, and even though I would treat him in an emergency situation, I am reluctant to do so under elective conditions. I admit that these answers are far from satisfactory and I would be grateful to any reader for suggestions of how the surgeon may wish to disengage in order to protect himself or herself while, at the same time, not hurting the sensibilities of the patient. I fear that the patient would understand all too well the motivation for saying "no." Aside from the legal repercussions that might ensue, the thought of hurting a patient who is already in a profoundly painful condition, emotionally and physically, would be distasteful to most physicians.

Reasons to Reject a Rhinoplasty Patient
I am considering here the patient who does *not* have AIDS or is *not* HIV positive.

Earlier I have discussed the kinds of patients who may represent trouble postoperatively. I have stressed, perhaps overstressed, also that the male rhinoplasty patient is apt to be more dissatisfied than his female counterpart.

Wright [286] offers four criteria for rejecting rhinoplasty patients: the presence of paranoid thoughts; symptoms of a delusional fixation; symptoms of surgical addictions; and the strong suggestion of malingering.

Although I agree with these unambiguous criteria of exclusion, I believe that many more patients, not fitting those indices, should not be candidates for rhinoplasty because of their potential for dissatisfaction. Wright [286] has acknowledged that

> the esthetic surgeon does have to diagnose psychic pathology in order to recognize the patient who is a psychological risk. One should remember that the primary diagnostic symptom of a risk patient is a surgeon's awareness of feeling intuitively uncomfortable. Even then, the surgeon should not abruptly reject the patient, but should either refer him or her for consultation or arrange a future appointment. Because the cosmetic patient tends to be distant and is not inclined to be open with others, a second consultation is often advisable. However, if on the second visit the surgeon still feels intuitively uncomfortable, he or she must refrain from performing surgery.

With every patient willing to have a rhinoplasty or any other operation, every plastic surgeon must decide on the patient's suitability according to his or her own perceptions and feelings. I tend to reject the patient at the initial consultation if I feel uncomfortable. Most likely I have detected something that a second visit may either confirm or negate. The possibility exists, however, that the patient during the second consultation might be cleverer than I in masking troublesome signs that were evident initially. I might then unwittingly consent to operate but later regret it.

In evaluating the rhinoplasty patient postoperatively, the plastic surgeon must realize that satisfaction does not necessarily depend on whether others recognize that the patient has had a significant change in his or her nose. It is what the patient thinks the change has been and what the patient thinks the change has done for him or her. Marcus' [178] study showed that the cosmetic rhinoplasty

> improves psychological or social well-being is not due to the many social advantages or greater physical attractiveness in our society; the unbiased, impersonal onlooker does not notice a significant improvement in the . . . patient's appearance. . . . The mechanism of psychological change for CR [cosmetic rhinoplasty] appears to lie in the patient's self-concept and the reduction of narcissistic self-absorption. With this reorganization of the narcissistic self towards a more modest degree of self-absorption, new energies are liberated which can now be used for increased psychological and interpersonal adjustment and participation. Indeed it would appear that a surgical operation has long-term positive effects by releasing previously repressed and inaccessible energies and allows the patient to develop a significantly different life-style. This sequence of events is analogous to Lichter's 'ripple effect,' namely the long-term generalized therapeutic advantage of removing a single persisting symptom which obstructs any genuine emotional growth. . . .

In this instance, the benefits of rhinoplasty are not in the eyes of the beholder primarily but in the eyes of the bearer—the patient.

What About the Chin?

In conjunction with rhinoplasty, a frequent procedure is chin augmentation, generally by means of a synthetic implant. The alternative is by osteotomy and advancement of the lower portion of the anterior mandible. If the patient has asked about fixing a receding chin, then, or course, the issue is clear; one should discuss it with him or her. Occasionally patients are unaware, at least consciously, of their chin, and the dilemma is whether to initiate its discussion. It is important not to talk patients into an operation for a problem about which they have been unconcerned. If something does go wrong, they would be rightfully angry not only because of the complication but what they perceive as the plastic surgeon's coercion.

With teenagers, sometimes it is helpful to call the parents and to mention to them that you had not wished to enter a discussion about the chin because you felt that it might worsen their self-image. Nevertheless, you believe that they would be helped by having a more prominent chin. You can then ask whether their child has mentioned this before. Sometimes it has been a passing thought and the parent needs only to raise the issue with the patient who will then assent enthusiastically.

Another alternative is to operate on the nose first and the chin later, should the patient desire it. Not every patient is prepared for changing both the nose and the chin at the same time. Again the surgeon should be careful not to overwhelm this type of individual with further feelings of inadequacy. I have heard a few plastic surgeons say that because it would be offensive to their esthetic sense and their reputation for a patient with a receding chin to have just the nose done, they would refuse to do the rhinoplasty. I believe such an attitude is imperious and inappropriately possessive about what is truly someone else's body.

Other surgeons may prefer to take photographs with the idea of discussing only the nose at the first consultation and then to have the patient return. On that occasion, with pictures, they can tactfully talk about the nose in relation to the rest of the face, especially the chin. The patient can then think about a mentoplasty and call the surgeon a few weeks later after having made a decision.

Since I do not perform advancement of the mandible, I will restrict remarks here to augmentation mentoplasty by the use of synthetic material.

The first point to make is that the operation may sound more simple than it really is. Getting the right implant into the right patient is the obvious objective. Too often small implants tend to give the patient a "Pharonic" look—a pointed chin with the rest of the lower mandible in an unpleasing contrast with it. Although infection is unusual, it can happen whether or not one chooses the oral or submental cutaneous approach.

The patient should also be told where you will make the incision—intraoral or through the skin under the chin.

In augmenting the chin of older patients in conjunction with a facelift, it is better to underdo it than to overdo it. These patients generally want a modest modification, not a spectacular change.

Any patient having a mentoplasty of any sort should be warned not only about the usual complications of infection, bleeding, faulty position, extrusion of the implant, but also about possible loss or change in sensation of their chin.

The Finances

I have previously alluded to a situation that should not be a problem but frequently is. This concerns whether the patient has a true respiratory obstruction from an internal nasal deformity. If, indeed, none exists, then it should not be invoked to gain insurance coverage. This basic concept seems to have eluded many plastic surgeons who become more crooked than the septum they call deviated. I have heard many patients say, "Dr. _____ told me that he would say on the insurance form that I had a deviated septum and trouble breathing so the operation and the surgeon's charges would be covered. After all, I have paid the premium for years and never had to use the insurance." My reply is that the patient has been fortunate to have had good health, and, further, I would never falsify any document. I usually add that I would not do it for myself and why should I do it for someone else? I then suggest that they return to that doctor. Usually they do not. They probably feel somewhat uneasy with a surgeon who would be willing to lie. If they had been completely satisfied with that surgeon, they would not have made the appointment to see me.

Dr. Michael Gurdin [127] once remarked, "No patient ever thanked me for saving him money." He meant that the patients want the best result, and to compromise standards to save a few dollars is usually a foolish exchange for both the surgeon and the patient. Furthermore, the patient, should he or she get a poor result, and if you have fraudulently written a report, then settlement out of court (blackmail) would be a very easy alternative for the patient to arrange.

It is important when discussing rhinoplasty with or without mentoplasty or any esthetic procedure to tell the patient and family whether you charge for a revision and the expected cost. If you do not expect a fee for your services, the patient should be told that they will have to pay for the operating room and other hospital charges if you do not have your own facility (see p. 348).

Fees for Adolescents
One should remember that adolescents are in that stage of life when they are trying to establish their independence as well as their identity. Almost always they have to depend on parents to pay for the operation. The issue of independence-dependence as well as the unresolved conflicts between children and parents may cause sparks to fly. To avoid getting burned, the plastic surgeon should keep a safe distance but not so far away to be out of touch.

Another aspect of fees for elective procedures in adolescents is that their collection may be difficult because of the prevalence of divorce. Many teenagers come from so-called broken homes. The mother who usually has custody of the child will say that her "ex-husband will pay for it since it is part of the settlement," a phrase that is glibly said but can present many problems. One should be very wary under these circumstances and insist that the husband be notified and that prepayment be obtained. Divorce, of course, affects the psyche as well as the financial status of children. The adolescent in front of you may be going through an extremely arduous time in his or her life.

Mother and Daughter Combination

Occasionally, a mother and daughter decide that they wish to be "done together." The surgeon may be flattered by the request and may actually enjoy the special situation, which will be discussed undoubtedly throughout the hospital and give him or her momentary and monetary pleasure; however, the negative aspect is that the father, if there is one, may feel that he has been a victim of an unholy alliance: daughter, wife, and surgeon. A more practical consideration is who will be home to care for both the daughter and the mother? Will the father, now disenchanted by their plans, be there to help his errant family? With the mother also recovering from operation, will there be that necessary support, emotional and physical, for her daughter?

Another problem, previously mentioned, is the decision on whom to operate first. Whoever it is, it is advisable not to let the other see the patient immediately after operation because of possible swelling, ecchymosis, bleeding, pain, nausea, or vomiting. An additional consideration is that the daughter will generally recover faster than the mother because of her age, and the mother might feel depressed by this difference. Unpleasant feelings of competition might be aroused. In short, I would approach this doubleheader with great caution.

The Second Consultation

I have already mentioned that I do not usually see a prospective patient for rhinoplasty more than once before operation as a routine. The reason, I admit, is a crowded schedule; however, some surgeons routinely schedule a second consultation. For example, Musgrave and Garrett [184] described their practice of taking Kodachromes and, at another appointment, projecting them for the patient and the family with more explanations about the proposed operation, with emphasis on its limitations. As a method of preoperative communication, it has proven effective for them and has diminished ambiguity and false hopes. Its disadvantages are the extra time for you and the patient as well as the expense for the patient to make a return trip or to lose a day or part of one at work. Sometimes it is impractical or impossible for the patient to return for another consultation if he or she comes from a great distance. The use of a Polaroid camera at the time of the initial consultation is a way of obtaining photographs that you can use almost immediately in the initial consultation with the patient. Other techniques to improve communication are to give printed material to the patient before the consultation or afterward, or both; to show prepared audiovisual films; or even to furnish their photographs on which they can then draw to give you (and themselves) a better idea of what they want changed. A problem with this tactic is the tacit implication that you will be able to produce surgically what the patient desires. Performing a rhinoplasty is not custom tailoring.

Despite the painstaking preparations and discussions, all of us recall patients whom we should have weeded out, principally because of their quest for perfection or for the unattainable. If the second consultation is to help one decide about the patient's emotional suitability for operation, you do have the opportunity for more personality probing. Yet this occasion may foster a bond, albeit tenuous, which should never have begun. Then it might be harder for you to say "no." You might have done better in following your intuition at the first visit.

Elsewhere, I have discussed the fact that despite the most careful preoperative discussions, along with written and visual material, patients retain surprisingly little and often only that which causes them the least emotional trauma. They screen out the unpleasant; some surgeons also relieve their anxiety through denial.

SECONDARY RHINOPLASTY

As long as rhinoplasties are being performed, secondary rhinoplasties will be done. The difference, however, is that it is not always the same surgeon repairing or attempting to repair his or her initial work. Although the average rhinoplasty today is better than it was a few decades ago, unfavorable, even disastrous results, continue to occur. The first important decision for any of us seeing a patient, perhaps our own, requiring revision is whether we can do it properly. If not, we should refer the patient to someone we think can. A second unsuccessful operation is not just one more failure; it has almost geometric adverse consequences for the patient anatomically and emotionally.

Patients

As mentioned, secondary rhinoplasty patients can be either yours or somebody else's. If the patient requires only a little more rasping of the dorsum or elevation of the tip, the task is relatively simple and the interpersonal relationship is minimally strained unless the patient, perhaps an adolescent, cannot emotionally tolerate local anesthesia. The prospect of general anesthesia escalates fears and costs. At that juncture, the family may well resent paying more money for an operation that they thought should have been performed correctly initially despite having been informed that this could occur. Even patients who have signed forms stating that they will be responsible for the hospital costs involved in trying to improve a result (see Appendix) are less than pleased to meet that obligation.

A worse situation with regard to finances occurs when it is necessary for you to refer the patient to somebody else whom you deem more experienced. Then the patient will undoubtedly face the reality of additional charges that will also involve paying the surgeon. It is too much to expect that with today's economic pressures a colleague will undertake the challenge without charge. Even if he or she should lower the customary fee, other costs would still have to be met. At this point, the mutual good will between the patient and you is liable to run out. Despite your most compassionate words, money occasionally becomes the ultimate consideration. The patient or his or her family may request that you return the fee so that they can put it toward paying for another operation. It would be wise to consult an attorney in that situation to be sure that your giving back the money is not misconstrued as an admission of negligence. On a couple of occasions, I have returned the money to the patient. In both instances, the result was by no means bad, but it was not good enough by my standards as well as those of the patient. The patient wanted to go elsewhere, and I consented to return my fee, with misgivings. No litigation resulted and I clearly dictated in my notes that I had returned the fee to spare them additional financial stresses.

In talking to colleagues, this matter of additional costs for secondary rhinoplasty if done by someone other than oneself may lead the patient to an attorney. In my experience, the financial matters involved in secondary rhinoplasty may be as difficult as the structural problems.

EYELIDPLASTY AND FACELIFT

Time was beginning to walk across the face.
Roger Kahn
The Boys of Summer

They aren't making mirrors the way they used to.
Tallulah Bankhead

There is a certain melancholy in seeing yourself rot.
Katherine Hepburn

Patients

Patients for these procedures are most likely to be white, middle- or upper-class women (approximately 1 in 10 is a man) between the ages of 45 and 55. Characteristically, they are active socially and professionally. The patient is not usually one of the "idle rich," a term that seems to pertain to fewer and fewer people these days. Having been considered attractive throughout her life, she fears losing what has been an important asset. One woman quoted her mother as saying, "A beautiful woman dies twice." Most who come for an eyelidplasty and facelift do not want to dissimulate their age but to reaffirm to themselves and perhaps to others that they are still youthful, optimistic, and effective. Many say that they do not desire to look much younger but want to avoid appearing much older than they should look considering how they feel. They still think of themselves as more youthful than they are chronologically. For some, a sagging face is symbolic of life's inexorable downhill course. They do not want to see their life contracting coffinlike around them; they are in your office to rid themselves of the daily reminders of decay.

Lenclos, a seventeenth-century French lady of fashion and epicure known for her beauty and distinguished lovers, wistfully remarked, "If God had to give woman wrinkles, he might have at least put them on the soles of her feet."

Many patients who come to rejuvenate their faces say that "suddenly I got older." That observation is akin to what someone else said, "You just wake up one morning, and you've got it." Of course, signs of aging begin subliminally for most people but inevitably reach the point of no escape. Goin and Goin [93] have written that "perhaps the most important aspect of the facelift operation is the time of life in which it is done: the years of the crises of middle and old age. This fact cannot be over-emphasized. The operation results directly from the ravages of time. It is done at a time of life when the patient has probably lost a number of loved ones." They then cite Webb and colleagues who found that 90 percent of facelift patients over 50 years of age had lost an important person during the previous five years. The losses may range from a separation, divorce, removal of a body part (mastectomy, hysterectomy), death of a loved one, children moving away, a home being sold, or even termination of psychotherapy.

Goin and Goin [92] emphasize the fact that motivations for the majority of women having facial rejuvenation are in some way directly related to feelings about aging. Burk and colleagues [35] found that the female cosmetic surgery patient is "a normal woman in terms of self-esteem who is attempting to remediate a consciously felt inconsistency between general and specific body-part esteem. Cosmetic surgery seems to reduce this inconsistency, which comes through in the remark about 'feeling younger than I look.' "

The fact that patients begin to look older when significant changes occur in their life makes it difficult to know precisely why they are having the operation. By that I mean that the patient does look older and that is a reality; however, the woman in her mid-40s or slightly older may be either in the menopause or facing it. The losses have started to overcome the gains: Her body has aged; her children have undoubtedly left her home; her husband's attentions may have waned; at work, she may feel excluded by those younger; less sand is in the hour glass now [102]. For some, the facelift is an active means of coping with life; they can have a facelift even though they cannot keep their children from leaving home or their husband content in their bed. The facelift may be a passport to a new pattern of living or to the resumption of an old career, perhaps interrupted by marriage and child rearing.

In our society and much of the world, the woman suffers from what Sontag [248] has called "the double standard of aging." Women are penalized more for aging than are men. "Aging means a humiliating process of gradual sexual disqualification. . . . Aging is much more a social judgment than a biological eventuality." I would disagree with that last sentiment: For some, aging is equally a "social judgment" and a "biological eventuality."

The process of aging is generally imperceptible on a day-by-day basis. It proceeds slowly but not necessarily at the same pace in different parts of the body. There are, however, what the French term *crises d'âge*, when suddenly a person seems to age rapidly. Some-

4 *Types of Operations and Types of Patients* 141

times this coincides with an emotional trauma. Many have correctly recognized that the tendency to aging is independent of life's events and seems to be more an inherited characteristic. They may resent genetic predisposition, especially if an older sister has escaped it or her mother has had it. Commonly I hear a patient say; "I dread getting to look like my mother." She does not like the unpleasant irony of beginning to resemble the person toward whom she has had such deep ambivalence.

Many women wish to appear young for professional reasons, as in the performing arts, or because of a liaison with someone younger. Statistically these patients are in the minority. Most seeking an eyelidplasty and facelift want to lessen the visible evidence of time's passage in order to improve their self-image with the hope that the reverberations will affect their performance.

The patient may feel ashamed about having cosmetic surgery and usually does. Often she has had to wage her battle alone. Friends may consider her foolish; her husband may call her "crazy"; and her family doctor may be strongly opposed. The following letter is typical of that kind of physician: punitive, rigid, and unsympathetic.

> Dear Doctor Goldwyn:
> When I saw Liza Albert [name changed] a few weeks ago, I was surprised to hear her express an interest in a facelift.
> She is a lovely, little old lady, rather childish in her behavior and lost since her husband's death several years ago, drifts from one relative to another, and is an extremely passive and dependent lady.
> As far as her medical history, there is no contraindication to the surgical procedure; however, it would seem to be a radical step to satisfy this masochistic need.

She did have a rhytidectomy and seemed very pleased with the result. A close relative, previously skeptical, reported that it "did her a world of good. I was surprised." Undoubtedly her doctor was also if he had the capacity to recognize the change and to admit it.

One patient called the entire process of obtaining a facelift a "lonely vigil." In a world where the haves are reminded of the have-nots, she may feel even more guilty because she is spending money (often her husband's) since esthetic surgery and the associated hospitalization generally are not covered by insurance. Nowadays, women are more likely to have a career but still they find it difficult to go it alone financially; if married, they usually seek their husband's tangible as well as emotional support.

Many patients apologize for taking the doctor's "valuable time" and for occupying a hospital bed "meant for sick people." In this regard, outpatient surgery is most appropriate for them in addition to its other advantages.

The patient considers the operation for improving the aging face to be an enhancement. She will accommodate to the "new look" since it is really the old look—the way she was.

Other patients, however, come for a facelift/eyelidplasty as a way of beginning life anew, the operation being emotionally a reparation for damages suffered. I remember a 42-year-old woman whose daughter had died following a four-year battle with leukemia. "Now I can do something for myself," she declared.

The Male Patient

As mentioned, male patients for esthetic surgery and, indeed, for facelift procedures are in the minority although rising—slightly. In my experience, they usually have a facelift because their wife or "significant other" looks younger or because they are in the process of trying to meet or having met someone younger.

Groucho Marx once cracked, "A man is only as old as the woman he feels." Although that may have been true for him and for others, many men do not like the discrepancy in age; they loathe being taken for their woman's father instead of husband or lover.

In contrast to men for rhinoplasty, males for facelift generally are satisfied postoperatively. I have found them to be less finicky than their female counterparts. In summarizing their observations about males for rhytidectomy-blepharoplasty, Edgerton and Langman [66] characterized them as occasionally having mild depression, "little psychopathology, realistic expectations from surgery, normal interpersonal relationships, pleased with surgery."

Despite these supposed advantageous features of having males for facelift and eyelidplasty, Flowers [77], in my opinion, rightfully states that "males are vastly more difficult patients than females [referring to the operation itself]. They tolerate stress less well and more uniformly have lower pain thresholds. Their cardiovascular systems are less stable, they are more prone to cardiovascular disease, and they require considerably more medication for anesthesia than do females. They become restless more easily, have less tolerance for lying still for long periods, and are generally more difficult patients."

In addition to these impressions, males do have more postoperative bleeding in association with rhytidectomy and they must have their incisions and scars carefully explained to them because of their being unable, generally, to use makeup for dissimulation. In addition, the beardline must be contended with, and male patients must be precisely briefed about where the incisions will be and what they can expect in terms of future shaving; e.g., the beardline moving back further toward the ear; their barber noticing the scars behind their ear (as others might also).

Vistnes and Jobe [263] have observed that "males tend to be more apologetic and embarrassed by their 'weakness'; they need more support during the events surrounding rhytidectomy."

A technical point—one that should be obvious but occasionally is forgotten—is that baldness or thinning of hair is much more common in men, and incisions as well as flaps must therefore be carefully planned, not only for the present but for the future with regard to scarring.

Although no patient theoretically should have to wait long to see any doctor, reality is different. Male patients, however, since they are usually in the minority in the waiting room, are particularly anxious and embarrassed about having had facial surgery. Therefore I make it a priority to see recently operated on patients, female and male, but males particularly, as soon as they come for their appointment.

Initial Consultation

At the first visit, it is essential for the plastic surgeon to know what the patient, generally a female, wishes and what type of individual she (or he) is. No matter what the gender, no matter who the person, those undergoing facial esthetic surgery will be more particular about their results than if they had a procedure on a more hidden area of the body, such as the back or abdomen. The breasts, obviously also, are an emotionally laden area. The point I am making here is that if the patient had not been concerned about his or her appearance, then that individual would not be in your office in the first place. To expect that they will be cavalier about their results would be absurd. For that reason, someone observed, and many would agree, that cosmetic surgery would be easy if it were not for the patients. By that, we are acknowledging the fact that technically, though this type of surgery is exacting, it does not require extraordinary talents given to only two or three in the entire country. The problem is that patients are usually demanding and fussy about results.

During the first visit I try to weed out the patient who cannot stand imperfection because, frankly, most patients after facelift and eyelidplasty, at least mine, will have imperfections; the flawless result is seen more often in slides at meetings and in articles in journals than in one's own office. I have reviewed the charts of my patients who have lingering dissatisfaction with the outcome of these procedures. Statistically, they represent about six percent of all patients, but emotionally in terms of their impact on the surgeon, myself, they seem to have been a much greater proportion. In every instance, my secretaries or I, or both, had a presentiment that this patient might be "difficult." Most were hard to please in other spheres of life; at least that had been my impression. What most surgeons do not know is how many emotionally difficult patients have fared well in our care. We remember the problem patients but forget those from whom expected trouble did not arise. We have very little way of tracking those whom we have rejected for operation because we thought that they would be impossible to please, when, indeed, they might have gone elsewhere and have been totally satisfied with the outcome; however, for some patients a home run—not a triple—is essential to success, and, more than that, the ball must be hit precisely in right center field. As I get older, I prefer not to accept such challenges. Unlike in fishing, the one that gets away in plastic surgery may be a blessing for you.

Baker [8] has said, "The object of the operation should be to improve appearance not to make the patient happy if she is sad to begin with. You both will likely end up sad." Yet, the reality is that many patients seeking a facelift or an eyelidplasty have as part of their "secret agenda" becoming happier [94]. Indeed, as I have mentioned before, happiness is an objective of esthetic surgery. A patient wants satisfaction with the result, but, in addition, she may want more than that: a more pleasurable state of being. She may have regarded a facelift procedure as a way of feeling better about herself, doing better in life, lessening or even erasing dissatisfaction and disappointments.

The history taking should of course involve inquiry about general health, including present or past psychotherapy, previous operations and emotional reactions to them, allergies, and medications, especially aspirin-containing compounds. Is the patient a smoker? If so, what and how much? What about alcohol? Again, how much? The inquiry should not be abrupt but low-key. Nevertheless, one should persist to be certain to get the information.

Physical Examination

As with rhinoplasty, I ask the patient to indicate, while holding a mirror, what she or he would like improved. Compared to men, women are usually more conscious of the skin redundancy and sagging of their upper lids than of their lower lids. Perhaps that is due to the fact that they use an eye-liner and are cognizant of the diminished or absent fold.

Frequently, the patient wants only her neck done, and even though she might benefit also from an eyelidplasty, it is advisable not to extend the scope of the operation beyond the neck and face. In that instance, the patient should be told that to get rid of the excess skin of her neck, it will be necessary to make an incision in front and behind the ear.

The patient's face, like every other body part, is hers (or his); she may allow us to operate, but we are not given a carte blanche to pursue our trade wherever we wish. The patient and the plastic surgeon do better to undertake less than to try for more. Future surgery is always possible, but one cannot take back what one has already done. Nowhere else in medicine are Aristotle's words more true than in cosmetic surgery: "It is not part of a physician's . . . business to use either persuasion or compulsion upon the patient" [6].

The procedure you might add to the patient's list may well be the one that will have a complication.

Occasionally, however, a true dilemma exists. For example, a patient, who wants only the upper lids done may thereby accentuate the aging of the lower lids (painting-just-one-room-in-a-house syndrome), making her face as a whole look worse by comparison; however, if carried to absurdity, an upper eyelidplasty would lead to a lower eyelidplasty, a face and neck lift, a mastopexy, an abdominoplasty, a thigh lift, liposuction, and, perhaps, topping it all, a rhinoplasty. The patient's desires and your common sense should establish the direction and limits of the surgery.

An important point in the preoperative examination of a patient for an eyelidplasty or a facelift is to note facial asymmetry, in repose and in smiling. Is there any evidence of weakness of a branch of the facial nerve? Did the patient have Bell's palsy? Whatever differences exist between one side of the face and the other, and there usually are some, should be shown to the patient by means of a mirror or reinforced with photographs, or both. Postoperatively, that patient might expect more symmetry than he or she has ever had or could ever have. It is interesting to observe how little imperfection patients can tolerate after an operation but how much imperfection they had managed to live with before.

Do not neglect the forehead. Is the action of the frontalis muscle equal bilaterally? Are the eyebrows at the same level both at rest or in elevation?

Although this book is not intended to be a text of plastic surgery, I think it is important to emphasize here the need for a thorough eye examination, if not by you, then by an ophthalmologist. One must be certain that the patient, especially if older, has had a complete evaluation within the past six months or year. I always write the eye specialist about the contemplated operation in order to obtain reports about his or her findings and suggestions. One should test at least gross vision in each eye: ability to count fingers or to read with and without glasses. Also one should evaluate the patient's lacrimal function in order to detect an actual or potential "dry eye." This is a difficult entity for most plastic surgeons to diagnose precisely; however, if the patient can wear contact lenses for several hours at a time, it is good evidence of sufficient lacrimation. If in doubt, a referral to an astute ophthalmologist is advisable. Every plastic surgeon should also be able to elicit chief points in the history: complaints about dryness of the eyes; necessity for using drops; poor tolerance of sunlight and wind; a "grainy" or "sandy" feeling in the eyes; frequent tearing. One should also note how much elasticity is present in the lower lid simply by pulling it outward and watching how well or how poorly, how rapidly or how slowly it retracts.

Wrinkling or Sagging or Both?

For someone whose face has the "Gucci bag" look, dermabrasion or chemical peel in addition to or instead of a surgical rhytidectomy may be what the patient needs, particularly if she minds the wrinkles more than the sagging. She might benefit optimally from both procedures, staged to avoid the application of phenol to skin just undermined. Occasionally a patient will refuse a chemical peel because she fears scarring, a remote possibility, or dislikes a permanent change in pigment, a likely event. For want of something better, you and the patient may settle for just the surgical lift. Despite your candid and thorough explanation of the limitations of the rhytidectomy alone and her declaration that she understands what you are saying but she will be grateful for "whatever you can do for me," you both will be sinking into the slippery and steep-walled pit that you have dug for yourselves.

E.N., a 63-year-old sales manager, widow, and former solarphile, had marked wrinkling of her cheeks and forehead, and around her mouth. She also had moderate jowls and prominent platysmal bands in her neck. Her principal concern, however, was her cheek creases, which, I explained, would be managed best by a chemical peel. When she understood that the procedure could be followed by scarring, although it was highly unlikely, and that she would have some changes in pigmentation, she decided against the chemical peel but opted for a surgical lift. It was not her primary concern, however.

She: Even though a peel and lift would be the best, a lift by itself would help me, wouldn't it?
I: Yes, but only mildly.
She: What would you do?

I: That's for you to decide.

She: You say that no one can guarantee that there will not be scarring?

I: Yes, but scarring is not common after a peel although it does happen.

She: But you also said that my skin may not keep the same color it has now if the chemical is applied.

I: True, but you will look better with many of the lines and wrinkles less prominent and some actually gone.

She: Well, I am a little bit afraid of the chemical peel now that you've explained to me what could go wrong. So I will have a facelift and will have to be satisfied with any improvement it will give me even though you say it's not as good as if I also have the chemical treatment.

A few weeks after an uneventful facelift and when the swelling regressed and the lines reappeared, she seemed subdued, evidently depressed, and said, "Even though you told me that I wouldn't get a fantastic improvement, I honestly thought it would be more than this. My friends can't believe I ever had anything done. In fact, one asked me when I was going in for my facelift."

I again offered her the opportunity of supplementing the facelift by a chemical peel, but she refused for the same reasons as before. Only now, she considers the small gain from the surgery as a loss because of her large outlay—physically, emotionally, and financially.

The lesson from this patient is clear, and it has relevance to all elective surgical situations, not just the instance of the patient with the wrinkled face: It is better to do nothing than something of dubious value, particularly when it does not center on the patient's primary complaint. It will not meet the patient's desires and expectations.

Malar Pouches

Although malar pouches occasionally can be lessened, they cannot be eliminated, at least in my experience. Judging from the number of unsuccessful procedures proposed to make these pouches disappear, other plastic surgeons have evidently had the same frustration. Although initially surprised at this limitation of the facelift, the patient must truly comprehend it. In fact, during the early postoperative phase with the generalized swelling, these pouches will look more prominent and the patient will need assurance that they will not be permanently worse than they were prior to operation.

CHIN IMPLANT WITH FACELIFT

Augmenting a retruded chin, which often the bony resorption accompanying aging has worsened, can decidedly improve a patient's profile. It is important to assess where the chin is deficient: at the very tip or in a larger perimeter? Usually the deficiency extends laterally, and the implant must take this into account. One caution: Sometimes the addition of an implant can cause slight webbing of the neck, making the profile worse unless measures are taken intraoperatively to prevent this unwanted phenomenon, such as approximating the platysma in the midline. Another caution: Do not overdo—use a smaller implant when in doubt [151]. Until I had learned that lesson, I replaced a few implants because of a "Mussolini look."

FOREHEAD LIFT

Within the past decade, the forehead or brow lift has become more popular. No longer a rare surgical event, it is a procedure about which patients inquire and plastic surgeons propose; however, it is important to examine patients very carefully to be certain that they will benefit from this procedure. In New England, fewer request forehead lifts relatively speaking than in California and in Florida.

Kaye [151], who has been an effective champion of the forehead lift, notes the verity that the forehead and brows "ultimately yield to the effects of time and gravity as does the lower two-thirds of the face." In his opinion, correction of the upper third of the face is just as important as improvement of the lower two-thirds. The primary indications for a forehead-brow lift are ptosis of the brows and lateral hooding of the upper lids. Kaye is correct in noting that an upper lid blepharoplasty does not adequately correct lateral hooding, which is due more to ptosis of the brows and forehead.

One should inquire whether the patient has had an upper eyelidplasty previously in order to prevent inability to close the eyes following a forehead lift. Patients must understand that forehead wrinkles will not be eliminated by the lift. In males, the procedure should be more conservative than in females, and one must take into account the man's hairline and hair, its thickness and distribution. The male patient preferably should have hair to cover the incision line, but they may later lose their hair, and the scar, once hidden, will now be visible.

Beyond my experience but certainly not beyond that of those skilled in craniofacial surgery are procedures to improve the bony structure of the face [199, 200, 272]. This merging of esthetic with reconstructive techniques will most likely become a routine part of the surgery of appearance to the patient's psychological benefit [215]. Future techniques will go beyond the mere chiseling away of the prominent orbital ridges that many of us now do.

Informing the Patient Having Eyelidplasty or Facelift, or Both

In a chronological sequence, I take the patient through the contemplated operation. For those wishing an eyelidplasty, I discuss the mechanisms of outpatient surgery (at the hospital); the use of local anesthesia with intravenous supplementation; the expected pain; the length of the procedure (about an hour and a half); the need for someone to drive the patient home; the regimen of bed rest, head elevation, and iced dressings to the eyes for 24 hours; the return visit to the office for suture removal in three to five days; and the expected resumption of normal activities—in the home or at the office—in three to seven days after the operation, depending on the nature and setting of the job.

With the patient holding a mirror, I indicate the incisions and inform him or her about the inevitability of scars but say that hopefully they will not be noticeable at conversation distance. I do emphasize, however, that wound healing is unpredictable and that scarring might be prominent, red, and thick. I also tell patients about the small probability of infection and hematoma. I inform them also about the much smaller chance of blindness in one or both eyes. The patient and the family must understand that although an eyelidplasty is not a major operation, like a gastrectomy, it is a surgical event subject to unpredictable occurrences—one of which is blindness. Admittedly, this event is uncommon, with a probability of 0.04 percent, like that of getting struck by lightning; however, despite the rarity of blindness, I never do a bilateral lower eyelidplasty in a patient with monocular vision.

With every patient I clearly stress the limitations of the surgery: not to expect every wrinkle to disappear but to anticipate significant lessening of skin redundancy and prominent bags. I tell each patient that swelling and ecchymosis will last two to three weeks, but that he or she must wait six to nine months for a near-final result. To the question of how long the surgical improvement will last, I say that the lift may stall the aging process, but it never halts it. In general, the worse the problem, the longer the benefit. Even the best-executed operation can produce only a minimal effect if the problem is minimal. The patient is told that aging and the surgical results vary from individual to individual, depending on genetic factors, past and present, and future health and other variables beyond human control. Some patients have the misconception that suddenly one morning they will wake and have their face "drop." This fantasy may reflect their guilt about trying to thwart nature.

For those having a facelift alone or with an eyelidplasty, I demonstrate the planned incisions around the ears, into the hairline, and possibly under the chin if something has to be done for the neck through this approach. I mention many of the things that I have already discussed for an eyelidplasty. In addition, I tell the patient about the possibility of damage to the facial nerve, a surgical event more often discussed than observed, but one that can occur, especially as the procedure now involves more being done to the fat of the cheeks and neck and to the platysma and to deeper structures. These patients must understand that they may feel an unpleasant constriction and numbness in their neck for a few months, but usually these sensations disappear.

Some patients may have excessively redundant skin of their lids, cheeks, and neck; I tell them that a secondary procedure may be necessary in six to twelve months to improve the initial results. Patients having a facelift want to know the length of the operation (three to four hours), the type of anesthesia (usually local and intravenous), the duration of hospitalization (overnight usually), whether their hair is shaved (no, except only to make an incision), when they can go to the hairdresser (six days for a shampoo; twelve days for color), whether they will go home with a bandage (no), when the stitches are removed (three to five days for the lids; seven to ten days for sutures in front of the ears and ten days for those behind), how long the swelling and ecchymosis will last (two to three weeks, but the final result will take six to nine months to be appreciated), when they can use makeup (to the face, around five days, but not over the incisions; false eyelashes, six days after operation). Various surgeons will answer these questions differently, but the important point is to answer them or to raise them if the patient has not thought of them.

I also tell patients that it is not unusual to have a mild, transient depression for a few days after operation. I say this because I have observed it in many patients having facial surgery, usually a rhytidectomy with or without eyelidplasty but rarely in eyelidplasty alone. The downward swing in emotions is due to many factors, not all understood. The patient is obviously disappointed in seeing herself (or himself) in a contused, unnatural condition; there is also the metabolic response to operation—initially euphoria followed by a downswing. Moreover, the fact that these operations are done under local anesthesia with intravenous medication does not make them "minor" procedures, as far as the patient's response is concerned. The challenge to soma and psyche is greater than the patient expects and the surgeon appreciates. Numbness and paresthesias will add to discomfort and depression. Again and again throughout the course of treatment, the patient must be reminded not to be "an impatient patient." Wound healing is not a question of days or even weeks but months.

The patient must be warned about hair loss near the incisions as well as a difference in the hairline in front of and behind the ear if you believe it will occur and you do not take intraoperative measures to avoid it.

Pigment changes in the skin are common and are usually the result of schemic changes from either dissecting the flaps too thinly or pulling them too tightly, or both. The argon laser for these problems is useful.

Brown areas and blotches over the sternocleidomastoid muscle may appear and may even be permanent in many patients. Sometimes the pigmentary alterations are the clue to someone's having had a facelift.

Even with the most thorough imparting of information regarding possible complications and unfavorable results, most patients often are as unwilling to acknowledge the possibility of their occurrence as they are to express their deepest motivations for undergoing the operation.

Fees, of course, must also be discussed—the cost of your services as well as those of the hospital, operating room, anesthesia (or of the office if the operation is being performed there). One should stress again if the patient does not already know that third-party coverage is usually unavailable for cosmetic surgery and for any complications such as hematoma and infection. The patient must be told that occasionally a revision may have to be done to improve the result and that will involve hospital costs (unless one has one's own facility) for which the patient is responsible.

Informing the Patient Having Forehead Lift

Patients having a forehead and brow lift must be aware of the possibility of hematoma, skin necrosis, hair loss, scarring, and the inevitability of pain. Furthermore, scars are not always invisible. It is extremely important to emphasize that they will likely have sensory loss, usually in the scalp posterior to the coronal incision. With time, numbness decreases but permanent loss of sensation is possible. In addition, the patient may have dysthesias, particularly annoying itching. These sensory changes may be permanent, but even if they disappear, it may take more than a year.

The patient must also know that it is possible to damage the frontal branch of the facial nerve so that he or she will be unable to raise the eyebrow(s). Even if the nerve has not been cut and not even directly injured, paresis, unilateral usually but bilateral possibly, can result from stretching the nerve, thus producing an inability to raise the eyebrow or wrinkle the forehead on the affected side(s). The patient must understand in addition that if the frontalis nerve has been cut on one side, loss of its function will occur, and late repair of the nerve is a difficult and not always successful procedure even though it may be attempted. A selective frontal neurectomy of the opposite side may have to be done to regain symmetry, a step not to be undertaken lightly.

As mentioned previously, many patients are asymmetric in their frontalis action, and photographs should be taken of them at rest and raising the eyebrows. I can remember occasions when I sorely wished that I possessed such documentation when the patient complained after the operation about a "difference in my eyebrows."

During the Operation

To the observer, patients undergoing rejuvenative surgery of the face seem relaxed and without apparent internal turmoil. This tranquil scene may be deceptive since some medications may make it difficult for a patient in discomfort to express his or her displeasure.

I had this recent experience with a patient who was having a facelift: When the coil to my headlight became entwined around my feet, I commented, "This is not right." The anesthesiologist indicated to me that the patient's blood pressure and heart rate rapidly increased and advised me to clarify to the patient that I was not speaking about her operation but about a mechanical problem relative to my headlight. Indeed, I did so and her vital signs returned to normal. Later in the office she recalled this incident and said, "I thought something was going wrong and didn't want to say anything because I thought it would only distract you and things could have gotten worse for me."

A word about dressings: Do not apply them too tightly, especially over a drain in the neck after rhytidectomy or over the forehead after a lift. An excessively tight dressing will not stop a hematoma, but it may cause skin necrosis, especially if bleeding occurs.

After the Operation

Patients must be told or given clear instructions about their care: when to remove the dressing, when to shower, what to do about suture line care, if anything, and when to exercise, have sex, and return to work. I stress that any activity during the first two weeks following any facial operation—facelift, eyelidplasty, rhinoplasty—should not be vigorous or bleeding will possibly result. Also, to aid healing, smoking should not be resumed for three weeks and hopefully not at all, but that might be too much of an expectation.

Although most patients having eyelidplasty and facelift will be satisfied if they have been properly selected, this does not guarantee that all patients will be beaming with gratitude. Those who have had the operation not just to look younger but to recapture youth will be disappointed. Their lease on life has not been extended. The plastic surgeon who carefully questions patients following the procedure will detect more depression than had been suspected or has been commonly reported. As mentioned, this emotional letdown usually passes, but it may persist. Despite what you have said, the patient may have forgotten that she would get depressed and despite your telling her not to expect too much from the procedure, she may have anticipated a miraculous transformation, an immediate turning back of the clock by 20 years—without swelling or ecchymosis. Almost universally patients expect to be fully recovered in just two weeks—no swelling, black or blue, numbness, stiffness—despite your having warned them about how long it does take to recover.

Immediately after the operation the patient probably hides from all but her closest friends and her hairdresser. One patient said, "I learned to sit in the first row in church so I could get out first and also to sit with my thumb under my chin" [hiding the incision].

For many women seeking a facelift or eyelidplasty, the surgeon is the hired hand. He or she has been asked to do a job just as she might have requested a mechanic to repair her auto. When the result is good, the patient is pleased but not grateful, unlike the patient who has had a musculocutaneous flap for a debilitating chronic ulcer of the lower leg or the patient who has undergone a much-needed reduction mammoplasty. Aside from their general disenchantment, patients may be greatly upset if a complication or unfavorable result ensues. Do not expect them to accept this turn of events with equanimity. Although you have told them about its possibility, most patients will not consider it seriously. If they did, they probably never would have pursued their request for the operation. Therefore, when a complication does occur, they feel wronged and may be extremely angry at what they consider your "incompetence." How to manage this trying situation is discussed later (see p. 246). A further difficulty is that since insurance does not usually defray the cost of complications, they feel even more unhappy and resentful. If we were in their position, we would probably react the same way.

If indeed the patient seems to have a severe postoperative psychological disturbance, do not wait long to call a psychiatrist. Schweitzer and Hirschfield [235] have reported a patient who became psychotic following rhytidectomy—a very rare event as they themselves note. More often it is a reactive depression that will pass, hopefully, with appropriate therapy or even with time alone. The problem is then how to get the patient who needs the psychiatrist to the psychiatrist.

In conclusion, the eyelidplasty and facelift as well as the forehead lift can be satisfying operations for patients as well as surgeons; however, remember that a principal objective of the initial consultation is to identify that patient who is a poor candidate for this procedure because of what she wants, what she has, or how she is. Again, my advice is to select that patient *who can tolerate imperfection* and truly understands the limitations of the operation.

The Opinions of Others as a Determinant of Postoperative Satisfaction
After eyelidplasty and facelift, perhaps more than anywhere in esthetic plastic surgery, the opinions of others, even strangers, may greatly influence the patient's satisfaction or dissatisfaction with the anatomical outcome. This is true to some degree after rhinoplasty with regard to the judgment of the parent, particularly the mother and peers. My observations suggest that the friends of the adolescent girl are usually more supportive than those of the middle-aged woman, who is extremely vulnerable to the opinions of her friends, especially those of the same sex. Their approbation or disapproval is usually more important to her than that of her husband. Because she may have undertaken her surgery with his opposition or grudging consent, his opinion is not important now since it never was.

Even though the patient sought the operation by herself and presumably for herself, she is very much aware of the reaction of those around her. Just at the time she desperately wants their support, her friends may impale her by their verbal thrusts:

> "You certainly are swollen. Will it ever go away under your chin?"
> "You really look funny."
> "Your eyes don't match."
> "How come Betty looks so much better than you, and you went to the same surgeon?" [Betty may be six months postoperative and your patient, only three weeks.]
> "I told you that you should have gone to somebody else."
> "After seeing what you look like, I'd never have it done."

How apt the line from the Old Testament is here: "I was wounded in the house of my friends" (Zech. 13:6). The patient's "friend" may resent her likely change for the better. Perhaps that friend may have wanted the operation but lacked the money or courage, or both. She may also fear that her husband will now find her rejuvenated friend more attractive than she. It is probably true that a good friend helps you in distress, but a better friend helps you in success.

The surgeon cannot insulate a patient from the barbs of those close to her; however, he or she can support her recovery from injury and can point out the possible psychodynamics responsible for a "friend's" behavior. It takes considerable control for you, as a surgeon, not to become angry at the patient's friends for making such remarks and for withholding much-needed succor.

Sometimes family members hesitate to be enthusiastic initially because they are unsure of the result [221]. They withhold their applause not because they are hostile, but because they are cautious and bewildered. The patient usually looks distorted—swollen, as for example, after rhinoplasty or a facelift.

When the patient is at a low ebb, she may not be able to deal with distressing situations that she has previously managed fairly well, for example, an unhappy relationship with her husband or a child.

A recent patient of mine four days after a facelift came to the office accompanied by her son, in his late 20s. He looked hostile and the patient said to me in front of him: "He's angry I had this done." Her son defended himself by saying that he opposed any unnecessary risks such as this type of elective procedure. His mother later told me in confidence that while that ostensible reason was true, her son said to her, "Without your big double chin, you don't look like grandma, and I used to snuggle up against her neck while I was young."

Aside from this particular and, perhaps peculiar, instance, for many children, no matter what their age, having a mother suddenly looking younger is threatening. Not only may it reawaken the conflicts of the past, but it is a reminder to children that parents do age and will die and that this will inevitably happen to them as well.

Many husbands characteristically joke, "She [the wife] looks so young that I'm afraid she'll run away with someone younger." As we know from Freud, much emotional significance lies even in the simplest humor, and the aging man's fear of losing his younger wife and now a younger-looking wife runs deep in our culture as well as in many other societies. Feminists will rightly interpret this also as evidence of the secondary status of women—being chattel or sex objects. Although I would not necessarily go that far in interpreting every instance in which the husband voices his fear, certainly the comment has a possessive tone. Love, however, does involve emotional if not actual possession for both the male and the female.

Any operation, and facial rejuvenative surgery is no exception, engenders stress for those concerned with the person's well being. The patient, in response to the operation itself or the pressures of interpersonal relationships at home, may complain of insomnia, pain in the face and neck, and even unhappiness with the result of her procedure. With regard to the last complaint, her criticism may be a response to the external stresses rather than the objective deficiencies of the outcome. By listening to the patient and not by running away from her (with the excuse that many others are waiting), you may be able to sort out the causative from the incidental factors. You may then be able to give the patient a perspective on her problems. Your reassurance will help restore her confidence and temporarily wounded self-esteem.

As Goin [89] has written,

> Many people who have esthetic surgery are those with high personal standards of performance, the need to deny their wishes to be cared for,

and an obsession with their independence. They feel guilty and down when they are not meeting these standards. Patients find they are not able to function at their preoperative capacity for a few days. If they were ill with cancer, this might seem acceptable, but following elective operation it is intolerable. The guilt about self-indulgence is already at a high level and consequently it is important to carry on at home as if nothing has happened. The mother of six feels it is important to be up and ready to go at 6:30 A.M., getting her children off to school efficiently, clean, cook, or, if she works, go off to work as usual. When she finds herself unable to tackle these tasks with her normal vigor, she is struck with a sense of inadequacy and guilt over inability and sense of depression.

Patients with that type of personality are most prone to depression, which sometimes the surgeon can relieve, but which occasionally does require a psychotherapist.

COLLAGEN INJECTION AND FAT TRANSPLANTATION

Though popular and remunerative, collagen injection and fat transplantation are of dubious value for facial rejuvenation. Absorption, liquefaction, infection, drainage, and undesirable contour may occur after fat transplants because of hypersensitivity (despite negative pretesting).

Physicians who enthusiastically recommend collagen and fat to their patients should give more consideration to their long-term results than the short-term remuneration. The argument that collagen and fat installation does little harm (unless you happen to be the patient) is specious. One would expect that when a physician recommends a treatment, it should accomplish something more than a transitory placebo effect. If we cannot do better than that, then why not instill saline to plump out tissue or administer vitamin B_{-12} to make the patient feel better? The fact that a patient requests a procedure or treatment does not mean that he or she should receive it. That decision has to be at least partly our responsibility as professionals.

In defending collagen injections and fat transplants, many colleagues cite the "few patients" who have benefitted. What they fail to emphasize, however, are the many who have not. They would argue, furthermore, that nothing lasts forever; even the best facelift fails against gravity, time, and ultimately death. This kind of nihilism does not excuse a physician from recommending medical or surgical treatment that is questionable, to use a euphemistic adjective.

It is disturbing that many physicians who have studied and trained many years and supposedly should have learned something about the scientific method should occupy the therapeutic fringe, dispensing nostra. That so much fat has been transplanted and so much collagen has been injected into patients over many years without rigorous documentation regarding results is extremely disappointing, to say the least.

Because of disillusionment with transplanted fat and injected collagen, some plastic surgeons, including myself, have used grafts and flaps of dermis with or without fat, fat alone, even rotated platysma or parts of the superficial musculoaponeurotic system, at the time of rhytidectomy to fill concavities or to heighten the malar areas.

BREAST AUGMENTATION

Despite the far from perfect results, augmentation mammoplasty is a frequently performed operation. Although it might not satisfy the esthetic criteria of the surgeon, it does answer the psychological needs of the patient.

Patients

From a psychiatric evaluation of patients undergoing augmentation mammoplasty, Gifford [87] concluded that many had

> unhappy childhoods, experience of loss or maternal deprivation and conflicts in identification with parents. They tended to make early marriages, in which they played a submissive or frankly masochistic role . . . many described longstanding feelings of inferiority or low self-esteem, and several described periods of clinical depression. The "typical" breast augmentation patient seemed to have reached an emotional turning point in her life, when she had decided against having more children and was seeking a new direction, increased self-assertiveness, some kind of personality change. In these women, the breasts had come to represent something more than sexual attractiveness, because their breasts were their representation of an ideal self, real or imagined. This was an image of themselves as they were at some former time or as they had hoped to

be, an ideal self which they had been deprived of or lost through hardship, childbearing or the vicissitudes of life. The operation represented the restitution of this loss, the restoration of an ideal or former self.

Other studies have documented depression, low self-esteem in general and as a woman in particular, as well as hysterical traits in patients requesting breast enlargement [243]; however, Shipley, O'Donnel, and Bader [240], who used control groups of small- and average-busted women, concluded that their patients for augmentation were psychologically healthy although they placed greater emphasis on physical attractiveness and "modern or revealing" dress. Their data did not support the findings of others that women wanting this procedure suffer from feelings of inadequacy and a generally poor body image. Also, there was no evidence of depression, social malfunction, or a higher incidence of either major gynecological surgery or psychiatric counseling.

Although controversy exists about the personality type of patients seeking augmentation mammoplasty [68], one thing is incontestable: These patients feel inadequate about the size of their breasts. When surgery gives them larger breasts, they are almost always satisfied with the result [14, 135, 182, 196, 243]. Thus plastic surgeons continue performing an operation that may produce an undesirable result because of unnatural firmness and contour. In 27 years of practice, I have been asked by only one patient to remove the implants. In this woman, the reason was not capsular contracture but religion, the fear that God would punish her by causing breast cancer for having altered her body. In her case, I had had enough misgivings before removal of the implant to ask for an evaluation by a psychiatrist whose advice was to proceed.

When one asks a patient why she wants augmentation mammoplasty, the usual response is that the small size of her breasts has always "bothered" her and "finally I want to do something about it." Some will complain that buying clothes is a "hassle." Passing through the mind of this male surgeon is the thought that taking the risk of operation with its attendant pain to change one's body shape just to buy clothes seems astounding. The real reason for having augmentation mammoplasty is much deeper and more important than the issue of shopping for dresses. Gifford [87] was probably correct when he deduced that for these women, their breasts were "their representation of an ideal self, real or imagined."

Occasionally a patient will say openly that she is upset because her "adolescent daughter is built better" than she.

Many patients who are married are frequently accompanied by their husbands, who seem perplexed by their wives' behavior, since the size of their breasts has never been a barrier to their physical attraction; however, in investigating this matter, one finds that the patient has usually complained to her husband about her embarrassment over having small breasts. Her husband has finally consented unenthusiastically to the operation. He is concerned justifiably with the danger of the procedure, its cost, and the possible adverse effects of the presence of implants on his wife's future health, specifically breast cancer. The husband is also hopeful but somewhat dubious that the augmentation will satisfy his mate's expectations and make her feel "good about herself." Only rarely does a woman seek the operation because of a request by a man. In that situation, it is unwise to be the surgeon who implements her acquiescence and masochism.

Frequently, women for augmentation mammoplasty, as well as many other types of esthetic surgery, are in transition—between marriages, affairs, or careers [232]. Some are undertaking augmentation mammoplasty to start life anew by correcting something that disturbed them emotionally for many years and that now might make them less able to establish a gratifying and easy relationship with a new man [14, 15]. In that regard, most plastic surgeons have been taught by psychologists and psychiatrists that the woman's self-image is the prime motivation, but in my experience it is a rare woman who, when contemplating augmentation mammoplasty, has not had at least some concern about its effect on an intimate either directly or indirectly, i.e., on the woman herself and thus affecting how she behaves and how this behavior might be received by another person, usually a male, whom she either knows or in her fantasies may meet.

The important point here is that the patient should not undertake breast augmentation to save or improve a relationship, especially if her lover seems to be tiring of her. Large breasts with respect to the patient never attracted that man initially and will be unlikely to anchor him ultimately.

As a group, these patients for augmentation are less perfectionistic than those for eyelidplasty, facelift, or rhinoplasty, at least in my experience. There is, however, a small subgroup who constitute a cause for concern; those who on physical examination have normal-size breasts, but who nevertheless insist that they are "too small." Under these circumstances, I suggest that they not have the operation until they see a psychiatrist, or if they do not wish to do that, I refer them to another plastic surgeon.

In taking the history, it is important for the plastic surgeon to assess what the patient expects to get from the operation. Usually, she will be aware that she wishes to feel better about herself—increased self-esteem. Patients usually are reluctant to air unrealistic expectations principally because they probably do not have them but also because discussing one's breast size with a male surgeon whom one has just met is not an easy thing to do.

The plastic surgeon should inquire about previous pregnancies and nursing, possible future pregnancies with nursing, family history of breast cancer, and recurrent pain or masses in the breasts that may have required biopsy. If the patient has had a breast biopsy, the plastic surgeon should try to determine as concretely as possible the diagnosis made.

Another point to find out is whether the patient regularly examines her breasts. Obviously, every woman should, and having had an augmentation mammoplasty does not change that admonition.

Physical Examination

That 1 in 12 women in the United States will develop breast cancer at some point in their life should be sufficiently sobering to the plastic surgeon to perform a thorough breast examination. In addition, for every patient 30 years or older, I order mammograms unless recent ones, within the past nine months, are available. In the examination, one should look for breast asymmetry and, if present, point it out to the patient. Its presence may change the usual operative plan and choice of implant. One should take particular note of whether the breasts are ptotic and whether the patient will have to have a mastopexy in conjunction with an augmentation.

The woman's build is also important, especially in the selection of the prosthesis size.

The patient should be examined and photographed not only from the front but from the back in an upright and flexed position to detect and document scoliosis and chest deformities, such as pectus excavatum.

While the patient is partially undressed, I take that opportunity (with a female nurse or secretary present) to indicate where the incision is likely to be: areola, axillary, or inframammary. The patient may have her ideas also, and one can then discuss the advantages and disadvantages of each approach.

Informing the Patient

Size

Most patients have a definite idea of what they want for size. Sometimes their expectations are unrealistic. For example, I recall one petite woman who wished to go from a 34-A to a 34-D. Not only did she lack sufficient soft tissue to harbor such implants, but the esthetic result would have been poor—even bizarre. Despite my explanation, including a statement that such massive prosthesis would almost predispose her to abnormal firmness and contour, she persisted. I then suggested that she consult another plastic surgeon who might comply with her wishes.

I have samples of the common prototypes of breast implants in my office and show them to the patient (soft gel, polyurethane covered, textured, gel-saline combination).

In general, I use a soft gel prosthesis, occasionally textured, in a subpectoral position and usually put in a 220 to 300-cc size. I realize that choice of volume and configuration varies with the habitus of each patient and it also varies with different areas of the country. It is rare in the Northeast, at least in my practice, for women to want overpowering breasts. Seemingly, the more intellectual the patient, the more anxiety she has about becoming too large. She is usually concerned that others will note a drastic modification. This sentiment is particularly true of high school teachers who fear the response from the males in their class. In 27 years of practice I have had only half a dozen patients who were disappointed because I had not made them larger. In a couple of women, I did make a mistake because I had not properly taken into account their height, the breadth of their shoulders, and the laxity of their breast. In those situations, I usually offer to exchange the implants at no charge, but they are responsible for the hospital expenses. Interestingly, all these patients declined further surgery because they did "not feel like going through the operation and pain again." Furnas' [82] suggestion to let the patient make the final decision about size by seeing herself in a mirror during operation is worthwhile; however, one must remember that she is likely to be under the influence of medication and the other possibility is that she might be under general anesthesia.

If a patient has had a strong family history of breast cancer and a past history of multiple biopsies, I would not undertake the augmentation. She may then go to somebody else, and that is entirely her decision.

I tell patients that at the moment no data exist to demonstrate that the presence of implants per se causes breast cancer. Yet, I also tell them that we do not know what future studies will conclude. They should be aware than an implant does make mammography more difficult, although with new techniques by people experienced with patients having had augmentation, the efficiency of the mammograms is about 97 percent in nonaugmented women.

The patient must also be informed—and on more than one occasion—that she still must have regular breast examinations, preferably by one physician, be he or she a general surgeon, internist, gynecologist, or a plastic surgeon.

Mammary Hypoplasia and Ptosis

I confess that the presence of ptosis along with hypoplasia is a condition that I have found difficult to treat and achieve consistently excellent results. In a sense, one is trying to do two things simultaneously that are diametrically opposed: create a sufficient pocket for the implant and tighten the skin (by excising the redundancy) in order to rectify sagging. Some plastic surgeons prefer to correct the ptosis in one procedure and then perform the augmentation; others do it in a reverse fashion. I usually do both together, and one of the major reasons is that the patient is reluctant to return for two procedures, each of them usually a strain financially.

In general, the worse the ptosis, the more difficult it is to manage along with an augmentation. If one places the implant behind the pectoral muscle, the initial results after augmentation may be excellent; however, when these patients are followed for five to ten years, the breast usually descends, leaving the implant as a mound rising superiorly.

The patient must understand that gravity and time as well as their constitutional predisposition to ptosis may create the condition again. This is particularly true if the patient is planning a future pregnancy along with nursing. In that regard, a patient who has that in mind for the short term—in the next year or so—should proceed with her family and then return, should she still desire, for her breast surgery.

It is important to inform the patient that with time, changes may occur but not necessarily on both sides to the same degree or at the same rate. The fact that her breasts are bilateral does not necessarily guarantee that their status postoperatively will be identical.

Breast Hypoplasia and Pectus Excavatum

For these patients, a decision has to be made about correcting the pectus excavatum or leaving it and augmenting only the breasts. Sometimes, a breast augmentation will make the pectus deformity more noticeable. In other patients, however, augmenting the breasts and placing the implants medially will help obscure the pectus. Some patients will require one operation for correction of the pectus and another for the augmentation; in others, everything can be done at the same time. Often a custom-made moulage for the pectus is indicated. With these patients it is important to consider their entire breast and chest as a totality and to realize that their surgical problems are not solved by the usual, relatively simply executed breast augmentation.

Hematoma and Infection

Hematoma and infection may follow any operation; but, in my experience, their likelihood after augmentation mammoplasty is about one percent. Because of the possibility, although small, of an expanding hematoma requiring immediate evacuation, I advise patients who live more than one and one-half hours drive from the hospital to stay overnight nearby. A hematoma is an unfortunate happening not only because it imposes more physical stress on the patient, but it can also add to a financial burden since most insurance plans will not defray the hospital charges for the treatment of any complication after a cosmetic operation that was not even covered initially. Needless to mention, the plastic surgeon's services should be free in the event of this complication. The patient may require general anesthesia for adequate management of her anxiety as well as for operating ease to remove the hematoma and to control bleeding—which can be a painful process. Also, a 24-hour hospitalization will likely be necessary. Surgeons who operate in their offices have an advantage since they can offer their facility free of charge, but mobilizing nurses and possibly an anesthesiologist at night might be impractical or impossible, and a hospital will still be needed. The patient must be told in the initial consultation that she will be responsible for the expenses arising from complications, a point already mentioned. One should discuss specifically the sequence of events should a hematoma occur.

Infection, fortunately, is uncommon, even less frequent than a hematoma [57]. The patient should understand that it can happen and that it is not always susceptible to antibiotics. The implant may have to be removed, and a later attempt at augmentation will be required.

Incisions, Placement of the Implant, and Scars
Whatever the plastic surgeon's approach to insertion of the implant, the patient must understand it. She must be told of the possibility that her scars might be red and thick, even though usually they are not. Bad scarring does happen in the axilla, although it is not frequent. If, indeed, the approach is around the areola or immediately inside its edge, the patient should know that, and, as mentioned, I use the opportunity of the physical examination to indicate what approach I prefer. The patient and I can then discuss that either during the examination or when the patient is more at ease, after having

dressed, in the consulting room. The patient should also know where the implant lies in relation to the breast—under or over the muscle. This information is important for her to relate to other doctors who may be examining her.

Ability to Nurse
I have had many patients nurse following an augmentation mammoplasty performed either through the inframammary or the intraareolar approach. Some patients, however, especially if they have had no children, prefer the inframammary incision because theoretically it should disrupt the breast tissue less than an operation via the areola. These preferences should be heeded even though data are lacking to support that contention. If a patient is planning to become pregnant soon and wishes to nurse, it would be wiser to defer operation until the child has been weaned.

Type of Implant
Most plastic surgeons have chosen from the bewildering assortment of implants available one or two types that they prefer for most patients having symmetrical mammary hypoplasia. I show the patient a prototype of the gel implant I use, taking care to state that "this will not be your size," since it usually is not. I use sizers during operation to determine the proper size. I also have used inflatables, but less so than in the past because of late deflation, but I do discuss this alternative with patients since many have heard that the inflatables give a softer breast, and, indeed, several studies have confirmed this impression; however, I emphasize that no prosthesis can give a predictably normal breast in every instance. Discussions these days center around the polyurethane-covered implant and the textured implant. I discuss the advantages and disadvantages of each type, although admittedly the long-term data are remarkably scarce despite the many operations performed utilizing these implants.

Firmness and Abnormal Contour
Firmness and abnormal contour are the principal problems with augmentation mammoplasty. In my experience, about 30 percent of patients had unusual firmness and capsular contraction in one or both

breasts postoperatively if the implants were not placed under the muscle. With the subpectoral position, capsular contraction and significant firmness have been decreased markedly, less than 10 percent.

The patient must understand that thick capsules and spherical contraction can occur, no matter what or where the implant or who the surgeon. I tell patients that steroids or antibiotics or both, may be instilled into the dissected pocket, but their value is controversial. I also say that occasionally steroids may cause skin atrophy and descent of the prosthesis.

Patients want to know what can be done about abnormal firmness if it occurs. I explain that manual compression in the office can improve them but only permanently in about 30 percent of patients. Surgical release of the capsule is possible, but I inform patients that many women may still have remaining firmness even after one or two surgical capsulotomies.

I tell the prospective patients that many women who have had firmness have chosen to live with it, unless they are bothered by it, particularly if they are unable to lie flat on their abdomen, if they have discomfort during intercourse, or by their general feelings of disappointment with the abnormal shape and feel of their augmented breasts. The prospective patient is told also that since augmentation mammoplasty appears to give women satisfaction as a result of the increased size of their breasts, only a small percentage of patients who have firmness will elect to have more than a manual capsulotomy, and some may even refuse that.

The patient must understand also that since one cannot guarantee a normal flowing and feeling breast, a man might know that she had "had something done" even if he does not see the scars. For some patients a photograph of a woman with moderately severe bilateral and unilateral capsular contracture after augmentation mammoplasty is necessary to get one's point across if one senses that the patient cannot comprehend this kind of problem.

Coldness
Many patients have complained that they were not properly informed about the fact that their breasts would feel cold, particularly during the winter and while they are skiing. This has more relevance, of

course, for those in New England than in a tropical or subtropical climate. Although this sensation of cold is not usually a primary complaint, it may become more important when other things have gone wrong after augmentation. Having been forewarned the patient will obviate a later apology or an accusation of being insufficiently informed.

Sensation
For many years, it was not generally appreciated that augmentation mammoplasty altered sensation of the skin of the breast, the areola, and the nipple. Usually the problem is mild and transient hypoesthesia, yet I have had patients who admit, if questioned carefully, that they still are "numb" over their nipple and areola, and objective testing with a voltimeter confirms it. Usually, however, their erotic responses may even be heightened because they feel more secure about themselves and more relaxed during sex. These changes in sensation have occurred in equal frequency with the areola and inframammary approach [55].

Pain
Since patients vary in their tolerance for pain, one must establish whether a particular patient can be operated on under local anesthesia (with intravenous supplementation) as an outpatient. In my experience, about 90 percent of women can be managed in this way and prefer it; it allows them to almost immediately resume their usual life-style; to preserve relative anonymity by going home and not meeting friends in the hospital; and, of course, it significantly lowers costs; however, some patients may be very needle shy and susceptible to physical pain. They should be given general anesthesia on an outpatient basis, if indicated, and not be made to feel inferior because they cannot tolerate or do not want local anesthesia. To allay their feelings of guilt about more expense and their sense of inferiority, perhaps long-standing because of their small-sized breasts, I point out that each human being has his or her own strengths and weaknesses and that she might tolerate emotional stresses of another sort far better than other patients and some of her friends, for example.

Not everyone is or even should be a Spartan. In general, women who have had natural childbirth or practice yoga or transcendental meditation are good candidates for outpatient operations and local anesthesia.

I confess that when a patient is under anesthesia I am more relaxed and the operation seems easier. With shorter-acting anesthesia agents, augmentation mammoplasty can be done very well with general anesthesia.

With regard to discharging the patient from the hospital the day of the operation, it is important to be sure that someone takes her home and also remains with her through the night. I do not advise patients who have had this procedure or any other operation of significance, such as a facelift, to return to an empty house. In the event that the patient suddenly bleeds or becomes faint or falls, perhaps even fracturing a hip, she will be completely helpless.

The patient who is having augmentation mammoplasty understandably would like to keep this information confidential, but it is even more important that she be properly cared for after the operation. Although one wishes to accede to the patient's request for privacy, one should not place her in danger. You and she are liable to suffer the consequences: you legally; she medically.

Possible Future Breast Cancer

Most patients, certainly their husbands, will ask about possible carcinogenic effects of augmentation mammoplasty. I have stated that no current data have shown a carcinogenic effect of the implant. Mammography, however, will be more difficult. I wish to emphasize here that the patient has a responsibility, and you should reinforce it, to continue her periodic self-examination and her visits to her doctor. After operation, the patient who was once so preoccupied with her breasts may now refuse to think about them and will actually avoid going to her gynecologist because she does not wish to divulge her augmentation. If the plastic surgeon senses that the patient will not go for periodic breast examinations, he or she should offer to do them, at least at first. Later, after the patient has overcome her anxiety about others knowing, she might be amenable, and usually is, to return to her regular physician or gynecologist or may even request a name from the plastic surgeon who, she thinks, knows physicians who are familiar with this procedure.

Closed Capsulotomy
Closed or external capsulotomy is a relatively simple procedure, but occasionally complications arise, such as hematoma, rupture of the implant, or asymmetry from a differential splitting of the scar tissue around the implants. In the last instance, the breasts, though softer, may not match so well. One should inform patients of all these possibilities prior to doing an external capsulotomy. In addition, the patients should understand that they will have pain. Most of them can endure it without any medication, but oral or intramuscular Demerol may be advantageous. If one is giving intravenous medication, such as diazepam (Valium) in the office, one should be prepared to treat cardiac and pulmonary arrest.

If you charge for this procedure, the fee should be discussed prior to the manipulation.

Another consideration is that if the implant ruptures and silicone extravasates, you as well as the patient must be ready to remove and replace the implant. Sometimes, of course, the amount of silicone that extrudes is minuscule, but it may be a larger and worrisome amount.

Although this book focuses on the patient as having a complication, in the instance of closed capsulotomy, the plastic surgeon may also sustain a lasting injury—to the collateral ligaments of the thumb. To spare the surgeon's hand, devices have been developed—some of them rather fearsome in appearance. I cannot comment on these because I have not used them.

Following capsulotomy, the patient must understand instructions regarding massage if one believes in it. I do but it may not prevent recurrence of capsular contraction—a possibility about which the patient must also be informed prior to the procedure.

Instructions
Following augmentation mammoplasty every patient must know her postoperative regimen precisely: activity at home or at work; ath-

letics; sex; dressing changes—if so when; massage, if you advise this. Some plastic surgeons have mentioned that patients may be reluctant to massage their breasts because of fear of rupturing or dislodging the implant and because they are shy about what they may consider a form of masturbation.

Many patients ask specifically whether the implant can rupture, and the answer is "Yes, but only very rarely." The usual question is "Will it rupture if I am in an auto accident?" I say that it probably will not, but if it did, it likely would have saved her life by protecting her from severe thoracic injury.

Many patients today have heard about "leakage" from the implant—not saline but silicone. I tell them that this is a phenomenon and that it occurs in usually small amounts. I also tell them that no data thus far show that it is harmful to their health unless there is a significant rupture with release of the silicone.

I usually mention to patients that there have been scattered reports about the association of augmentation mammoplasty with rheumatoid arthritis or other types of collagen disease. These reports, I go on to say, are, as yet far from conclusive, but, nevertheless, data are still being gathered, and this issue is by no means resolved.

CORRECTION OF BREAST ASYMMETRY OR AGENESIS

Unilateral or bilateral agenesis of the breast or marked asymmetry is usually very distressing psychologically to the woman so affected. Many say that they have been ashamed of their condition to such a degree that they have kept it a secret from their parents, siblings, and friends. Some girls may have told their mothers of the problem but have not allowed them to see it.

Those who seek correction of this abnormality obviously have not adjusted to it; however, they may not be representative of all those with mammary agenesis or asymmetry. Many whom I have treated have shown extremes in their heterosexual behavior, either avoiding all contact with men or promiscuity, the latter seemingly to prove to themselves that they still can be women despite their deformity. Illegitimate pregnancies and abortions are also common—again a reaffirmation of their feminine capability. One patient with almost total absence of one breast said to me, "I couldn't wait to finish high school so I could marry and have children and nurse them." Pointing to her deficient breast, she announced proudly, "What a great surprise to see milk come out of that little thing!"

Like the husbands of patients for augmentation or reduction mammoplasty, the spouse of a woman with mammary agenesis or asymmetry does not think that his wife has to undergo the operation since he is not turned off sexually by his wife's anatomical problem. With a few patients, my impression was that some husbands not only tolerated the deformity but even may have enjoyed it, not perhaps in a sexual way but in terms of power because they felt more secure about having and keeping a wife who was insecure about her physical abnormality. These women's quest for reconstruction represents a step toward independence and may cause marital strain, whose ramifications for one of my patients and her husband led them to psychotherapy following the operation; fortunately, the outcome was successful, anatomically and maritally.

As one takes a history, it is best not to focus exclusively on the breast problems with treatment in mind, but one should attempt to understand its emotional meaning to the patient and those close to her.

Physical Examination

Look carefully for abnormalities of the chest wall, pectoral musculature, and spinal column (scoliosis). Compare the breasts as to relative location, volume, shape, areolae, nipples. Observe what type (and size) of bra the patient is wearing. Does she use a prosthesis?

With asymmetry, always ask the patient which breast, if any, she likes. Occasionally, the patient may want the larger reduced, or the smaller augmented, or something done to each.

Many patients want either their mother or husband present during the examination. This helps to ensure that all concerned will know your findings and surgical plans. Sometimes the presence of someone else in the room, even a female nurse, is very upsetting to the patient. Be sensitive enough to recognize these differences and preferences.

It does not harm to ask directly, "Stephanie, would you want your mother to be present when I examine you, or would you prefer to have us discuss things with her afterwards?"

Informing the Patient
At this time in the consultation one should know what must be done: reduce or augment, or both; inflatable or gel prosthesis or moulage, or a combination. Remember that what you think is not the sole consideration. Make certain that you know what the patient wants. Is it possible to achieve it? If not, tell her. Spend time also to emphasize the impossibility of reconstructing a breast to precisely match the opposite [47]. Stress that the operation will give improvement, hopefully, but seldom perfection. As with augmentation mammoplasty, the patient and family must understand the possibility of infection, hematoma, abnormal contour, and firmness. Indicate where you will make the incisions and what the expected scars will be.

Before the Operation
Many patients feel sufficiently embarrassed by their problem that they may prefer a private room if they are to be hospitalized and may be willing to pay for it. In my experience, third-party payment is not usual for the correction of mammary agenesis or asymmetry.

After the Operation
In addition to your usual care of any patient or those after breast surgery, be especially attentive to the psychological reactions of these patients. Usually they are very happy with the improvement; however, an occasional patient may find readjustment difficult. Previously, her breast deformity was the reason (she told herself) for her avoiding normal social contact. Now she no longer has that excuse. It may be many months before she is willing to expose herself to a man. Be careful that you do not browbeat her with questions about this aspect of her life. She will feel more overwhelmed and inadequate. Most patients will let you know subtly or even openly that they have crossed the Rubicon.

MASTOPEXY

A pure mastopexy is a facelift of the breasts. It is an entirely cosmetic procedure, and the patient will judge her result by esthetic standards. I have discussed correction of breast ptosis under the subject of augmentation mammoplasty (see p. 165).

Patients

Patients for mastopexy are usually in their 30s and 40s, white and middle class. The majority have had children, and many attribute their sagging breasts to pregnancy or nursing, or both. Another commonly invoked cause is rapid, significant weight loss. Patients say that the wilted appearance of the breasts depresses them. A common remark is, "I am only 40 but my breasts look like those of a 60-year-old." They may ask to have their breasts restored to what they once were—a size B or C. By that remark, they have introduced another aspect and that is breast volume. In taking the history, the plastic surgeon must determine whether the patient wishes not only to have her breasts raised but to have them enlarged. As with the patient for augmentation, these women seek the operation for themselves; the man in their life is usually perplexed by their persistent unhappiness with their breasts.

A thorough history should include information about general health, previous breast problems, if any, and familiar predisposition to mammary malignancy.

Physical Examination

The surgeon must now assess whether the patient's problem is ptosis, and if so, whether it is severe enough to warrant an operation. In some patients, the condition is so mild that the scars for its correction would surely disturb them more than their ptosis.

It is important also to establish whether the patient needs not only a breast lift but also a reduction or augmentation. By raising the breasts with tension on the skin (your fingers or adhesive tape), you can let the patient judge by looking in a mirror whether the volume of the elevated breasts satisfies her. The breasts may be atrophic or hypertrophic as well as ptotic.

Your examination is not only to determine the type of procedure that will give the best appearance; careful palpation for possible masses is mandatory. These women generally are older and the possibility of breast cancer is greater.

Informing the Patient

This discussion with the patient must necessarily concern what is to be done: nothing, a mastopexy alone, or a mastopexy in conjunction with an augmentation or a reduction.

The patient must understand that any operation will leave permanent scars, even when the procedure is performed by a circumareolar incision whose resultant scar frequently widens. Do not underestimate this reality.

The principal decision usually for you and the patient is whether to do an augmentation. Adding a prosthesis to a markedly atrophic and ptotic breast without correcting the sagging will give a grotesque result. When a mastopexy and an augmentation are needed, the patient must understand that she may be subject to all the problems of both procedures but in particular those of the augmentation, especially abnormal firmness and abnormal contour. Many patients whose breasts are mildly or even moderately atrophic may elect to have only a mastopexy rather than run the risk of artificiality from a firm, unnatural breast. Many women worry that the presence of the prosthesis will interfere with subsequent breast examination and radiographic analysis—not an unreasonable fear. In my experience, doing the mastopexy first and the augmentation later is cumbersome planning; it makes the patient go through the operation twice, it increases cost and anxiety, and it does not produce a better result than the single-stage mastopexy/augmentation.

Some patients who describe their problem as sagging breasts actually have large, pendulous breasts that require a reduction. A few will ask to preserve the volume but elevate the breasts. I remember well one woman to whose wish I grudgingly acceded. The result was a bulky breast whose areola and nipple projected displeasingly, pushed out by the excessive tissue. She later required the removal of breast parenchyma under the areola.

Patients for mastopexy alone must be told about possible changes in sensation, particularly around the nipple and areola, although in my experience these have been negligible, much less than after augmentation or reduction.

The major focus for discussion is to inform the patient that her scars will be permanent, but the lift will probably not be: Time and gravity are likely to lower what you have so carefully raised. Most patients will ask how long the effects of the procedure last. You must honestly reply that you do not know since individuals vary in their wound healing; skin elasticity; genetic predisposition to aging of tissue; future health such as illnesses or pregnancy (with or without nursing); and weight fluctuation. You can point out that a sagging breast is somewhat like a sagging face; another surgical correction may be necessary. Since most patients know about repeat facelifts, they will better comprehend the problem through this simile.

For most women having mastopexy with or without augmentation, it can be done under local anesthesia with intravenous supplementation, on an outpatient basis. Some patients, particularly those requiring reduction, will do better with general anesthesia and a one- or two-day hospitalization, for which most will have insurance coverage only if the reduction is of sufficient magnitude to be considered functional. A scanty removal of skin and breast tissue does not justify calling the operation a reduction mammoplasty in order to obtain third-party payment. Insurance companies are right in being wary of these shenanigans.

After the Operation
As with every procedure, information to the patient must be clear and complete. With mastopexy, wearing a bra constantly for many weeks would seem advisable, although as far as I know, no objective study has been done of the value of the bra in these circumstances. When an augmentation has been done in combination with the mastopexy, the dilemma is that you wish to free the patient from constricted dressings and to begin massage to keep things loose, an objective at cross-purposes to maintaining tightness of the repair.

Finally, all women must have periodic breast examinations by a physician in addition to self-examination in order to detect any malignancy. After a year, the breast, if not augmented, will become soft; the more deeply placed scar tissue will not interfere with palpation.

In patients 35 years or older, baseline mammograms are helpful to serve as comparison should a future nodule be detected. In that circumstance, when the patient is beyond the immediate postoperative period, never hesitate to do a biopsy. Procrastination and false attribution of the nodule to "a stitch" or "scar tissue" could be disastrous.

REDUCTION MAMMOPLASTY

Reduction mammoplasty, which is being performed with increasing frequency, combines features of both esthetic and nonesthetic surgery [116]. Although there may be controversy about how to classify reduction mammoplasty, few would contest the observation that most patients are pleased with the results of their operation. Indeed, if the macromastia, more severe, usually the patient is happier postoperatively unless a complication has occurred. Recently, however, as this procedure has become more popular, patients come with lesser degrees of hypertrophy. Some are in your office not primarily for a breast reduction but for a correction of ptosis. They may exaggerate their physical complaints—neck and back pain—in the hope of securing insurance coverage. For the surgeon, the difficulty is that they might judge the results by standards of appearance rather than by those of function. One might comment sentfully that any good surgeon should be prepared to have his or her work appraised by "cosmetic" criteria. This type of patient, however, might become upset by minimal scarring, whereas another person requiring a significant breast reduction might be indifferent to the scars.

The age of patients wanting this surgery ranges from adolescent to postmenopausal. The older the woman or any patient, usually the more information you must know or will extract. Most women with very large breasts consider their condition a deformity [128, 137]. They feel conspicuous and resent being singled out for this aspect of themselves. They will complain that men fixate on their breasts to the exclusion of their personality or intellect [71]. Buying clothes is a frustrating and expensive experience. Unlike patients with small breasts who can hide their problem with a padded bra, patients with very large breasts, even with the most ingenious brassieres, still remain an object of scrutiny.

A common story is that patients will avoid athletics or going to the beach in a bathing suit. One woman said, "I dread each summer." In addition to these psychological problems, their macromastia may have had physical consequences: pain in the back, neck, and shoulder-strap areas; kyphosis; intertrigo; and obesity. Some patients consciously or unconsciously gain great amounts of weight, perhaps in an effort to make their breasts seem smaller in comparison. A psychiatrist who referred an 18-year-old girl for breast reduction told me that the obesity was a way of repulsing men to avoid an intimacy that would lead to exposure of her breasts. This low self-esteem is a frequent finding in patients with severely enlarged breasts.

Many patients will describe futile consultations with male pediatricians and family doctors who never suggested that surgery was possible, warned them against it, or advised them to adapt to their large breasts because later men would like them. They have become long-suffering victims of male ignorance and chauvinism.

Often the younger patient is accompanied by her mother, who has also had to bear this problem without relief. The father is usually not present because he is "completely opposed," as the mother usually says, to the procedure. At best, fathers agree to the operation only with great reluctance.

Physical Examination

The surgeon who treats the female breast is dealing not only with an organ of appearance and function but with one subject to carcinogenesis. He or she should always be aware that the patient could have or develop a carcinoma, and every means must be taken to rule out its presence. Remember that the outer quadrant is the most common location for carcinoma. A systematic breast examination should include palpating for cervical, axillary, and supraclavicular nodes, the last being an often neglected but frequent site of metastasis from primary breast cancer. Because of the large size of the breasts, physical examination is difficult but should nevertheless be performed thoroughly. Each breast should be inspected with the patient's arms at her sides, elevated, and behind her head—with the patient sitting and supine. Look for skin dimpling, surface flattening, and nipple pointing (toward an adjacent tumor).

To detect curvature of the spine, the patient should be instructed to bend forward and to flex laterally while you are standing behind.

Note grooving and irritation of the shoulders from brassiere strap pressure. Sometimes, there is a decrease in sensation and motor power in the ulnar nerve distribution of the hand.

With the patient disrobed (and a nurse or family member present), I outline the incisions for the surgery. I then take photographs: front, side, oblique, and back.

Empathizing with the undressed patient, I suggest that she put on her clothes and then we can discuss the procedure more fully and with her more comfortable. The patient and the family must understand that reduction mammoplasty is major; it usually involves general anesthesia with approximately three to four hours of surgery, moderate pain, a two-to four-day hospitalization, and definite scarring. In addition, there is a possibility of infection (unusual), hematoma (uncommon), and ischemic necrosis of the nipple-areola complex as well as of the skin. No matter what the technique, there is always a chance of partial or total loss of the nipple and areola. The fact that you have done an operation 95 times without this occurrence does not mean that it will not happen later. Statistically, partial or total ischemic necrosis of the nipple-areola has an incidence of one to five percent, depending on the series of patients reported. When you use the term *loss of nipple* with the patient, you must explain it since she may think that you have simply mislaid it. The greater the weight of the tissue to be removed, the more frequent the complications.

Until recently, it was little appreciated that patients have altered sensation in the nipples, areolae, and breasts following reduction mammoplasty. Preoperatively, the sensitivity of some patients with considerable hypertrophy is less than normal, and postoperatively, their tactile sensitivity may improve. In the majority of instances, the sensation after surgery will be less. I have at least four patients whose appreciation of touch has not returned to one nipple and areola after three years. I tell patients that for erotic purposes, they will usually have adequate sensation in their nipple and areola. Although objectively their appreciation of touch may be diminished, because they will feel better about themselves, they will be more relaxed during sex. It is important to speak openly and directly about these issues. Many patients will be too shy to raise the subject.

The surgeon must know the patient's expectations regarding size and shape. Although most women in my practice want to be a size B, some may specify an A and others a "good C." In this connection, discussing the procedure with the man in that patient's life is wise. Some men will sit in your office with obvious sullenness and hostility, angry that they will lose one (or two) of their prized possessions. To squire a woman with large breasts in our culture enhances the self-esteem of most men. Talking to the unhappy man before the operation may be helpful to avoid being in the middle or the focus of a squabble after surgery. I have had a few patients who have complained that their husband or boyfriend "has not come near me since the operation." Unconsciously or consciously, the man is retaliating in a passive-aggressive fashion. Occasionally, this situation has required a psychotherapist. A few women relate that the scars repel their partners. Often this obstacle can be overcome by suggesting to the patient that she wear her bra during intercourse for a few times.

Obesity

The obese patient is generally more likely to have a complication than someone of normal weight. Ideally, it makes sense to wait until the patient has lost all or most of the weight she intends to shed before modifying her profile; however, in my experience, the breast reduction provides the best stimulus for weight reduction. Many patients feel that whatever they do to lose weight will make little difference so long as they have large, unwieldy, and unsightly breasts. Furthermore, this deformity acts as a barrier to their exercising, especially in public.

Autologous Transfusion

Most patients undergoing reduction mammoplasty will not require blood transfusion, a hospital event they fear in this era of AIDS. For the general population, however, infection by the hepatitis C virus is a much greater possibility, infecting approximately two to five percent of recipients [190]. A new antibody will soon be available to detect the virus and will thereby reduce if not eliminate the chance of hepatitis spread.

In more than 25 years I have never had to give a blood transfusion to a patient having an elective procedure; however, if I perceive that someone is very anxious about the remote possibility of receiving blood, I suggest autotransfusion. Every hospital has a blood bank, and one has to follow their rules, which vary among institutions. A method of decreasing the need for transfusion is using epinephrine, a practice that I abandoned a few years ago when I found that with careful electrocauterization, I could decrease my average blood loss per breast to 150 ml. In addition, experimental evidence exists to suggest that epinephrine may adversely affect a flap, and all transposition techniques of reduction mammoplasty embody the nipple–areola-bearing flap.

Insurance Coverage

In most states and with most insurance plans, reduction mammoplasty coverage depends on the weight of the tissue removed. Sometimes it is difficult to know whether the stipulated amount will be reached. In that situation, one should communicate with the insurance company, perhaps providing them with photographs, if permitted by the patient, to get a preoperative judgment about coverage. If a patient is of particularly short stature, less weight may have to be removed in order to obtain insurance backing.

Most insurance companies will ask for the operative note, and, to my distress, I have heard reports of surgeons who have increased the weight of the tissue removed by injecting saline into it. This is fraudulent and is poor medicine as well as poor ethics.

Mammograms

In every patient 30 years or older, I obtain mammograms prior to reduction. One might argue that mammograms should be done in every instance because of the fact that undetected malignancy of the breast can occur in patients even under the age of 20. Yet, unless a compelling family history of breast cancer exists, from a practical point of view and from the reality of the breast density in young women, mammograms done before the age of 30 are usually of little value.

About a year after reduction mammoplasty, I again obtain mammograms, which then will serve as a baseline for possible future detection of a breast abnormality.

After the Operation
In general, most women having reduction mammoplasty are pleased with the result and enjoy increased self-esteem and a less distorted body image; however, not every woman is ecstatic immediately after her procedure. It is important that you do the first dressing change. Despite the considerable discussion that you may have had with the patient about ultimate breast size, she may react to her new look with surprise, dismay, and even denial. Some patients will declare, "I don't even want to look at them." Usually, however, they do sneak a glance and are pleased or unhappy. Few are indifferent. Some actually become weak and dizzy. Some say, "They don't look like mine and they don't feel like mine." Or, "Will they ever look like breasts?'

You had expected gratitude for relieving her of deforming burdens; now perplexed and disappointed, you stand uneasily at the bedside. Before you become angry and stomp out of the room, remember that she had to make a major adjustment to her body image. Unlike the patient after a facelift who remembers when she was young, the big-breasted patient, especially if middle-aged or older, may never recall having a normal bosom. Moreover, if she is obese, following reduction her breasts may appear especially small compared to the rest of her. If she had intended to lose weight, gently remind her that you have gauged her surgery to match what she will look like (if that is what you truly did). Your statement to her brings to mind the exchange between Pablo Picasso and Gertrude Stein, who said, after she saw his portrait of her, "It does not look like me," to which Picasso replied, "It will."

Reassure the patient that her feelings of bewilderment and depression are common and ordinarily pass in several weeks after she becomes more accustomed to her new breasts and body contour. Psychological adjustment only occasionally requires psychiatric help if she has your support and availability as well as an understanding family and friends, especially the male members. You can do much before operation and afterward to prepare her intimates to deal with these new problems of adaptation.

I usually remove drains on the second postoperative day. I send the patient home in her old bra without stays or underwires or in a bra that I give her (Sears catalogue #78495, cups C—D). The patient is responsible for her dressing changes, which should be done preferably by herself or by a friend or a member of the family. I usually advise patients to wear a bra day and night for four to six weeks. With normal healing, she can resume driving at a week, sex at two weeks, and athletics four weeks after operation.

As doctors, we have a responsibility to the patient beyond the immediate operation. The fact that someone has had a reduction mammoplasty does not confer immunity from breast cancer. Any suspicious lump should be biopsied and not simply ascribed to "scar tissue" or "stitch reaction." Many patients request that you periodically examine their breasts because "My doctor says he is not used to checking breasts that have had this kind of surgery."

Aside from the oncological value of doing the breast examination, long-term follow-up will give you important information about your results. You will then be better able to evaluate the technique you used, and you will be more knowledgeable when informing patients about what they can expect from this operation. Frequently the patient is more pleased than you. You will note unattractive scarring, slight asymmetry, unwanted fullness, elevated nipple, or altered sensation. Resist the temptation to proclaim, "Mea culpa." Expressing your dissatisfaction may make you feel more honest but will also make the patient more unhappy. Being a good physician also requires knowing when to remain silent. Inwardly record your observations so that you may do a better procedure for the next patient. But remember also that variations in technique will not necessarily give a perfect result.

Pathology Findings
Every plastic surgeon who does reduction mammoplasty should carefully read the report of the pathologist. The microscopic examination may give an indication that this patient, unknown to herself or you, despite a good history, may be at high risk to develop breast

cancer. The patient should be informed and properly followed, usually not by a plastic surgeon but by a general surgeon or gynecologist familiar with breast disease.

I have heard of an instance in which the plastic surgeon neglected to tell the patient that an incidental malignancy (small focus of intraductal carcinoma) had been found. The patient later developed a mass and the diagnosis was finally made. A settlement out of court was also made. The importance here is less the legal risk for the doctor but more the medical risk and survival of the patient. With a patient in whom an occult breast cancer has been found, it is advisable to speak to a surgeon in order to have a plan of treatment and not simply tell the patient that she had the incidental finding of a breast cancer. Even under the best circumstances and with the greatest compassion and psychological skill that you can employ, that news will cause emotional devastation. The patient who has probably disliked her large breasts for a number of years has just been given breasts that she finds much more to her liking. In the midst of her joy comes the savage intrusion of breast cancer. I have had this unfortunate situation in only two patients, one of whom required prolonged psychotherapy in an attempt to adjust to the reality of the cancer, but even more to the subsequent mastectomy. Although I did not do the mastectomy, I had performed the reduction mammoplasty, and the patient so associated me with it that when I wanted to do follow-up studies on patients having had reduction mammoplasty, she refused to return to the office, saying that even though she had "nothing personal against" me, she wanted to avoid the emotional trauma that would be reawakened by a follow-up visit.

INVERTED NIPPLE

The patient with an inverted nipple is generally a female bearing a congenital problem and has not had a previous operation to rectify it. As we know, the inverted nipple can be unilateral or bilateral. Ostensibly it should be easy to correct, but the fact that there must be at least 100 procedures for its amelioration should be sufficient testimony to its difficulty. Failure with recurrence of inversion is distressingly frequent.

In discussing the proposed procedure to correct an inverted nipple—whatever the specific operation you choose—it is obviously crucial to emphasize that results are not predictable, at least in my experience. I tell the patient that the failure rate as judged over a period of two years can be as high as 20 percent, and it can occur on one or both sides, if, indeed, the patient has a bilateral problem. I also emphasize that she will have scarring and may have decreased or absent sensation. I make clear that should she wish to nurse in the future, she may find it impossible.

I have used the nonoperative suction method, but unfortunately I have not found it successful. This is not the place to discuss the relative advantages and disadvantages of the various techniques, but it is the place to emphasize that one should clearly record that the unpredictability and shortcomings as well as the complications of any procedure have been discussed in detail with the patient. I say this with particular vigor because I have had the experience of a patient who accused me of not having properly informed her of the possibility that the nipples would be scarred and have altered sensation. In that instance, I am pleased to report, when the patient's attorney—and she tried to hire more than one—looked at my records, the case was dropped. It is interesting that this particular patient instituted charges of malpractice five years after the operation at the time of her divorce. Perhaps she thought that her inverted nipple was a negative stimulus leading her husband to go elsewhere. My attorney, less Freudian and more practical, said, "Naw. She just wanted the money."

CORRECTION OF GYNECOMASTIA

Correction of gynecomastia is one of the few cosmetic procedures sought exclusively by men. In essence, however, the operation performed for correcting gynecomastia is a bilateral subcutaneous mastectomy.

Patients
Usually in their teens or early 20s, patients for correction of gynecomastia are acutely embarrassed by the feminine appearance of their chest [233]. In an effort to rid themselves of the stigma, they have

done thousands of push-ups and hoisted tons of steel. They may have taken anabolic steroids, obtained illicitly. The unfortunate result is a hypertrophy of their pectoral muscles and an increase in their mammary projection.

In your history taking, it is important to find out whether the patient has received testosterone injections from a physician for associated hypogonadism. I have had two such patients in whom occult cancer was found in their resected breast tissue.

Unlike patients for rhinoplasty, who are frequently accompanied by both parents, these patients, if adolescents, usually come with only one parent, the one more sympathetic to their problem. Often, these patients and their families have never been informed of the possibility of surgery; rather, the boy has been told that his gynecomastia will disappear when he is older and if he loses weight. The patient with adiposogenital dystrophy (Fröhlich's syndrome), or simply the "fat kid," may never grow out of his problem. Subjected to a multitude of laboratory tests, endocrinological evaluations, and testicular examinations, he looks on surgery as a relief, and once he knows that he can have it, he wants it as soon as possible. He does not wish to suffer through another summer, avoiding the beaches, making awkward excuses for not going swimming or for wearing his T-shirt on a scorching August day.

There may be a family history of gynecomastia, but uncovering this information may embarrass the father, if present.

Physical Examination

You should examine the breasts carefully for discrete masses. Check the axillae for palpable nodes and the abdomen for an enlarged liver. Does the patient have a normal male escutcheon, and are both testicles present and normal? (Hopefully, this will be the patient's last genital exam in relation to gynecomastia.)

Be certain to distinguish the patients who have only apparent gynecomastia; their problem may be simply hypertrophy of the nipple. Obviously, a more minor procedure is indicated for this problem than for the usual gynecomastia. Are the patient's breasts too large to get rid of the excess skin via an areolar incision and a subcutaneous mastectomy?

Informing the Patient

Most patients with gynecomastia essentially require a bilateral subcutaneous mastectomy, as mentioned, unless the breasts are very large. In that situation, inframammary incisions have to be made, and although patients may consent to them, once they see that the scars are prominent and "ugly," they may say they had not fully understood the implications of what you had proposed. I try to avoid an inframammary incision, and I have never made one in a patient who has had only gynecomastia (not a transsexual).

The main complication with the usual operation for gynecomastia is postoperative bleeding, despite careful hemostasis. Seromas following removal of the drains (suction) even after four to five days can occur, and although not serious, are annoying. Also, the patient who notices the swelling may be very anxious because he fears that he will still have the same problem despite your reassurance otherwise.

Infection, although always a possibility, is unusual.

Changes in sensation do occur, but only one patient, who was married, said it was disturbing because his nipples had long been a focus of pleasure for him and his wife. In a year, sufficient sensation returned to allow them to resume their usual activity, but even after two years, the sensation was less than it had been before operation.

Although you may be justifiably concerned about causing a concavity from excessive removal of tissue, the patient will object more to a convexity from an insufficient procedure. I recall a 19-year-old whom the resident told that I would do the procedure very carefully so that there would be no noticeable indentation. When I later saw the patient, he was very worried that I would do less than he wished. "I don't care if I get a hollow there," he said, "just get all of it out. I don't want to go around with these [breasts] anymore."

Payment

In almost every instance, correction of gynecomastia is cosmetic. An admitting diagnosis such as *mass of the breast(s)* or an operating title such as *mastectomy* is usually a ruse to obtain third-party coverage. This practice does little to enhance the status or reputation of medicine in general or the doctor in particular. Aside from such lofty considerations, not telling the truth by falsifying insurance forms is fraudulent and illegal.

At the Operation
The plastic surgeon must remove sufficient tissue so that the patient does not have residual gynecomastia, by taking away too much will produce the unwanted dishpan deformity. The use of liposuction allows better contouring to give a better final result; however, some men want to be flatter than may be esthetically advisable or anatomically possible. I have had two patients who have consulted me with their desire for correction of gynecomastia not having told me that they had already had the procedure. They thought that not enough had been removed, and they wanted to see whether I would simply schedule for correction of gynecomastia. Fortunately, in both patients, I did not find sufficient breast tissue present to advise operation.

After the Operation
You will relieve the anxiety of most patients by telling them immediately prior to the operation that when they awake, they will have bulky dressings. If you do not mention this, they will be extremely upset by their chest appearing even larger than it was before surgery.

Unless complications ensue, patients stay in the hospital for just two days. Their drains can be removed in your office.

You must tell the patient how much and what sort of physical activity he is allowed. It is a rare patient who does not ask you repeatedly whether the swelling "will ever go down." These patients must be seen and reassured frequently because of their concern that you did not "take enough out."

For a comparatively simple operation, you will generally have a most grateful patient if you do not make the mistake of doing too little.

RECONSTRUCTION AFTER MASTECTOMY

Gradually the medical profession has recognized the needs and rights of women for reconstruction after mastectomy. The overwhelming preponderance of men in medicine just two decades ago may have accounted for the unfortunate attitude that breast reconstruction was unnecessary and frivolous. Length of life—survival—was obviously much more important, and quality of life was given relatively minor attention. Consciously or unconsciously, the sentiment was that breasts are an adornment, something once there for species preservation but now present for sexual gratification. This chauvinistic stance happily belongs more to the past than the present. It did not take into account what a woman's breasts mean to her. Notman [193], a psychiatrist and a woman, wrote:

> For a woman they [breasts] represent an important component of her femininity, combining nutrient maternal potential with sexual attractiveness. Her capacity to nourish and to give is important not only in her actual functions as a nursing mother or in the role of a lover, but in creating the sense of worthwhileness and adequacy which underlies self-esteem. . . . The significance of her breasts to a woman goes beyond realistic considerations alone . . . the symbolic importance of the breasts remains throughout life.

Since breast cancer occurs in young women even though its incidence increases with every decade until 80 to 89, patients having had a mastectomy and wanting breast reconstruction range widely in age. In my series, the youngest has been 19, the oldest, 74.

Not every woman who has had a breast removed wants a reconstruction, but almost every patient having had a mastectomy must deal with the threat to her life, the physical and emotional trauma, and the interpersonal consequences: her fear and anxiety about the loss of her breast, her mutilation, her concern about her sexual attractiveness, her dread of metastatic or recurrent cancer or new cancer in the opposite breast [90, 227, 288]. Additionally, women after mastectomy have practical problems, such as buying and wearing clothes and being in a bathing suit. Their freedom is constrained. One will frequently hear such patients say, "I can never be just in a housedress. If anyone comes to the door, he will see that I am lopsided." External prostheses are cumbersome; they slip and macerate the skin. Furthermore, the woman never internalizes them since, in reality, they are not internal. Putting on the special bra and prosthesis in the morning becomes a despised ritual.

These women, especially those without a family history of breast cancer, have likely asked themselves, "Why me?" With regard to reconstruction, they now are asking, "Why not me?" and why not immediately after mastectomy or as soon as possible afterwards? For many women, the impasse to having a breast made is not their psyche but how the possibility of reconstruction, immediate or delayed, is presented to them by the surgeon who did the mastectomy. A decade ago I remember many surgeons, usually male, who advised against rebuilding the breast. They cited reasons that sounded as if they were medical (e.g., possibly stimulating or hiding recurrence), but, in reality, what they advised had less to do with scientific data than with their own puritanical and punitive views: Restoring a breast is self-indulgent and vain; the patient is lucky to be alive, and she should not complain about a minor matter. Unconsciously, the male surgeon may have felt that the patient should pay for her survival with suffering. Fortunately, with the pressures from patients, the articulate voice of the feminist movement, the increasingly sympathetic attitude of the press and the media, and the convincing experiences of other patients, women now find strong support in their quest to be restored to normal [21]. In addition, more surgeons are capable of reconstructing the breast, and these surgeons are not exclusively male; many are female, and the younger surgeons of both sexes today, in contrast to those a generation ago, have more empathy with the woman and her plight.

The male surgeon should realize that the patient wants the reconstruction for herself primarily and not as a way of pleasing a sexual partner. A frequent story is that she desires the reconstruction, but her husband is opposed to it because he thinks it is unnecessary (he loves her anyway), he is afraid of the risks, and he does not want his wife to go through more pain and hospitalization. Many women frankly admit that their husbands want to have sex with them, but they, even in a bra, feel "deformed" or "freakish" and back away. That the reconstruction of the breast is a family affair is evidenced by the usual presence of the husband or fiancé or important other when the woman comes for the consultation. Often she has been so depressed by the mastectomy with its many implications that she has ceased to function adequately in her role as a mother and wife at home or as an effective doer at work. Frequently the family urges reconstruction in the hopes that it will lift the heavy cloud from their home.

The psychological benefits of breast reconstruction, having been well documented, are by now well known [141]. Wellisch and colleagues [269], for example, have listed them as reducing the woman's preoccupation with the life-threatening disease, facilitating choice of wardrobe, elevating dysphoric mood and diminishing anxiety, enhancing body image, and improving sexual responsivity. Teimourian and Adhan [256] found that of 100 patients evaluated, 45 found that it increased "sexual expressiveness," 91 considered the result "acceptable" or better, and 92 would have had the procedure again.

Timing of Reconstruction

Although more breast reconstructions are now being done months and years after mastectomy, immediate reconstruction has now gained many adherents. Its advantages are that it spares the patient another hospitalization, another induction of anesthesia, and another interruption in her life; it also produces happier patients. Stevens [252] studied 13 women who had immediate reconstruction and 12 who had delayed reconstruction. Those who did not have to wait had a "lower incidence of psychological morbidity postoperatively," something that I have previously observed also.

We plastic surgeons have also changed our attitudes toward immediate reconstruction. Our fear was that the patient who had not lived with the deformity would be hypercritical of the result. This has not proven to be true.

The principal reasons for postponing reconstruction in the past were to be sure of the patient's prognosis on the basis of breast tissue and nodes removed at mastectomy, to allow time for ancillary treatment, such as chemotherapy and irradiation, and to observe how the patient fared. It has been found that a reconstructed breast, whether by implant alone, expander, flap, or a combination, does not interfere with subsequent irradiation and chemotherapy, although it may delay these treatments a few weeks. Since the prognostic implications of local recurrence are identical to those of distal recurrence, most patients with local disease will also have systemic spread. unfortunately. Because the rate of local recurrence after mastectomy is less than 10 percent, more than 90 percent of women will not have cancer in their reconstructed breasts. Those who argue for immediate reconstruction believe that if a patient remains apparently free of disease, then waiting for six months to six years will have been needless. If she dies of her cancer in six months or a year, her last months may have been happier because of the reconstruction.

The Consultation

When I see a patient for a breast reconstruction who is accompanied by an intimate, male or female, I am relieved, because I know that the patient is also likely to be relieved that she is not alone. The isolated woman having to face breast cancer by herself, without support, has much to overcome, not the least of which may be the feelings of loneliness and abandonment. Patients after mastectomy vary in their reactions to their malady as do other human beings. Some patients even with support are devastated; some without obvious emotional buttressing seem self-sufficient. The reality of today is that many women are separated or divorced and live far from parents. The appearance of breast cancer can never be at the right time in anyone's life, but sometimes it coincides with a disruption in a marriage or a deep relationship, making the ordeal even worse.

History

In taking the history from a patient who has already had a mastectomy, one should know the precise diagnosis and operation, the pathology report with regard to the axillary nodes, and the patient's subsequent course: irradiation or chemotherapy, both or none? For the patient who is to have a mastectomy with either delayed or immediate reconstruction, one should also have information concerning the microscopic diagnosis.

One should also inquire about family history since this information may determine the management of the opposite breast. In the focus on the breast, one should consider the rest of the body: allergies, previous operations, cardiovascular and pulmonary status, current medications, smoking history.

Physical Examination

Your examination of the patient who has undergone mastectomy may tell you about the presence or absence of local recurrent disease, the state of the scars and soft tissue (thick, atrophic, mobile, fixed). If the patient has had x-ray treatment, are signs visible on the skin? Is the pectoral muscle present in its entirety, or has it been partially removed and denervated?

One should obviously appraise the opposite breast and note its size and shape, particularly whether ptosis is present. Will it be difficult to match? Since the chance of malignancy developing at some time in the opposite breast is about 10 percent, one should examine that breast very carefully. One must palpate for axillary nodes bilaterally. Is lymphedema present in the arm or hand secondary to the mastectomy or the irradiation, or both?

Observe and record body proportions, which are relevant to the reconstruction.

While the patient is undressed, it is a good opportunity to photograph her and to explain in so doing the reasons for the photographs as well as to discuss what types of reconstruction are available and which specific one you would advise. This can be done fairly quickly but only as a preamble to a much fuller discussion in the office with the patient clothed.

Since being only half clothed is justifiably upsetting to most patients, it is wise to have the patient dress and then to finish the consultation in detail with the patient comfortable and attentive, not embarrassed and trying to shield herself from your scrutiny; however, sometimes the patient becomes confused when dressed as one tries to discuss the various reconstructions, most especially the one contemplated. It is most helpful on occasions if the patient has an intimate—possibly a female friend, or perhaps the mother—with her in the examination room so that the anatomic realities can be easily appreciated.

Informing the Patient

Whether or not the patient is to have an immediate or delayed reconstruction will significantly alter the course of the discussion. A consultation with a woman who has the prospects of mastectomy in a week or two has an urgency that reverberates to affect the plastic surgeon also. In many instances, the patient and her family are still trying to cope with the dread diagnosis and the unwelcomed operation of breast removal. She can barely sort out the pros and cons possibly of a modified mastectomy versus a partial mastectomy with irradiation or chemotherapy, or both, following her mastectomy. Under these circumstances, it is hard for the patient and her intimates to be dispassionate about the reconstruction and to retain the complex information that she will receive. Many have had the diagnosis so abruptly made that they have not had time to read about breast reconstruction.

Furthermore, the options for reconstruction are many and bewildering to most patients. Sometimes it is even hard to explain the various procedures to medical students and residents who rotate for the first time on a plastic surgical service. The patient tries to keep in mind the difference between an implant and an expander, the meaning of a flap, and also the advisability and possibility of nipple-areola reconstruction—when and how? The following comments are not the only ones that the patient hears, but I have chosen them to emphasize important areas for discussing breast reconstruction with a patient [96].

Implants
Because of the great abundance, perhaps overabundance, of various kinds of implants, both the patient and the plastic surgeon may be confused about which to use and where and why. One should be prepared to explain the reasons why one prefers or does not favor a subglandular or subpectoral placement of an implant that is gel, saline only, saline-gel, or a polyurethane-covered or silicone-covered implant. Most patients and their families will likely ask whether the implant by itself will hide or promote recurrence (data seem to indicate that it does not) or will itself cause cancer (the patient may be confused by reports in the media of the association of the silicone prostheses with sarcomas in rats). The plastic surgeon who is honest and self-searching will find it difficult to be positive in his or her preferences for a particular prosthesis because, in reality, sufficient data are still lacking.

Expander
The expander is a useful technique, but the patient should realize that even if it is done carefully and even if it involves successful fillings over a period of months, the final result may not be what either you or the patient wanted. She may have a breast that is not as big or as shapely as she had expected, and the breast may actually be distressingly firm, an outcome that she thought she could avoid, as did you, with the expander. Furthermore, the process of expansion may cause pain, a symptom not sufficiently emphasized in articles dealing with this technique. The obvious way of avoiding it is to instill less over a longer time.

At present I try to avoid using an expander in patients who have had irradiation.

Flaps
The disadvantages as well as the advantages of any flap must be discussed in detail with the patient. Usually the patient is willing to exchange a scar on the abdomen or back for a rebuilt breast, but only if the scars are what she considers reasonable. Sometimes the scar, though expected according to your standards and experience, is not what the patient had anticipated. She may fault you even though it is not your fault. I have seen many patients in consultation who have complained about the scars in their donor sites when, in fact, these scars appear only slightly wider than desirable; of course, the bearer of the scar is the one who has to live with it continually.

A patient who once felt deformed and now feels better about herself and still wants more is a tribute to the value of reconstruction; however, it may be difficult for the plastic surgeon to hear about the deficiencies of his or her work. One should never forget that were we in the patient's position, we would want the best available and even the best not yet available.

If the choice is the latissimus dorsi flap, the patient must be warned about stiffness in the shoulder and back, which can last many months and even years. Although she may not be limited in her shoulder motion (a general decrease in function of about 5%), she may still find exercising uncomfortable and early morning stiffness annoying.

If a rectus abdominis flap has been used, the patient must understand that she is likely to have decreased abdominal strength and the possibility of a hernia. At the present time, many plastic surgeons refrain from using the rectus abdominis flap in a patient who plans to become pregnant. Follow-up information on women having children after rectus abdominis myocutaneous flap breast reconstruction is meager.

Nipple-Areola Reconstruction
Patients may ask (and if they do not ask they should be told) at the time of the initial consultation if it is possible to reconstruct the nipple and areola. My preference is to do this at a later stage, on an outpatient basis or with an overnight stay, approximately three months after the breast has been reconstructed. I can then site the nipple with more precision. In my practice at one time only 2 in 10 women actually had nipple-areola reconstruction. This has changed significantly in the past several years. The addition of the nipple gives the patient a sense of completeness [165]. As one woman said, "It is like putting the crown on the queen."

Wellisch and colleagues [268] found in their patients that the "nipple-areola addition appears to change the patient's sensory and visual perception of the entire breast reconstruction outcome. This is indicated by the significantly greater self-rated satisfaction with the size of the reconstructed breast and sense of softness. These attributes, in themselves, are obviously not changed by the addition of the nipple-areola complex." The difference was in the patients' perception of their breast as being more like their real breast—soft and sensate.

Until the time of nipple-areola reconstruction, the patient may wear a paste-on nipple-areola; some have even a realistic tint and almost realistic texture.

Limitations
Every patient must understand that the reconstructed breast is only an imitation; it does not have normal sensation and texture; it may

lack normal color and may be asymmetric with respect to the opposite breast.

I would urge anyone doing breast reconstruction to remember that the procedure begins as reconstructive but ends as esthetic. By that I mean that the woman initially may consider it a reconstruction and may not have or express desires for perfection, but after the reconstruction, the complaints may come forth about how the "scars are too thick and show too much," or "the breasts don't really match." Comments like these, despite the fact that the patient was informed about the shortcomings of the procedure, tend to be exasperating, as previously mentioned.

Stories in the media fuel unrealistic expectations on the part of the patient because excellent results are usually the only ones shown by plastic surgeons eager to appear before the public to demonstrate their prowess. Their preoccupation is less for the public knowledge than for their self-display. They market more than they inform, exaggerating the results usually achieved in most of the patients. A few surgeons, I grant, may have been merely misled at meetings and in journals by speakers and authors who show only their best, pretending that these outcomes are the average and without complications. Long-term results are too infrequently shown [115]. Although we should expect the truth from our colleagues, we unfortunately do not always receive it. This fact leads us to expect to achieve more with a technique because its originator or proponent has not told "the whole truth and nothing but the truth." A plastic surgeon who does not know reality is not likely to pass it on to a patient—and so this deplorable cycle continues.

The Opposite Breast

The breast is a paired organ. Consequently the patient will compare her reconstructed breast with the other. Usually symmetry is lacking.

What to do with the opposite breast is a major decision. Occasionally, depending on the shape and histology of the opposite breast (normal breast tissue or premalignant or *lobular carcinoma in situ*), the decision with the patient may be to remove the opposite breast. In that regard, I prefer a total mastectomy (simple) and would avoid subcutaneous mastectomy, which gives less prophylaxis but certainly can be associated with many complications, or to elevate it if it is only ptotic, or to leave it alone. Some women might prefer a breast that is larger but normal, without scars. Before anything is done with the opposite breast, it is advisable to confer with the surgeon who has performed the mastectomy and the other physicians involved in the patient's care, particularly the oncologist.

The patient, however, is the one to make the final decision and hopefully will do so on the basis of the best information available—facts more than impressions [73, 74].

No human being and certainly no plastic surgeon or patient under stress can be totally objective. The patient, however, may be unaware that she has been advised to have an implant because the surgeon knows more about prostheses than about flaps; or conversely, she may have received a recommendation for a flap when another way, perhaps better, would have been an expander with an implant. On occasion a patient may be advised to have a free flap because of its advantages of a hidden donor site (such as the gluteus) but may not fully comprehend the extent and nature of such a procedure, particularly if she has to have a bilateral reconstruction.

I am not trying to advocate one procedure over another but simply to emphasize that decisions are made, even by the most well-meaning surgeon, not so much on the basis of fact but on preference, whim, or even fantasy.

Another matter with regard to choice of breast reconstruction relates to scheduling. I have heard more than one colleague say that they prefer an expander because it takes less operating time and does not disrupt their day as much as with a more lengthy reconstruction by flap. Sometimes the surgeon does not know himself or herself well enough to sort out the true reasons for his or her preferences. If a surgeon would engage in more self-scrutiny, he or she would soon realize that we are far less objective than we think we are in our treatment of patients—not just in the instance of breast reconstruction.

Complications
The patient must be informed of the common complications associated with various types of reconstruction, especially the one con-

templated. For example, she should know that abnormal firmness and displeasing contour, even when an expander has been used, can develop in the reconstructed breast. The patient who is having reconstruction by a flap should understand that ischemia is possible. In that regard, she must be told to stop smoking at least a month prior to operation. This may not be possible if she is to have immediate reconstruction in the next two weeks. Although some plastic surgeons would refuse to operate on a patient under these conditions, I find it difficult, truly impossible, to refuse. I am willing to take the risk if the patient is. I need not emphasize that one's records should contain the details of the conversation with a patient who cannot stop smoking in a sufficient interval before operation.

The patient and the family should also understand that breast reconstruction can be followed by any complication that might occur with any operation and general anesthesia, e.g., death, pulmonary embolism, infection, bleeding.

Other Information
The patient should understand and hopefully remember information relative to the specific method of breast reconstruction. She should know the nature of the procedure, the approximate length of the operation, whether she should donate blood (I have never needed to transfuse a patient who has had breast reconstruction even immediately after mastectomy), what type of pain to expect, when she is likely to be discharged from the hospital, and when she might be able to resume work. I recommend no driving for about a week, no tennis or golf for about four weeks following an implant, and a two-month wait before vigorous exercise if a flap has been used. Whatever the regimen, this is the time to outline it to the patient, who must arrange for coverage at work and in her home, particularly if she has young children. She will probably also need this kind of information at various times during her treatment because she will undoubtedly forget some of it.

Showing Photographs
The media have made the public aware of breast reconstruction, and this may account for that patient's being in the office. It is equally

likely that the patient has heard about breast reconstruction from a newspaper or television show rather than having seen the result in a friend; however, as mentioned, because many articles exaggerate the esthetic result of the reconstruction, the patient as well as her family may have unrealistic expectations. These patients are one of the few groups (reduction mammoplasty being another group) to whom I routinely show photographs of average results as well as of certain unfavorable outcomes, such as capsular contraction and asymmetry. In this regard, I tell the patient and her family that she will look better in a bra, and I have photographs that illustrate this fact. The purpose of the pictures is not to sell the operation but to document graphically its limitations so that the patient will not be dissatisfied afterward.

Although many patients' satisfaction with the result usually exceeds the actual anatomical attainments, not every woman will be pleased and grateful with your best. Sometimes you can see the expression on her face as you show a result that you think is excellent. To paraphrase Sam Goldwyn (no relation), "Include them out" at your initial consultation.

Fees

Although breast reconstruction in general is covered by insurance, procedures to improve the result and to match the reconstructed breast by reducing the opposite breast are usually not covered or, at best, are covered only after a prolonged battle with the insurance company. The patient must understand her financial obligations with respect to you as the surgeon and to the hospital. An occasional patient, once pleased with her surgeon, may become angry because of the fact that the surgeon who had accepted payment in full for the initial procedure now is charging the patient because of lack of insurance coverage.

The Patient's Family and Intimates

By necessity, the person having the breast reconstruction is the focus of therapy and attention. Although this is logical and appropriate, too often the husband or "important other" as well as the patient's children and parents are apt to feel useless, forgotten, and unimportant. As one husband said, "I feel like the proverbial fifth wheel." One should not just peremptorily inform the husband periodically; one should take care that he not feel like an unwanted observer or perhaps even a jilted lover if the patient's physicians and surgeons at this time in her life are all male. I do not make this observation lightly. The husband remains long after we surgeons, male or female, have left the scene. We should take every means to be sure that we have not left obstacles to their getting their life back in order again. Furthermore, the husband who feels the support of the plastic surgeon, in turn, will be able to give more support to his spouse. Of 30 husbands interviewed, Wellisch and colleagues [269] found that about one in four wished that they had been more involved in the process. However, as Goin and Goin [93] have observed:

> The reactions of spouse or lover to a woman's mastectomy play an important part in her feelings about herself but they rarely influence her decision to have a breast reconstruction. Warmth and support from the important people in her life are crucial to the psychological healing process. Similarly, rejection by a loved one at this time provides a critical stress. However, the woman's decision to have a breast reconstruction is usually based on her own intrapsychic wounds, which cannot be cured entirely by the warmth and support of others. If a spouse does play an important part in the decision, it is much less likely he is the one who is pushing her toward the operation. Instead, the husband, often wishing to protect her, is urging her to reconsider and hopefully to dismiss the idea of subjecting herself to another operation.

Nevertheless, no patient, unless completely isolated, can remain impervious to the reactions of an intimate, especially a family member. The surgical act—the operation—has repercussions beyond the patient herself.

Since a major reason for the patient to have breast reconstruction is to be less preoccupied with cancer, it would be unfortunate if the reconstruction, now having been performed, sets the stage for another focus of great concern and obsessive thinking—now with regard to the intimates in her life. Besides her husband or lover, the patient may have children. If older, they will comprehend the nature of the operation; if younger, they will certainly notice the mother's absence and will probably hear that she is in the hospital. Teenage daughters will get some solace from knowing that their mother's breast can be reconstructed. In fact, some patients have undertaken the operation as a means to reassure their adolescent daughters that should they develop breast cancer and have to have a mastectomy, reconstruction is possible. Teenage sons, who may be exploring the breasts of girlfriends, may find it difficult to separate what may be for them a pleasurable part of the opposite sex from what has obviously been a hazard to their mother's life. All these psychological dynamics taking place do not warrant special psychotherapy, but the situation does entail understanding and sensitivity on the part of the plastic surgeon as well as all the physicians caring for the patient.

If the patient does have daughters, one should *gently* inquire whether they see a physician regularly for breast examination. Most patients and their own surgeons have already attended to this aspect.

The Psychological Preparation of the Patient

Throughout this section on breast reconstruction, I have directly or indirectly considered the psychological effects of mastectomy and reconstruction on the patient and her family.

The psychological preparation of any patient for any procedure is rarely perfect, frequently poor, but hopefully adequate. Some determining factors are the type of operation, the personalities of the patient and the surgeon, and the urgency. A 50-year-old woman with long-standing symptoms of chronic cholecystitis who finally has the diagnosis made and is scheduled for cholecystectomy two months later is likely (not always) to be better prepared emotionally for that operation than if she had breast cancer identified during a routine annual mammogram and the diagnosis confirmed by biopsy—with mastectomy strongly recommended within the next three weeks.

Matheson and Drever [179] have noted that "just as the amputation of the breast is traumatic, the reconstruction of the breast has its own psychological effects." They, like others, have recognized that the patient's expectations for reconstruction include "regaining wholeness, improving sense of sexuality and femininity, improving sexual and marital relationship, personal or professional success or both." One would add, as already mentioned, the practical matter of more ease in buying clothes and getting rid of a cumbersome, annoying, and often skin-irritating prosthesis as well as eliminating a deformity that is a daily reminder of cancer with its feared consequences of incapacity, pain, and possibly death. Also involved in the patient's thought prior to reconstruction may be the opposition or apprehension both of the husband or lover and the patient's own possibly unrealistic expectations and hopes. The astute plastic surgeon and those significantly involved in the patient's care—oncologist, internist, surgeon, radiation therapist—may recognize these expectations and concerns. Unfortunately such insight does not always occur. The major reason why it does not, I believe, is not due to the obtuseness of the physician, whatever his or her specialty, but the unwillingness to spend sufficient time with the patient, simply listening and being empathetic.

Although Matheson and Drever [179] have written about preparing their patients for the reconstruction by providing them with written and prerecorded material as well as hypnotic relaxation, I do not believe that all these measures are necessary in most instances. The benefit to the patients in this series reported by Matheson and Drever may have been less the kind of protocol employed but more the time spent with the patient who perceived their commitment not just to the proposed procedure but to her emotional needs. In short, the patient wants not just an expert plastic surgeon, oncologist, or radiation therapist but would like each to be a friend as well. In that situation, would we not want the same?

Pressures on the Plastic Surgeon

Aside from the usual stresses on us to do good work and to be committed and available to the patient, the plastic surgeon will have less choice in the decision to operate when the patient sitting across from him or her is to have a mastectomy soon and then an immediate reconstruction. Frequently, I find myself agreeing to operate under conditions that are not the way I would like them to be. In a patient, for example, who is a smoker or has unrealistic expectations, I would defer the operation if she were seeking a delayed reconstruction. Perhaps I would then be able to convince the patient to stop her smoking or maybe the patient would be able to readjust her expectations, either by herself, after consultation with other plastic surgeons, or after another visit or two with me; however, postponing the reconstruction or refusing to operate is not easy when the patient has already been scheduled or is soon about to be. Yet, I must admit that many patients about whom I had my doubts in terms of their postoperative satisfaction turned out to be grateful and even enthusiastic about their results—perhaps more enthusiastic than an objective assessment might allow.

After the Operation

The first dressing change may be a pleasant or unpleasant experience for the patient. Generally, with time, the reconstructed breast projects more than it does initially, when its shape is amorphous. The patient must be reassured about this, and that is why your presence will be valuable support to her. It is wise to instruct those close to her, such as her husband and friend(s), to support her emotionally during this early phase. You and they must urge her not to expect the final result within the first couple of weeks.

I remember one patient, a 48-year-old city planner, who became very depressed just after her reconstruction. I thought the reason was her dissatisfaction with the shortcomings of the procedure. In fact, she did say that she had expected "something more" than what she saw at the first dressing change. She did acknowledge, however, that she had "quite an improvement." A few days later in my office, she analyzed her emotional state as being due to "a reawakening of all the feelings I had at the time of my mastectomy four years ago." At my suggestion, she called the psychotherapist who had helped her then. With time and after talks with him by phone (she had moved from the Midwest), her mood returned to what it had been before the operation.

Some patients become depressed after any major surgical procedure; their reactive depression probably has a different etiology, perhaps biochemical, than that in the patient just described, who had gone through operations other than on her breast without subsequent depression.

As with any other procedure, the patient after breast reconstruction must know what she should do about dressing changes, exercising, driving, and housework. Sending the patient home in a brassiere helps immeasurably to restore her self-confidence. It is important also to give specific advice about when to resume sex, since this might be the patient's unvoiced yet ultimate test for the operation's success. Generally I suggest that after two weeks, intercourse is allowed. My reason for being so specific is that I was once awakened in the middle of the night by a patient whom I had not instructed but who asked me, "Is it all right to go ahead now?"

Postoperative care includes continued vigilance for recurrent cancer or new malignancy in the opposite breast. The fact that the breast has been reconstructed has not eliminated that woman's cancer potential. We need to be certain that the patient is being adequately evaluated at regular intervals, preferably by her original surgeon or oncologist, or both, as well as by you.

The plastic surgeon must fight the temptation to admire the breast that he or she has reconstructed and must take care to elicit a proper history from the patient or give her a thorough examination that might indicate recurrence or spread of the cancer. I recall well a patient whose breast reconstruction was above the average in terms of result but who complained of low back pain "just like what I usually get from time to time." Fortunately, she had already been scheduled with her referring general surgeon who had performed the mastectomy (she had had an immediate reconstruction by means of a rectus abdominis flap) who, being more suspicious than I, ordered a bone scan although one 3 months before had been negative. Unfortunately, her disease was now metastatic.

The fact that women who have had breast reconstruction think less about their cancer may extend to the plastic surgeon who, having rebuilt the breast so well, is reluctant to recognize that the patient can still die from her disease.

LIPOSUCTION

I hope readers will forgive me for using the term: *liposuction*. Others might prefer something different, perhaps more elegant, such as lipolasty, liposurgery, suction-assisted lipectomy, or body fat reduction. Whatever we call it, I doubt much ambiguity exists concerning what I mean.

About 20 years ago, while doing a facelift, I used suction to get out the fat. I am sure that many others of my vintage did also and then proceeded to do what I did: nothing further. Why we did not pursue what should have been obvious is the story of many discoveries: bringing an idea to fruition takes more than mere thought; the gap is as great as between dating and marriage.

Like many others who first read about liposuction and then saw it performed, I thought it crude but it did get the job done, an observation akin to what George Bernard Shaw said about copulation.

Now as a confirmed and practicing liposuctionist, I can loudly and honestly state that it is an excellent procedure in properly selected patients, and their satisfaction rate is very high. A testimony to its success is that liposuction is the fastest-growing and most frequently performed esthetic operation in the United States. The media's fascination with this procedure has promulgated its description and nature so that many patients who come to the office seeking the operation will say that they already "saw it done on TV."

Patients

Patients who come for liposuction include men as well as women, whose ages range from very young to quite old; however, in general, in patients older than 45, the skin may have lost its turgor and elasticity and will not be able to contract without wrinkling following removal of the fat. Liposuction is sought in many areas of the body, wherever a person thinks that he or she has too much fat: from a small area under the chin to a large expanse in the abdomen, with the most frequent areas of concern being the neck, hips, buttocks, thighs, calves, and upper arms. Since the cannula can reach almost anywhere in the body, patients request liposuction for surprising areas: elbows and even big toes (both of these patients I refused).

Although this is not the place to detail the indications and techniques of liposuction, I should emphasize what others have also stated: Liposuction is no substitute for weight reduction; liposuction generally gives results that are satisfactory, even excellent, that meet expectations of most patients, but the essential point, as in every elective procedure, is proper selection of patients. When I initially began to perform liposuction, I thought that I would have many dissatisfied patients; in actuality, most are very enthusiastic about the results and tend to refer their friends for the same procedure.

History
One should inquire in detail about previous illnesses, in particular anemia, and previous symptoms of coagulopathy—ready bleeding. One should know whether a patient smokes or takes any medicines that may affect her postoperative or even intraoperative course, especially aspirin-containing compounds and antihypertensive agents.

Physical Examination
The chief point regarding physical examination is to know precisely what areas annoy the patient and whether or not they can be significantly improved. Skin elasticity, just mentioned, is critical in deciding on liposuction for the patient's problem. If the patient is older and if her complaint is fatty inner thighs, one should evaluate the turgor of the skin. Will it shrink after the fat has been removed in a way that will not cause an accordion-like appearance? The plastic surgeon should also know how much of an area is involved. If it is large, then autologous transfusion may be necessary and should be arranged.

One area in which it is easy to make a misjudgment is under the chin, particularly in men, where it is hard to know what one will achieve by liposuction alone without the necessity of a rhytidectomy. Occasionally, I confess, I have used liposuction in the neck and later did a facelift, which I thought I could have avoided by the first procedure. The patient should be warned about that possibility as well as the possibility of having puckering in the neck with excess skin surrounding it.

One small piece of advice relates to taking photographs. Covering a woman's genital area with a throwaway bikini is much welcomed by the patient. I have heard more than one patient complain that she was not "properly covered while he took photographs." How would we male plastic surgeons feel about having a woman photograph us in a similar situation?

Informing the Patient

The patient should know where you plan to direct the cannulas, where the incisions will be made, how much improvement he or she can reasonably expect, and that complications can arise. Teimourian [255] has emphasized that the complications after liposuction can be similar to those with any other kind of surgical procedure, anything from hypotension, anesthesia mishaps, thrombophlebitis, pulmonary embolism, fat embolism, and the ultimate, death, which is very unusual.

Based on a 1988 survey of 2,695 members of the American Society of Plastic and Reconstructive Surgeons, with a response rate of about 35 percent, Teimourian and Rogers [257] found that the complication rate for major suction lipectomy was 0.1 percent, for dermatolipectomy 0.9 percent, and for abdominoplasty 2.0 percent. Of the 15 deaths from all these procedures, pulmonary embolism was the causative factor in 9 (60%). These authors concluded that suction lipectomy "had a low complication rate and is a reasonably safe procedure."

The patient may urge the surgeon to do more than he or she feels is safe. One should remember that when liposuction is combined with abdominoplasty, care must be taken not to interfere with the blood supply of the flaps, which, when stretched for closure, may undergo necrosis, especially if their vascularity has been compromised.

If one expects to remove a very large amount of fat, autologous transfusions may be necessary.

Pertinent to the area undergoing liposuction, the patient develops unevenness, severe ecchymosis, infection, bleeding, pain (particularly if the lower extremities and flanks are being done), numbness, and dysesthesias [54], these last sometimes taking months to go away. Since liposuction is done on an ambulatory basis, the plastic surgeon should determine whether a patient going home will have someone available to provide care. If not, the patient should spend the night in a nearby hotel or in a hospital.

One of my colleagues told me of a patient who had liposuction on her thighs and buttocks and was sent home to an empty house, where, during the night, when she tried to go to the bathroom, she fainted and fractured a hip but could not reach the phone. Fortunately, one of her children came over in the early morning, found her, and was able to expedite her admission to the hospital, where she later recovered.

The plastic surgeon should be realistic with the patient regarding length of time out of work. How long should the patient have someone available to care for children and to prepare meals? Patients will generally be angry if, having been told that they will be able to return to work in a week, they find it impossible and even at two weeks have difficulty in walking or doing things without experiencing pain. It is easy for the surgeon to underestimate the pain the patient will experience and the degree of disruption in his or her routine. Although most patients, when younger, recover rapidly from liposuction on whatever body area, other patients, especially those older, may have less resiliency and may not be able to resume their normal gait or work for three weeks and, in some instances, even longer.

The Operation
It is better to have a patient return to remove more fat than to have suctioned too much and then be left with a concavity. One will likely have to resort to transplanting fat, which is far from a proven and predictable procedure.

Although some of my colleagues attempt mega-suction, I am still fearful of it and prefer to make the patient come back on a couple of occasions, or even more, rather than suction away 8,500 to 14,000 cc of fat and blood. Even though excess fat may be disturbing to the patient, perhaps even disfiguring, it should not become the surgical equivalent of Mount Everest. Even Hilary did not do it all in a day.

ABDOMINOPLASTY

Many patients who would have had an abdominoplasty can be managed by liposuction; however, the need for abdominoplasty still exists, and the procedure is worthwhile for patients, especially those who have lost a considerable amount of weight and cannot exercise away the remaining apron of skin and fat. The majority of patients, in my practice, are middle-aged women and men or younger women who may have a lax abdomen because of a major weight loss or, more frequently, because of childbearing, with perhaps one or more caesarean sections. Slender patients commonly say, "I really hate myself in the summer. I want to wear a bikini." From such an expression, one might conclude that they are undertaking the surgery for a frivolous reason. Compared to submitting to coronary bypass, it may be. But a clue to their true motivation is not the last part of their statement—the desire to wear a bikini—but the first part—their negative feelings about themselves. To them their skin redundancy is disagreeable evidence of the effects of aging and mothering. Instead of a badge of self-fulfillment, the crinkly skin has become a reminder of their body's decline [123]. Many patients who have recently been divorced or widowed want to start a new life. Recently a widow remarked, "I wish that I were a snake so I could get new skin." Another patient, a divorcee, commented, "I feel like a used car when I see myself without clothes." What she might have said is that she felt like an *abused* car, since she thought that her husband had treated her badly and that she had given him and the children "her best years without any appreciation."

Because an abdominoplasty, even if minimal, involves hospitalization, general anesthesia, and approximately a three-hour operation, it certainly cannot be considered "minor," if, indeed, any operation ever is. Abdominoplasty demands a thorough past history and system review. You should also inquire about the patient's plans for more pregnancies, an event that theoretically might worsen your surgical result. If the patient is planning to have another child in the near future, it would be better to postpone the abdominoplasty.

Physical Examination
The purpose of your examination is to determine whether or not the patient will benefit from an abdominoplasty and, if so, to what extent.

How much skin laxity is there? Does he or she have a diastasis recti or a hernia? Does the patient want the operation as a shortcut to losing weight? Should the patient shed poundage before undertaking surgery?

Some patients will still look as if not much had been accomplished even with a well-executed abdominoplasty. They are pudgy with thick skin and fat and often lordotic. They should lose weight and tighten their back and abdominal musculature before an accurate prognosis can be given about the benefits of abdominoplasty.

Informing the Patient
Unfortunately, the public may consider abdominoplasty a "tummy tuck," and some plastic surgeons may reinforce this misconception by minimizing the extent of the surgery and the type and degree of complications. The patient must be told and must understand that fatalities have occurred and that pulmonary embolism, infection, hematoma, and loss of skin from ischemia and dehiscence are possible [122]. The incisions used should be explained again (the first time should be during the physical examination) and the patient must realize that the scars will be permanent, hopefully not prominent, but possibly thick, red, and ugly. Do not neglect to mention the scars around the umbilicus. Also do not forget to discuss altered sensation of the abdominal wall. Occasionally, the patient may be bothered by numbness and paresthesias. Theoretically, there may be a difference in the localization of abdominal pain because of the shift of the abdominal wall tissues.

Patients must know the degree of expected improvement in abdominal contour. It is seldom more than they expect; it frequently is less. For example, unless an incision is made around the waist, the fatty, redundant lateral tissue will remain. Most surgeons do not do a torsoplasty because of the resultant scars, but the patient may expect to be transformed from the usual 40-year-old into a supple ballet dancer. In this regard, men generally have fewer expectations, overt or covert.

Female patients will usually ask whether the striae will disappear. The answer, of course, is "no," but they may be decreased by the skin excision and improved by the resultant tightening.

Abdominoplasty involves more pain and discomfort and more time for complete resumption of all activities than does a rhinoplasty, for example. Patients, especially mothers, want to know when they can begin carpooling, baby lifting, shopping, and housework.

Since most insurance policies do not include this type of surgery, its cost must be borne by the patient. Do not underestimate the length of hospitalization and the charges for the operating room, the anesthesia, and the admission studies, including an electrocardiogram and chest x-ray films.

It is helpful to be able to discuss all these aspects with the patient's family—spouse, parent—or even a friend. The principal reason is to be certain that all concerned realize that an abdominoplasty is a serious venture.

Since abdominoplasty is often done along with other procedures, most commonly augmentation mammoplasty or correction of breast ptosis, the surgeon and the patient must decide how much should be planned for that particular day. Although doing more than one procedure in one session on a patient may be attractive from a time-cost point of view, it sometimes boomerangs to the disadvantage of both the patient and the surgeon. Occasionally the second procedure is not done so carefully as the first unless the surgeon is fast and unless there is another team available. This does not mean, however, that you should not schedule an abdominoplasty with, for example, augmentation mammoplasty, but you must know how much you and your patient can tolerate. Prepare the patient also for another possible postoperative discomfort: having an indwelling catheter for a couple of days. This can be an unpleasant surprise for a patient awakening from surgery who has not been informed. Also notify the patient of the flexed position of the hips after operation and explain its rationale.

Insurance Coverage

Generally insurance does not defray abdominoplasty; it may defray a panniculectomy if the patient has lost a tremendous amount of weight; however, prior approval is advisable under these circumstances. To ask the insurance company to pay for correction of a diastasis recti by calling it a hernia is fraudulent.

THIGH AND BUTTOCKS LIFT

The thigh and buttocks lift, once a popular operation, is much less so because of the advent of liposuction; however, some patients, after having lost a considerable amount of weight, still do benefit from removal of the redundant skin of their thighs and buttocks. In an effort to streamline themselves in association with their weight reduction, most patients have made a fetish of exercising with an emphasis on cycling or an exercise bike, as much as 50 miles a day, with the result of adding more muscle to their thighs and buttocks but still not significantly reducing the sagging. Massage, "cellulite" treatment centers, slenderizing parlors, and friction belts may help some, but the patients in one's office have tried them all without success; you are their last hope.

Many women with heavy thighs and buttocks never wear shorts. They dislike their thighs "rubbing together," assuming others think it is unattractive; it may also irritate their skin. They also may say that for many years their "secret desire" has been to get into a pair of jeans.

Some patients have excess tissue in other areas besides their buttocks. Bernard Berenson [20] recounted the incident of a gloomy lady who was asked why she was sad. "How would you feel if, like me, you had to pass the rest of your days between a big bosom and a bigger behind?" For such people, a program of weight loss by diet should precede any consideration of weight loss by surgery.

Because a thigh and buttocks lift usually involves a hospitalization, general anesthesia, and three or more hours of surgery, you must inquire about the patient's past health, history of allergies, and current medications, if any. Compared to an eyelidplasty, a facelift, or a rhinoplasty, this surgery demands a longer recuperative period.

Physical Examination

The patient should indicate to you during the examination what bothers him or her. You can then determine whether the operation will meet expectations.

Depending on the specific areas of concern, the degree of laxity of the skin, and the amount of fat, the problem of the thighs, for example, sometimes can be resolved by only a medial excision of tissue; other patients require a lateral approach as well, and still others are best served by no operation. This last group comprises those who are squat, with thick, firm tissue and muscle and heavy bones.

Since this tissue does not sag, there is little to lift. An operation will give them discomfort, expense, scars, and disappointment. Another type of patient from whom to stay your knife is the person whose complaint is the gathering of tissue at the knees, particularly medially. Surgery by the usual incisions in the inguinal and gluteal areas will cause only a mild improvement distally. A direct attack on the problem with a vertical medial incision is usually unwarranted unless there is an enormous amount of tissue to remove, and even then, the resultant scars may make this operation unacceptable to the patient as well as to the surgeon. Sometimes, a patient will notice the beginnings of aging and its consequent minimal sagging. In that situation, surgery will do little for him or her. By pinching and pulling on tissue at various sites in the buttocks and thighs, you can give a patient some idea of what the prospective operation can do.

Examine the patient carefully for scar potential by scrutinizing preexisting incisions. Ask also about possible family tendency to keloids.

Informing the Patient

As mentioned, a thigh or buttocks lift, or both, is a major undertaking, and the spectrum of possible complications includes dehiscence and death. Infection and hematoma may occur, but the principal problems are the limitation in improvement and the permanence of scars. If only a modest (a euphemism for "negligible") benefit can be anticipated, I discourage the patient from surgery. Frequently scars will descend with time to a visible level even when you thought you had placed the incisions sufficiently high. Patients will then have to wear a longer bathing suit to cover your surgical tracks.

Patients having more than just a medial thighplasty should be told that they will walk stiffly for about two or three weeks because of pulling at the incisions. They will also have difficulty in dressing, climbing stairs, and getting in and out of bed. They should not expect to sit comfortably or to drive for seven to ten days or to play golf or tennis for about three weeks. To some patients who expect to get a noticeable improvement, these facts are not a deterrent.

In my practice and that of many others, the number of patients having thigh or buttocks lift, or both, has decreased, largely because the improvement is not always significant; the scars are real and lasting; and time and gravity can only lower what you have raised.

As with patients for abdominoplasty, you should inform them that they will be on urinary catheter drainage for a few days. If your preoperative and postoperative routine is a low-residue diet, notify them also about this.

CORRECTION OF PROMINENT EARS

Patients

Reduction otoplasty is unique in the list of esthetic operations because it generally attracts two disparate types of patients: young boys and older women. Therefore, the need for this operation crosses barriers of sex and age. In addition to the concern of human beings about their appearance and their desire not to be singled out because of what society considers a displeasing feature, a factor leading patients to seek the surgery is hairstyle. Until recently, little boys, unlike girls of the same age, did not wear their hair long enough to cover their prominent ears. The older woman, who, when younger, may have obscured her unsightly ears with lengthy tresses, may now want to wear her hair short. Overall, however, requests for reduction otoplasty have decreased, about 15 percent over the past decade, as judged by a recent survey of members of the American Society of Plastic and Reconstructive Surgeons.

Children in your office for reduction otoplasty may be there at their request or that of their parents. Occasionally, parents may bring a child to you when he is only two years of age. Surgeons differ concerning the timing of surgery. I prefer to wait until the child wants the operation, usually between the ages of four and six years, when playmates are quick to fasten on a deviant physical characteristic. The child, whose name the parents have carefully chosen, now becomes "Bat Ears" or "Elephant Head" or something equally inelegant.

If the parents bring the child to you before he realizes that his ears are disagreeably visible, he will feel that the hospitalization and surgery have been imposed unfairly on him. His willingness to cooperate will be less than if he had asked for the operation himself, and his psychological trauma may be more intense. The parent understandably desires to spare the child peer abuse; perhaps the mother or father had a similar problem for which he or she may have had surgery.

One of the parents may still have prominent ears and may say that "I want the operation to be done now in order to spare him what I had to go through." Occasionally a parent will have a reduction otoplasty soon after the child has had his.

Be certain to know the child as an individual, not only his medical history, with possible allergies, but his interests, i.e., preference for TV programs, sports, and so on. It is too easy to forget that this small patient is a person and not just a member of an amorphous species called children.

The older patient, usually a woman, may now want to "set the ears back" because, as mentioned, she may wish a different hairstyle. Usually, the patient will say something like, "I have hated my ears since I was a kid. I'm tired of wearing my hair like this and now that my children are older, I thought I would do something for myself." Compared to facelift, eyelidplasty, rhinoplasty, breast augmentation, and breast reduction, this procedure does not evoke much response in the spouse. He may be concerned about the cost but not about her safety or his reactions to the physical transformation. The ears are a sexually neutral area of the body. Of course, with more sex manuals appearing each day, one cannot predict the next focus.

Physical Examination
Since not all ears are alike, even those on the same individual, your examination must determine the specific aspect for correction. Note the presence or absence of cupping and asymmetry. Test also for gross hearing so that you could not be accused of causing an auditory impairment. This is not the place to list the numerous abnormalities that can occur among the many hillocks and valleys of the external ear. You should know, however, what operation you will do before you get to the operating room; for example, reduce the concha or retroflex the antihelix, or both, or something else.

Informing the Patient

For the young child, reduction otoplasty usually requires general anesthesia on an outpatient basis or intravenous medication as a supplement to local anesthesia. Occasionally an overnight stay in the hospital may be necessary, but the tendency today is to perform this procedure without hospitalization. In the older child or adult, the operation is almost always done under local anesthesia on an outpatient basis.

The patient and family should not expect absolute symmetry but should expect no more abnormal projection to the ears. If, in your experience, two or three percent of patients have recurrence of their condition, inform the patient and the family. Infection is uncommon, as is hematoma, but each is possible.

Scars are generally imperceptible, but keloids do occur. The sharp edge of the antihelix upsets the surgeon but rarely the patient or family. What truly causes disappointment and anger is not getting the ears back far enough.

The patient and the family must know what type of pain to expect. This procedure causes some discomfort; because it is far from life-threatening, this operation may be passed off to the patient as minimal, and the patient will be surprised by the amount of pain he or she might experience.

Also tell patients how long they are expected to wear a head dressing and whether you will also require them to have an ear-head band at night (and for how long). The bulky, warm dressing around the head can be very uncomfortable during the summer, when many children (not at school) and adults (vacation time and their children away at camp) have it done.

In some states, not the majority, insurance will defray the bills of the surgeon and the hospital. The patient and the family must clearly understand their financial obligations, particularly if there is no third-party coverage.

Many surgeons have the impression that the popularity of this procedure is declining, perhaps due more to the current hairstyles than to the incidence of the condition, the economic realities of our society, or social indifference.

In dealing with children, one should explain the procedure clearly;

one should not overwhelm them with details, but one should not minimize or omit unpleasantries. The child, like any patient, will want to know about pain. You may reassure the child that he or she will not experience pain during the operation but afterward, and that medicine can make it better. If hospitalization is necessary, the child should be told enough about a hospital to know in general what to expect. One should always offer to answer questions from the child after you have finished talking, and you should tell him or her that should there be further questions or any worries, you would be happy to talk to the parents or even to the child. It is important to talk directly to the child and not only to the parents, thereby excluding him or her—the patient—from the process.

The Operation

Although this is not a textbook of plastic surgery, I would like to emphasize my own bias: The important objective is to get the ears back (not unnaturally) and to avoid recurrence if possible. I admit that I would rather have a sharp edge to the helix than even a five percent chance of recurrence with the use of other methods (such as the mustardé method) since a recurrence will necessitate reoperation, another hospital experience, and obviously additional costs (even if you do not charge for the correction).

Techniques that restore normal ear contour in a child are not so easy in the adult whose cartilage is stiffer and resists gentle retroversion.

SCAR REVISION

> *He jests at scars that never felt a wound.*
> William Shakespeare
> *Romeo and Juliet*(II.ii)

Some might argue that scar revision is not "cosmetic" but "reconstructive," "restorative," "rehabilitative." Whatever its designation, the presence of mandatory seat belts (as well as mandatory seat belt use in many states) and shatterproof glass in cars certainly has significantly decreased the incidence of severe facial lacerations and the number of patients wanting revision of facial scars. The dog seems to have replaced the auto in causing scars of the face, particularly in children.

Patients

The majority of patients for scar revision come at the instigation of an attorney or claims agent. Always in the background is the question of legal proceedings. Sometimes the scar(s) is so small that you think "only in America" could this stir such a tempest. Other patients, however, have such ugly scars that you wonder how they ever adapted to their condition.

History taking should be precise, not only because it is better medicine but because you will probably have to send a letter to the patient's lawyer or insurance company. Frequently, the circumstances are unclear and the patient's reporting is biased. Record all that the patient says; do not attempt to unravel the skein, since that is the job of the attorneys or court. Inquire about previous treatment: when, where, by whom? Were there associated injuries: bony, visceral, cerebral? Was there subsequent infection in the repaired lacerations? What has been the interim management: steroid injection, massage with vitamin E or cocoa butter, further surgery? If the patient has had other consultations, it is helpful to obtain these reports in addition to the operating notes and hospital records.

The patient should be questioned specifically concerning the scars: physical or psychological pain, functional impairment, particularly with scars around the mouth and eyes or on the extremities. Answers to these questions may not always be honest because the patient or family, or both, is aware that the greater the complaint, the larger the financial settlement. Your business, however, is to record, not cross-examine.

Sometimes the patient is in your office because the insurance company has recommended an "impartial" consultation. The patient and the family may be accompanied by their lawyer and may consider you a hired hand, retained by the insurance company to give an opinion unfavorable to the patient. I always say that I do not work for any insurance company (the truth), but I have been asked to provide an objective evaluation, which I will communicate in writing. I also make it clear that I am not trying to displace another physician in the care of that patient. After these declarations, the wariness and hostility noticeably decrease.

Physical Examination

For your records, as well as for those of the attorney and insurance company, you should state the location of the scars and their appearance (color; whether raised or depressed, thick or thin), as well as their dimensions. Give a mirror to the patient, who can then indicate to you a scar that has faded well or one that is hidden, as on the scalp. At the same time, you can ask the patient whether the scars have improved and, if so, which ones? This will give you information about a scar that might be ready for revision.

By palpating the scars, you can judge their thickness and tenderness and, occasionally, you may find a foreign body, perhaps a piece of glass. In the face, it is important to record changes in sensation as well as the action of facial muscles, especially whether the frontalis is working normally. Some patients have a natural asymmetry of this muscle, unrelated to the accident. You should also palpate the facial bones for residual deformity if there has been a fracture. Occasionally, you may detect a fracture of which the patient is unaware.

With a child, you must rely on the observations of the parents. Sometimes, as mentioned, they may exaggerate the problems, perhaps because of their concern or desire for a more favorable recompense.

Letter to the Attorney or Insurance Company

I usually do not send a report to the attorney until I receive payment, since it is cumbersome to carry open accounts for the years that may pass before the case is concluded. You or your secretary may tell the patient that he or she can pay for the report, and presumably the settlement will refund him or her, although there is no guarantee. Unlike law offices, insurance companies generally send an immediate payment as soon as you bill them; therefore, I do not ask for prepayment.

In your letter to the attorney or insurance company, give the history that you obtained and your findings on physical examination as clearly and precisely as possible. Also discuss the patient's symptoms or lack of them: altered sensation, and emotional reactions to injury.

Make certain that you state that if a scar revision were to be done, you cannot guarantee the result but hopefully there will be an improvement. You might also declare that the scars are permanent insofar as you can judge at this time. With certain patients, you may have to withhold judgment because their injury is too recent, and a better evaluation can be done in three to six months.

The attorney or insurance company will want to know what operation you might do and what it would cost. Again, you may have to defer such information until you are certain that the scar will benefit from revision. If you know that an operation is necessary, state your fee and the expected hospital costs. This is a good time also to mention that one or more operations might be necessary, if that seems likely.

Informing the Patient

Patients for scar revision may expect too much from that operation, and they must understand, emotionally as well as intellectually, that you cannot eliminate a scar but hopefully may make it better. They should also realize that six months to a year must elapse before they will see the true results of your surgical intervention. The patient and the family should know that scars in general, and scar revision in particular, have better outcomes in older persons than in adolescents. Parents usually have the misconception that the opposite is true. You must take the time to describe in detail your plans for scar revision. It is helpful for the patient to look at the scar in a mirror while you draw your lines for revision, such as a Z-plasty or W-plasty. Other myths to shatter are that we plastic surgeons do invisible mending and that we always use a skin graft or something plastic. Give the reasons why a skin graft is usually not the best choice (looks forever like a patch), and stress again that once a scar, always a scar.

You should also discuss the circumstances under which you will do the scar revision. Most uncomplicated scars in adults and older children can be managed with local anesthesia on an outpatient basis.

Occasionally, however, a patient, usually very young, may have been so upset emotionally by having been awake at the time of the original repair that he or she cannot tolerate the same conditions and may request and merit general anesthesia.

Patient Permission for Transmittal of Information
You must obtain the patient's permission in writing to send your report to the attorney, even when the attorney is the patient's. Once I inadvertently corresponded with the lawyer for the opposite party—an unfortunate gaffe! In the case of a minor, a parent or legal guardian must give permission.

The Question of Payment
Probably no area of surgery causes more confusion than scar revision with regard to payment. What I have found practical is a form that the patient or parent signs to affirm their responsibility to pay you no matter what the decision of the insurance company or the court. Lately, in fact, I have insisted on prepayment. If you do not do this, you will wait years before recovering your fee. When I was first in practice, I was more bashful and invariably regretted it. You can be a good doctor and still get paid. For the patient who is not financially able, you will make whatever arrangements you wish. For those in a university setting, having the patient become a resident's case and then assisting with the surgery is a good solution since the patient will not be charged for your services and may have to pay only a minimal hospital bill, particularly if it is an outpatient procedure.

Photographs
As with every patient, it is wise to take two sets of photographs. Almost certainly the attorney will ask for one, which you can furnish at a moderate fee.

When to Operate
This is not a textbook on plastic surgical care, but many scars, even at six months, need maturing. Some scars are ready for revision much sooner than the usual three to six months' dictum. And, finally, some scars are better left alone, allowing time to do its scarless revision.

Beware of patients who have had a minimal scar for many years. They will probably expect more improvement than you can produce and will think that the red scar from the revision looks much worse than the old one that had many years to fade. Some patients with mild scarring will be surprised at your disclaimers—your refusal to guarantee a result. They will have heard about or even know someone who had "terrible scars" and had a plastic surgeon give them a "fantastic improvement." The point to emphasize is that it is easier to go from bad to good than from good to better. These are not simply semantic distinctions.

DERMABRASION OF ACNE SCARS

The popularity of dermabrasion may exceed its value; the reason is lack of something better and the shared hope of patient and doctor that the result will justify its doing.

Most patients for dermabrasion have acne scars whose presence has bothered them emotionally for many years. Women may have had the benefit of makeup, but they complain of the nuisance of applying it and the necessity of using many layers.

Almost every patient at some time has been under the care of a dermatologist; usually, but not always, the acne is no longer active. Today most patients have heard conflicting reports about the efficacy of dermabrasion and they are in your office to get information. They want to know whether the procedure will help them, how it will be done, whether it will be painful, and how much it will cost. Some patients, however, have already decided that they want dermabrasion and are seeing you to make definite arrangements.

For every patient, a thorough inquiry into general health, past illnesses, and allergies is necessary. Do not neglect to find out whether the patient had previous irradiation treatment and dermabrasion and with what results. Ask female patients whether they are taking oral contraceptives, since some types may produce hyperpigmentation after dermabrasion.

Physical Examination
With the patient holding a mirror, ask him or her to indicate which areas he or she would like improved. Usually it is both cheeks,

perhaps the chin, maybe the forehead—sometimes all these areas. Occasionally, it is not an area that looks bad to you, and it is wise to know this before you talk about treatment.

Note whether the patient has active acne. Frequently, the patient's skin looks unattractive not so much because of scarring but because of fresh acne eruptions.

Informing the Patient

You must now decide how much you believe dermabrasion can improve the patient's condition. I usually tell a patient that "on a scale of 0 to 10 (10 being the most improvement), you will get a 3, 4, or 5," for example. The patient must understand that you are not filling in the scars but planing down the surrounding tissue—not building up the valleys but leveling the mountains. The patient must realize that dermabrasion does carry the danger of unwanted scarring; milia (explain what that is to the patient); and uneven pigmentation, usually increased in some areas, most often transient, but occasionally permanent.

Another complication is herpes simplex, which is likely to occur in patients who have had it frequently before. Whether to give an antiviral agent, such as acyclovir, as prophylaxis may be advisable but is still debatable.

I tell patients that the most common unfavorable result is unhappiness from anticipating more improvement than is possible. Unfortunately, those patients with cystic acne scars need help the most but benefit the least. One patient, a male psychologist whom I discouraged from the procedure, showed me a Garfield cartoon in that morning's paper. A cat is saying, "Tomorrow I'll be two years of age. That's the human equivalent of fourteen . . . cats have it good. Adolescence without acne." For that patient, of course, for whom nothing could be done, the situation was not humorous.

For some patients, in whom I am doubtful about the result, it is useful to select an area on the face to test dermabrade. This can easily be done in the office, and the patch, about the size of a quarter, can then be observed for several months before deciding about further treatment. By this measure, the patient does not become committed, nor do I, to a larger, more expensive and unpredictable procedure perhaps without benefit.

Patients will usually ask about repeat dermabrasion—whether it is possible to do the procedure again should there be an improvement. The answer is that it can be done, but it is usually better to see what the dermabrasion can accomplish before deciding on more treatment.

Since most patients do not have insurance coverage for dermabrading acne scars, they will have to pay the costs. This is true even when some pits have been excised in association with the dermabrasion.

SKIN LESIONS

For those doing general plastic and reconstructive surgery, cutaneous lesions constitute a large proportion of their work. They are the bread and butter of a practice, especially for a beginner. To the surgeon, most of these skin growths are minimal problems, but to the patient or the referring doctor, or both, they are major considerations; otherwise that person would not be in a plastic surgeon's office.

For the young doctor who has just completed his or her residency, the facial lesion may be the test case, whether or not he or she knows it. The referring doctor and the patient will judge the young surgeon's performance in this minor situation before entrusting him or her with something of greater magnitude, such as a breast reconstruction or a facelift. They will evaluate him or her not only by the final scar but by the physician's personality. Treating these modest lesions thus is a means of becoming known in the community. In the same amount of time as required for an augmentation mammoplasty, for example (which involves only one patient), you can remove growths from five patients. Furthermore, patients who have facial lesions excised will discuss you and the operation with less reticence than they would if they had had a breast augmentation or a facelift. This form of advertising is appropriate and represents the safest base on which your practice should rest—patient referral.

In many instances, your removing a cutaneous lesion may save someone's life; for example, with malignant melanoma or invasive squamous cell carcinoma. Remember that when you tell a patient that he or she has a skin "cancer," the patient will be understandably frightened by the dreaded word. Just because an epithelioma might be routine to you, do not expect a patient to be equally placid about it—far from it. Many patients can remember a relative or friend who died of "cancer"—in some cases of a skin cancer. Take care to explain, if the circumstances warrant it, that a skin cancer such as a basal cell carcinoma does not have the same lethal potential as a cancer of the lung, breast, or stomach. In some instances, it is wise to telephone the patient's spouse or parent to give reassurance on that point. With regard to a small, untreated basal cell carcinoma, you should emphasize that the probability of cure is about 98 percent and that the patient probably will not be severely disfigured or scarred from the disease or your treatment. Obviously, these statements can be made only if they are objectively justified. With a malignant melanoma, of course, the situation is different, and undiluted optimism would be misleading.

In general, the surgical care of these lesions is excision under local anesthesia, on an outpatient basis either at your office or at the hospital. Usually the patient's insurance will pay for the procedure. If the patient is a subscriber to a group Blue Cross/Blue Shield plan, in many states you are not allowed to bill beyond what you are paid. Though these rules may seem unfair, especially if the recompense has been small, they must be honored.

Biopsy

Until recently, I did an excisional biopsy if I suspected a basal cell carcinoma unless the lesion was located in a difficult area of the face, such as the eyelid or nasal tip; however, because of legal considerations, I now obtain an incisional biopsy of large lesions so I can explain alternatives of treatment to the patient, who then knows the precise diagnosis. Some patients emotionally can never tolerate a scar, no matter how fine it is. For them, radiation therapy may be a good alternative. I arrange a consultation with a respected therapist so the patient will get information about the advantages and disadvantages of the method as well as about the number of sessions necessary over what length of time, about the possibility of recurrence, and about radiation changes in the tissues, from loss of pigmentation to necrosis.

Patients must be warned that occasionally a wide excision of an area diagnosed by biopsy to be a basal cell carcinoma will not show malignancy [118]. Unless the patient understands about the "disappearance" of the epithelioma, you will be accused of unnecessary surgery.

For every benign lesion, the surgeon and the patient should ask themselves why excision is being considered. Frequently, no operation should be done, for example, for a harmless-looking nevus or growth on the sternum or cheek. Beware of the patient who wants it removed for "cosmetic reasons." Although this is understandable as a motivation, the patient might be disappointed by the resulting scar. It is interesting and sometimes surprising that the person who has lived with an ugly lesion may have great difficulty in adjusting to a scar—even a good one. One must be certain to tell the patient there is no guaranteeing what type of scar he or she will have and that it will take several months to determine whether the scar is favorable or unfavorable. One also must be wary of operating on parts of the body that have an inclination to form hypertrophic scars or keloids: the sternum, the tip of the shoulder, or the neck—particularly in an adolescent. One also sometimes has to make the difficult decision as to how many nevi to remove; since most Caucasians have 10 to 30 "moles" on their body, it would be foolish to attempt to excise them all. Occasionally, to allay your anxiety and that of the patient and the family about not doing enough, a consultation with a dermatologist is helpful.

Be careful also of the patient who is having a lesion removed to please someone else. I remember a 25-year-old woman who wanted me to excise a small nevus of her chin. It was so inconspicuous that I asked her why she wanted this done now. The reason, she said, was that she was to be married in two months and her fiancé, a photographer, "couldn't stand the looks of it." In probing, I elicited other instances of his making her feel insecure about herself. Tearfully, she admitted her concerns about this aspect of their relationship. Of course, I refused to operate but did suggest that she rethink her decision about matrimony.

Preoperative Considerations

Underestimating the Problem

The Russian proverb, "More drown in puddles than in the sea" is apt here. Removal of a skin lesion may seem simple surgically, but occasionally closing the defect may cause you consternation and embarrassment. A flap or graft may be required, a possibility that you had not contemplated when you initially saw the patient; you may not have properly informed him or her then of this eventuality. Therefore, think carefully about any patient with a lesion and avoid the unpleasant situation of being unprepared in the operating room.

Another error is to subject patients to excision on an outpatient basis under local anesthesia when, in reality, they should have been admitted and operated on either with local anesthesia and intravenous supplementation or with general anesthesia. For the elderly or anxious patient, outpatient surgery may not be advisable. In taking the history, inquire about the patient's reaction to previous local anesthesia. Often, patients will tell you frankly that they cannot stand needles and faint whenever they go to the dentist. Sometimes these patients can endure local anesthesia on an outpatient basis but frequently they cannot. You must ask also about previous cardiovascular disease, palpitations, and current medications. It may be necessary for you to consult the patient's cardiologist or internist before deciding that the operation can be done on an outpatient basis with local anesthesia containing epinephrine, even in reduced amounts. Some older patients with facial lesions look healthy, but you may find out that they have not had a thorough physical examination in many years. You then must either refer them to an internist or family doctor or examine them yourself and then order a complete blood count, urinalysis, chest x-ray, and electrocardiogram.

Almost every patient with a facial lesion worries about the scar and may think that you, the plastic surgeon, can do scarless surgery. The reality will be an unpleasant shock. With the patient looking into the mirror, demonstrate the excision you plan by outlining it with a skin marker. If the lesion is a basal cell carcinoma, you can explain to the patient why it is necessary to remove a larger area than the apparent growth. You also can outline a flap that you might be using. Indicate also where the scars will be and reiterate that they will be permanent.

Many patients believe that plastic surgeons either use plastic or a skin graft so there will be no scarring. Disabuse them of these misconceptions by pointing out that a skin graft will always look like a patch, most likely depressed and of different color than the surrounding skin; and that ideally the best closure is bringing the edges of the skin together if there is sufficient tissue. If necessary, a flap may be chosen to supply skin, and you can discuss its advantages: a better match in color, contour, and texture than a skin graft.

A skin graft, however, may be indicated. Inform the patient as to the location of the donor site, how it will heal, and what type of scar it will leave. Be certain the patient understands that there is a chance the graft will fail and another procedure may be necessary a couple of weeks later. Because grafting is a common procedure for us, do not forget that it is unusual for patients. They have probably read about it and consider it mysterious and magical.

Some patients with basal cell carcinomas of their nose for example may be better served, in terms of scarring, by referral to a radiation therapist, in my opinion. Other patients with recurrent epitheliomas should have Mohr's chemosurgery. The patient should be informed about those alternatives.

Instructions to the Patient
I tell these and all preoperative patients in words and in writing not to take aspirin or aspirin-containing compounds for 10 days before the operation so that they will have normal clotting.

Patients are also instructed not to eat or drink for eight hours before their procedure if it is to last more than a half-hour. The anesthesia departments in most hospitals have rules for outpatient surgery. Although many of their stipulations may seem unnecessary and excessive, the patient will be safer medically and you, safer legally if these rules have been followed.

During the Operation
Wherever the procedure is done, lighting and facilities must be optimal. Doing a small operation under unfavorable circumstances may convert it into an unpleasant big operation. Music usually relaxes patients; it also overcomes the sounds of surgery (e.g., scissors cutting). I tell patients to bring their favorite tapes, which I then play in the operating room.

Every patient should have vital signs taken initially and periodically; older patients should have cardiac monitoring and an electrocardiograph running continuously. These precautions may seem superfluous, but it is better to prevent a problem than suddenly to have to remedy it and occasionally to be unable even to do that.

Your operation will be better for all concerned if the patient is relaxed. Avoid any discussion that might cause worry, blood pressure rise, and bleeding increase. Since the patient is awake, he or she is aware of all stimuli. Try to minimize unnecessary noise and the parade of personnel in and out of the operating room.

As the surgeon, you are ultimately responsible for the lesion reaching the pathologist. If more than one has been removed, each should be labeled separately. Complete the pathologist's forms yourself or have a responsible person do it, but never assign this task to someone unfamiliar with the patient's history or with medical terminology.

After the Operation
Instructions to the patient should be clear and, preferably, written so the patient and family and friends can be certain of what you want and what they should do. The patient should be told about the pain to expect and should be given something to counteract it. Again inquire about sensitivities to medicines.

The patient should know about the care of the dressing: in general, not to wet it. If you wish it changed, give the patient those instructions along with supplies. If the operation was performed in the area around the mouth, you may not wish to allow the patient to chew for a day or two. It would have been wise to inform the patient of this possibility prior to the operation so that he or she could have made proper arrangements at home and also could have refused social invitations where those restrictions might prove embarrassing. Either make an appointment with the patient to remove the sutures, or have him or her call your office to obtain one.

How the patient goes home is an important consideration. At the time of the initial consultation, you should have discussed this aspect and instructed patients to have someone drive them home if you felt that they should not do it themselves. No matter how slight the operation, every patient has anxiety about it. In addition, the local anesthesia may have changed the patient's normal body responses. If, at the conclusion of the procedure, the patient is not perfectly fit to leave the hospital or your office, keep that patient until there is no question about his or her safety in returning home. You should also know who will be at home to care for the patient. Sometimes it is essential that the patient be closely observed, particularly if very young or old or if there is a history of a systemic problem such as hypertension, epilepsy, or diabetes. If you have concerns about the patient's being able to go home, do not allow it, even if you had not discussed this possibility when you initially saw him or her at your office. Do not make two errors. Admit that you had not paid sufficient heed to the patient's physical condition or the availability of supervision at home. About once every couple of years, a patient unexpectedly must remain overnight in the hospital. Although this decision may cause consternation for the patient and family, it is preferable to later mourning another lapse in judgment.

REDUCTION OF NASAL FRACTURE

The reader might be surprised by my including in this book the seemingly simple procedure of reducing a fractured nose. Perhaps because of its presumed simplicity, the patient may erroneously expect a perfect result unless properly forewarned by the surgeon. My contention is that this operation has more unfavorable results than are generally appreciated.

In addition to the specific anatomy of the fractures, several other factors are responsible: The surgeon called in to treat the patient with a nasal fracture never knows precisely what the patient's nose looked like before the accident. The patient usually claims that it was perfectly straight. Sometimes looking at the patient's photo on a driver's license or an identification card can give one some idea of the pre-existing shape of the nose.

Frequently the surgeon schedules reduction of the nasal fracture at a time convenient for him or her but not optimal for obtaining the best result. Many patients arrive in the emergency room at night and they are scheduled for reduction 24 to 48 hours later, when the swelling is at its maximum and is obscuring the anatomical landmarks.

Often the nasal fracture is reduced under inadequate conditions of poor lighting and meager facilities (lack of suction and proper instruments). One patient told me that she had gone to a plastic surgeon who "seemed annoyed that he had to fit me into his office schedule. He did it right there in his office but he didn't wait for the novocaine to work. The pain was awful and my nose is as crooked as it was before he tried to fix it."

The patient's tale does emphasize the fact that the least a patient should expect from a doctor is a caring attitude about the pain involved with any procedure.

Every patient must be told that after reduction, the nose may not be what it was prior to the trauma, and that another operation, perhaps six months later, may be necessary to straighten it [183]. I inform each patient and the family that I will try to put back what goes back easily but I never use "brute force" to align the nose for fear of distorting it or causing hemorrhage, or both. Occasionally, even when the nose has been properly reduced, bleeding can persist and may require packing and, in rare instances, ligation of the external carotid or anterior ethmoidal artery.

Always inquire about the patient's past history with regard to hypertension and medications such as aspirin and anticoagulants.

Using local and topical anesthesia is customary, but some patients, particularly adolescents, are quite anxious about the operation although they pretend otherwise. Intravenous supplementation is helpful, but it should not be given unless the patient has been without food or drink for at least six to eight hours. Of course, with smaller children, it may be necessary to administer general anesthesia, whose risks should also be explained to the parents.

OTHER FACIAL FRACTURES

I will not go into detail concerning the interaction between the plastic surgeon and the patient with fractures of the face in addition to that of the nose. I wish to stress here the need for awareness of any associated injuries as well as disruption of other facial bones, besides the obvious fracture. Furthermore, the treatment of facial trauma may require the convergence of talent: oral surgeon, ophthalmologist, otolaryngologist, and neurosurgeon, in addition to plastic surgeon. The patient should never be the victim of the unfortunate internecine battles among specialties.

Another point for emphasis is to tell the patient, if alert and comprehending, as well as the family, what your operative approach will be and its expected success. For example, in the instance of a zygomatic fracture, the patient should know whether you are planning a Gillies', or transantral reduction, or coronal incision or one into the cheek with direct wiring or plating, if indicated. In the press of an emergency, it is easy to forget to take the time to give adequate information. Rushing the patient into the operating room is seldom warranted and can cause catastrophe if, for example, there is unsuspected systemic illness or unrecognized damage to the eye or brain.

It is wise to state your disclaimers before the operation. You probably should warn the patient and the family that he or she may never have the same bony configuration or soft-tissue covering as existed before the accident. Furthermore, additional operations may be necessary. Once the patient has recovered from the emotional shock of having sustained facial trauma, the gratitude that you think he or she will exhibit may disappear in the patient's disappointment that things are not perfect. The unhappy patient might reason that "if plastic surgeons can put back arms and legs, why couldn't they get my face to looking like it was before?" If you are able to remind the patient and the family about the fact that you mentioned the limitations of the operation before you performed it, energies will not go into defending yourself but into helping the patient readapt.

HEAD AND NECK SURGERY

Most plastic surgeons in the United States are seeing decreased numbers of patients with tumors of the head and neck. The reasons are multiple: decreased incidence of the disease; different methods for managing malignancy, such as irradiation instead of surgery; fewer plastic surgeons who are able and wish to care for these patients; and the availability of other specialists to perform the surgery (otolaryngologists, maxillofacial surgeons, and general surgeons).

Patients with head and neck neoplasms may have either benign or malignant disease. Aside from those with parotid tumors, patients with head and neck malignancy usually are men who disproportionately come from the lower socioeconomic groups and frequently have a history of poor oral hygiene, excessive smoking, and alcohol intake.

In general, these patients are seen more often in hospital clinics than in private offices in contrast to those for cosmetic surgery. Patients with parotid tumors, however, usually go to private surgeons.

No one with intraoral malignancy can be treated so easily or reassured so fully as someone with a basal cell carcinoma of the skin. With the former, the morbidity, mortality, and deformity are significant. Even with the newest techniques of reconstruction, utilizing musculocutaneous flaps and microsurgical transfer of tissue, the patient's appearance is forever altered, always for the worse. Furthermore, speech and swallowing may be impaired.

In a private office, the patient is usually accompanied by a member of the family. At the clinic, he or she may be alone; this should make the surgeon realize that the patient will have to depend more on him or her for support since the emotional cushion of family or friends may not be available.

In taking the history and systems review, you must remember that the condition of the patient is potentially, if not actually, serious, and the treatment will be major. An operation such as a resection of the floor of the mouth and a portion of the mandible, with a radical neck dissection, significantly stresses that patient's soma as well as psyche. Since those with head and neck malignancy are in the older age groups, their general health will be the principal factor in the selection of their treatment and its success or failure. In addition, as mentioned, these patients tend to drink and to smoke excessively. Since their cardiopulmonary status may not be optimal, they must be properly evaluated for anesthesia and surgery. Inquire also about fatigue, weight loss, appetite, and social habit, including their work. As you are asking these questions, try to ascertain what impact the disease and treatment will have on all aspects of the patient's life.

Physical Examination
No matter what or where the primary lesion, your physical examination must be thorough with regard to the entire head and neck: presence or absence of palpable nodes, status of the facial nerve, and condition of the teeth. Indirect laryngoscopy is mandatory for evaluation of the mouth, pharynx, and vocal cords. Is there any other primary lesion? Since extensive surgery is being contemplated, these patients must have their blood pressure taken as well as their heart, lungs, and abdomen examined.

Informing the Patient
If you think the patient will require surgery that you rarely do or are uncomfortable in performing, now is the time to refer (see p. 343).

You must inform the patient of your tentative diagnosis. Perhaps the diagnosis is known; maybe a biopsy is needed. If you believe that the patient will definitely require an operation, discuss it in detail, but do not suddenly overwhelm him or her with a statement such as, "This means that I will have to remove half your face and jaw." The same information can be given gradually and gently. Place yourself in that patient's position of fighting for survival while trying to preserve features as a human being. Sometimes it is better to defer telling the hard facts if you sense that the patient cannot take it all at once or if he or she is alone in your office; a better occasion may be when a spouse or sibling, for example, can be there. Offer to see the patient in a day or two when his or her usual source of support can be present.

If you believe the best treatment of the lesion is irradiation and surgery or irradiation alone, arrange for the patient to see the radiotherapist. Perhaps the patient should be evaluated by the oncology group at your hospital. These are useful maneuvers. The patient and you will usually gain from other opinions and a discussion of possible alternatives. The patient will then be able to accept your recommendations, feeling that you have not neglected anything or anyone in attempting to help. It also will give you more assurance for the course you are taking. Immediate reconstruction by free flaps of tissue and bone is now common. What these procedures entail, with specific reference to the donor sites, should also be well understood by the patient.

Allow time for the patient to ask some questions. Basic to the inquiries is a pervasive concern that the resulting deformity will be so great that even if he or she is well, the patient will no longer be welcomed in society and will be an embarrassment to family and friends. Sometimes the surgeon can call on patients who went through similar procedures and have offered to see other patients facing their type of surgery. Laryngectomy groups, for example, are extremely helpful. Hearing it from others who have been there before can be a tremendous source of confidence for the patient and his or her family. Remember that the face is sacrosanct: It is basic to the self-image of each of us. In every other situation in life, we instinctively try to protect our face. In this instance, the patient must sacrifice a part of it in order to live. The fact that you have done 250 extensive head and neck procedures does not lessen the impact for the patient, for whom this is the first such operation [250].

Almost every patient with a serious cancer, not a basal cell, however, feels a stigma. For most people, healthy or with malignancy, cancer means death, excruciating pain, something stealthy and dirty. This "metaphorical thinking," as Sontag [247] calls it, tends to isolate the person not only because of the reactions of others but also his or her own; the afflicted one withdraws through guilt, shame, and fear as if to spare his or her social circle the task of dealing with a deviant. The doctor, of course, must do everything possible to prevent the patient from becoming a pariah. If, indeed, a patient who has had hidden cancer treated (e.g., cancer of the colon removed by colectomy) experiences depression and a desire to run away, one can get some idea of what the patient with a head and neck cancer must endure. That individual has to bear the visible signs of the exorcism of this dread disease. Despite the tremendous stress that a head and neck malignancy imposes on an individual, the incidence of suicide is very low, less than 0.05 percent [52]—a tribute to the courage and adaptability of the human being [22, 68].

Before the Operation

Be meticulous about your preparation of patients for surgery. Warn them not to take aspirin or aspirin-containing compounds. Perhaps they will need a high-protein diet in preparation for the ordeal. They may also require determination of blood gases and chest physical therapy because of many years of cigarette smoking and the presence of emphysema and bronchitis. A consultation with the anesthesiologist before the patient is admitted to the hospital may prevent a frustrating night-before cancellation because of insufficient workup.

In the Hospital

Although many things could be discussed here depending on the procedure, the major consideration is your responsibility to help patients accept themselves and their new appearance, as well as perhaps altered speech and swallowing. Be there at the first dressing change. Do not abandon them at this critical time. Help them to look in the mirror and support them through the shock of seeing somebody new in the mirror, somebody who looks ugly and foreign to them. Most patients' immediate concern is appearance—not function, not survival, even though you may think it should be otherwise. Be careful of the patient who says, "My appearance doesn't really bother me." Perhaps this is true, but more likely the patient is trying to hide deep concern from you. Such a response may be a result of guilt about expressing displeasure with appearance when you have tried so hard to save his or her life.

The presence of sympathetic nurses is important to any patient. For a man, a female nurse or doctor will be the first woman to see his new face without dressings. If they do not grimace or turn away but relate calmly to him, this will considerably strengthen his self-esteem. In World War II, McIndoe knew well the value of this kind of social reintegration when he provided female companionship (a euphemism) for his facially burned RAF pilots.

The patient who has had extensive remodeling of the intestine, for example, after a Whipple procedure, cannot see what the surgeon has done because of the fortunate covering of the abdominal wall. The patient who has had serious head and neck surgery eventually must go unveiled.

Follow-Up

Your responsibility to the patient continues for his or her lifetime. The issue is not just survival at 5, 10, or 15 years, but resumption of normal living and relationships. A clue to how things are going at home is whether there has been a change in sexual relations with the spouse. Have they been able to get together? If not, why not? Sometimes the partner is willing but the patient feels worthless. Your intervention or that of a skilled family therapist may make a considerable difference in the lives of the entire family. In many ways, it is easier for a physician when the cancer is the only enemy. After surgery, the battle must be waged against more elusive opponents, sometimes harder to defeat. With more reconstruction, the patient's appearance can be improved, but ultimately there is a limit. At that point, the patient hopefully has been able to adapt. If not, referral to a psychiatrist or support groups of similar patients, or both, might rescue him or her from the downward spiral of depression.

Another point to mention is the necessity of an adequate postoperative follow-up. Too often, these examinations are perfunctory. Unconsciously, the surgeon does not wish to find recurrent or new disease; however, there is no point in examining that patient unless the surgeon is willing to find what is there and to act on it. Periodic evaluations by the local tumor group or the oncology group may be a helpful supplement to your care of the patient; however, the primary responsibility for your patient's management should not be shifted to someone else unless there is just cause. You have become, and should remain, that patient's doctor.

THE PEDIATRIC PATIENT

This heading was carefully chosen since the stages of infancy, childhood, youth, and maturity are arbitrary and indistinct, not only chronologically but physically and emotionally too. Presently most of my patients are adults, but I once had a brisk pediatric practice.

The pediatric patient is not an adult in miniature any more than an elderly patient is an aged child. A child has characteristics common to all children but also traits that are unique.

From a practical viewpoint, what is special about treating pediatric patients?

1. They usually do not come of their own volition. Parents or surrogates bring them.

2. In general, the earlier a deformity is corrected, the better the psychological effects (perhaps also the anatomical results) in a child. This axiom relates to the important aspects of body image and self-esteem. Quality of life for someone with Apert's syndrome, for example, would be significantly enhanced if the disfiguring abnormalities were improved before 2 years of age rather than at the age of 14. Of course, this surgical objective is not always attainable. We should remember also that the importance to psychic development of being different is not restricted only to facial features; any part, especially if abnormal, may be emotionally important to a particular person: webbed fingers, asymmetric breasts, a conspicuous nevus, or hemangioma of the trunk.

3. Very young children cannot verbally communicate their symptoms or concerns. Even when children can talk, their speech is not so elaborate as that of adults; however, in a few stark phrases, they may convey more that is meaningful and true than a 44-year-old, who has learned to dissimulate feelings and to bury anxiety and hostility under a cloak of words. Compared to an adult, the child rationalizes less. Whereas children are affected by what they may have seen on television or read in books, adults more frequently describe themselves and their sentiments in terms of what they think they should be or feel.

To reach the core of a child is easier than to reach that of an adult, who has a much thicker carapace. For many adults, one is tempted to ask, "Will the real Mrs. _____ stand up?" This is not so with a pediatric patient, although children can be devious in action and speech. More commonly the surgeon who is used to adults may be caught off guard by a child's direct expression of feeling, such as tantrums, crying spells, and sudden physical and emotional withdrawal.

A child, however, may be a better reader of body language than an adult. Perhaps this comes from a child's having to look so often at big people and having to judge quickly, for self-preservation, what that person may do either to harm or to help him or her. We might get a sense of that vulnerability by imagining ourselves in the company of the entire Pittsburgh Steelers team.

The more "intellectual" the adult (and being intellectual usually takes years), the more labyrinthian his or her thought. Adults may pride themselves on their subtlety and on their ability to emit double-entendres, to be clever with a forked tongue. Generally this is not so with a child, who is always on the important side of the decimal point.

Think straight, talk straight, and act straight should be our maxim with all patients, especially with children. One can be direct without being abrupt or uncaring. Telling a child that a needle stick will not hurt and is "like a mosquito bite" (rather than a bee sting) is a foolish lie. This breach of the truth may make the child distrust everything you subsequently say or do. Far better to inform the child that there will be momentary pain that is necessary for you to help with the problem.

4. Just as adults do better in a hospital with other adults, children fare better with other children in a pediatric hospital or ward. The staff are more familiar with their needs. Children feel secure knowing that they are in an environment dedicated to them. Not all doctors or nurses or all adults enjoy being with children, and children sense their irritation and hostility. Another advantage of a pediatric unit is the decreased likelihood of errors in medication from personnel more accustomed to managing adult patients.

5. When contemplating surgery in children, one must think in terms of future growth and development; whereas in adults, the consideration is aging.

For the child with a cleft lip and palate, the surgeon must question whether the procedure will interfere with normal maturation. When performing a facelift, the surgeon hopes that the procedure will interfere with the normal sequence of aging.

The variables of growth and development can surprise the surgeon: A result that looks good in an infant may look bad when the person is a teenager. Occasionally, the opposite occurs, particularly with scars.

6. Follow-up examination may mean something different to a child than to an adult. A boy, for example, who has had a cleft lip repaired at three months of age may not wish to see his surgeon every year because he fears another operation. The parents, in some instances, may not even have told the child that he had a cleft lip but attributed the scar to a fall when he was a baby. The child who knows about the cleft lip may become self-conscious with an excessive number of follow-up visits, especially if his result is good and awareness of the problem is minimal.

An older patient, however, after a breast reduction or augmentation or after an eyelidplasty or facelift may welcome return visits because they are reassuring and also offer the occasion to ask for more surgery. In fact, as was mentioned earlier, for this reason, some surgeons do not wish to follow their patients for a long time; they want to avoid expressions of dissatisfaction and pleas for touch-up operations.

7. Pediatric patients, in general, are less capable of following directions or performing their own dressing changes than adults. A 4-year-old child, for example, cannot be expected to remember to take medication or to change dressings alone. Most children are fortunate to have parental reminding and assistance. Also, children who are normally active may make a shambles of a dressing or a cast; that situation in an adult occurs less often.

8. Because the relationship between children and parents is generally close, it is rare for a child to pursue an operation without parental support. This is certainly not the situation with older patients, who may seek surgery against the advice and wishes of their family. The teenager, however, is in a revolutionary phase of life and may act in much the same way as the older, so-called liberated woman. The problem is that the older patient has society's support

as well as its legal sanction to proceed with treatment, but a child or a young teenager does not.

Although it is unwise in most surgical situations with adults not to have an operation become a family affair, it is almost impossible to avoid this when a child is concerned. That is why the surgeon with pediatric patients must be very much attuned to family dynamics.

Many hospitals have programs to make surgery less anxiety-provoking for children: preadmission tours, even parties, and films allow parents, siblings, prospective patients, and their friends to become familiar with what will happen during their hospitalization. Pediatric patients, like many adults, have a particular fear of anesthesia, and the opportunity to talk to an anesthetist, to see and examine the equipment, markedly reduces their anxiety. Having facilities to accommodate a parent is also a major plus or should be for the child and for you. Occasionally a parent, by his or her presence, may increase the child's fears. Frequently also the nursing staff may resent what they consider to be the intrusion of the parent in their province. Of course, it is the parent's child, not theirs, but this type of proprietary thinking on the part of a nurse has a positive side: It may be responsible for laudatory dedication to the welfare of those in his or her care.

A common mistake of many physicians is to attempt to reassure a child by hugging and kissing when you do not know each other. The child will instinctively retreat from this inappropriate and overwhelming advance. Proceed slowly but gently. In any relationship, it takes time to build trust.

THE PARAPLEGIC PATIENT

I have known a gentleman who was paralytic to a deplorable degree, enraged to a perfect use of all his limbs while his anger predominated.
Tobias Smollett
On the External Use of Water

The purpose of this section is not to describe the many procedures used for resurfacing a decubitus ulcer, rather, it is to share some thoughts concerning the management of paraplegic patients.

The most common error made by plastic surgeons treating a paraplegic patient is to place too much faith in a flap and to pay insufficient attention to the psyche. Commonly, we consult on an individual who has had numerous episodes of sacral breakdown and many previous reconstructive procedures. At this time, the use of musculocutaneous flaps is popular, but we must resist the temptation in our residents and ourselves to do this operation without understanding the etiology of the ulcer. I am not referring to the question of pressure or shearing force but something more fundamental. Has the patient been self-destructive? Do the repeated incidents of breakdown reflect a depression, an escape into alcoholism, a desire to re-enter the hospital because the outside world is too much to confront? Having been a consultant on a spinal cord injury service, I was impressed that some patients, fortunately only a small percentage, returned repeatedly to the hospital after having left healed; in every instance, the fault was not with the flap but in the mind of the patient. It is fruitless to expect that a new flap will provide indefinite protection when the patient refuses to cooperate in his or her own care. This type of patient needs counseling or group support and, frequently, prolonged psychotherapy. If the patient had seen a psychiatrist early in the course of his or her overwhelming disability, then some of these later psychological problems either might not have arisen or might have been less severe.

Often when we are called by another physician to see these patients, they are lying on their abdomen, and seldom do we go to the head of the bed to look at their faces and to talk with them before snatching off their dressing and outlining a flap. We treat them as an ulcer, not as a human being. Our attitude reinforces their low self-esteem and their hostility toward themselves and the world. It would be naive to assume that a plastic surgeon—even the most compassionate, understanding, and skilled—could reverse a damaging psychological sequence; however, at least he or she need not add to it. The plastic surgeon who comprehends the patient as a human being will avoid surgery that is doomed to failure. During the time that an ulcer is cleaning up [191] or healing in, an effort should be made to view and treat these patients globally so that subsequent surgery will not be a mere technical exercise for which the duration of success will be just a few months.

THE PATIENT WITH FACTITIOUS DISEASE

The crux in the management of this difficult type of patient is to recognize the diagnosis. So accustomed are we to relieving patients of an unwanted disease that we may easily overlook the possibility that someone may wish to have an illness. The patient, of course, has a psychological sickness in addition to the one that is simulated [194].

Psychological classification of such patients, termed by some to have Munchausen's syndrome, is difficult and controversial [187]. In my experience, patients have usually been women, 20 to 50 years of age, with a disproportionately large number in the medical field— nurses and technicians [110]. A plastic surgeon will usually encounter such a patient because of failure of the wound to heal or recurrence of a local cutaneous infection. Since many patients are one of our medical core, we are reluctant to consider the factitious nature of the problem. They may be attractive, intelligent, and seemingly desirous to get well. Some may flatter you by saying that you are supposed to be "the best" and that is why they sought you. For some, their relationship to the physician becomes the center of their life and gratifies their prodigious dependency needs. This attachment may perpetuate their conscious or unconscious repeated simulation of physical disease. The physician is always uneasy in confronting a patient with evidence that he or she has manufactured illness. Yet, at some point it may be necessary to do so, but only after psychiatric consultation and approval. These patients are notoriously refractory to treatment [63], and some may die in the course of causing their disease. Suicide by another means is also a possibility. Curing a recurrent wound breakdown, for example, may not solve the major underlying problems since another focus may be chosen, one that may be even more dangerous to the patient's health.

A simple rule is to think of factitious disease whenever a patient repeatedly fails to respond to standard treatment for a relatively simple condition [208]. Sometimes, you may have to intervene to treat the patient because of the disease that he or she has caused. Try to keep your interventions simple. Do a graft rather than a flap, if possible. Do not delude yourself with your own competence and your faith in the knife. Remember that the principal problem is cerebral, and even if you are fortunate to "cure" the ostensible illness, your success may be short-lived. For the surgeon, these patients present the modern equivalent of a Hobson's choice.

THE DISSATISFIED PATIENT

There are days and there are other days.
André Gide
Autumn Leaves

Nothing can ruin your day like a dissatisfied patient [72, 109]. He or she is as much a reality of surgical practice as the satisfied patient [117]. Although fortunately in a minority, the unhappy patient generally has a great emotional impact, albeit unpleasant, on us. No picture of the surgical landscape would be complete without showing somewhere—usually in the foreground—the patient whose expectations we have been unable to meet.

Although the dissatisfied patient need not be one of the proverbial triad ("everything unusual or bad in medicine occurs in threes"), one can easily have a succession of failures. Ward [265] vividly understood this phenomenon: "Regardless of how much experience, care and expertise has been invested in the operation one finds from time to time that everything one touches turns black and drops off. It leads to fatigue, disillusionment, depression, self pity and imminent alcoholism. However . . . although recurrent, it is a temporary phenomenon and that for some extraordinary reason a new day dawns from when everything goes smoothly once more."

As physicians, we seek to help others and to obtain their approbation. It is terribly distressing to have to deal with a person whom we not only have failed to help but possibly have made worse; who, instead of being grateful, is hostile; and who, instead of applauding our motives and talents, openly accuses us of greed and incompetence.

A plastic surgical residency, like most other educational experiences in our culture, does not usually equip us to manage the unpleasant side of our metier. As residents, we took care of the grief of somebody else's efforts, and even when it was our own patient, when we were chief residents, we had the glimmer of hope in the fact that the rotation would soon be over and we might even be leaving town in a few months to begin our own practice. But now, as professionals, we are all in a position so well described by Harry Truman as "The buck stops here."

The first task for the surgeon is to know when and why a patient is dissatisfied. Usually he or she will remove all ambiguity by a strong, unequivocal statement of complaint, but if this is not forthcoming, we should be alert to veiled discontent—a sullenness, an irritability, or some form of passive-aggressive behavior such as not keeping appointments or not paying the bill if, unwisely, we asked no prepayment for an esthetic operation. In some ways, it seems easier to let the patient leave the office, and we feel relief because he or she did not verbalize the unpleasantness we would then have to confront. But sooner or later the seamy side of surgery will have to be faced. We must not become so unreceptive that the patient's resentment will reach the proportions of a lethal abscess. Before this occurs a helpful comment might be, "You don't seem too happy today. What is troubling you?" Then step back as Pandora's box opens!

Some patients seem more unhappy than they are. Unless they have told you what bothers them, sometimes asking them if there is anything that they like about the result may elicit a more positive response than you had thought possible. This becomes a good foundation on which to build the ensuing discussion.

For many patients dissatisfaction disappears with reassurance that is justified by circumstances. For example, someone who is concerned two weeks after eyelidplasty about swelling can be told it will subside as healing progresses over the next few months. A patient may worry about the bulkiness of a recently turned flap. Here, too, reassurance about progressive flattening will be comforting.

Occasionally, postoperative unhappiness centers on the minimal or the nonexistent. In this situation, it is important to probe into "why this now?" Is the person depressed and guilty about having an elective operation or about something else? Has there been a recent loss such as a divorce or death? I remember a 35-year-old married woman who had a very good result following a rhinoplasty and chin implant but seemed depressed a few weeks later. Her girlfriend next door, she told me, had "kept away" and finally confessed to my patient that she feared rejection because she thought that my patient, now better looking, would need her less. Occasionally the culprit in postoperative depression is the family physician, who may have said to the patient soon after a facelift, "You went through all this to look like that?" This unkind and destructive remark may have been prompted by the patient's not consulting him or her about the surgery or proceeding without advice. In addition, the general practitioner or internist may feel that the surgical fee is excessive compared to what he or she receives for the care of that same individual. Envy and jealousy, although not usually openly discussed, are relevant when managing a dissatisfied patient.

In this regard another factor to consider is the spouse or lover who may have enjoyed the personal dominance that resulted partly from the mate's feelings of inferiority about a disliked feature. Since the patient is now rid of it, the partner may feel less secure about the leverage he or she formerly possessed.

What about the patient who complains legitimately about an undesirable result, for example, infection, asymmetry, or bad scarring? To detail the spectrum of complications is beyond the present task and unnecessary for the purpose here [112, 117]. The point is that if the patient's dissatisfaction has an objective basis, it, like any reality, deserves the surgeon's attention and respect, and the patient merits our sympathy [281]. Someone who has had esthetic surgery, for example, frequently has sought it against the advice of family, friends, and other physicians and may have had to pay for it personally. When something goes wrong, he or she feels foolish, ashamed, guilty, and angry. The patient may believe that this complication is divine recompense for vanity that led to risking health for a "frivolous improvement" that now has become a distinct liability.

Admit the Reality
As surgeons, especially since most of our results are favorable, we instinctively turn away from the adverse outcome, but the sooner we accept it, the better we can manage it [31, 112]. To become angry at the patient because of our ego's bruise will only succeed in increasing hostility. The duet will soon become a duel. It is much better to recognize the reality and to work together to correct it. An unfavorable result happens not just to the patient but also to the family, to the surgeon, and, I might add, to the surgeon's family. Do not distort reality by accusing the patient of incorrect observation. The patient is certainly capable of judging nipple asymmetry, for example, or a bulbous tip or a "keloid" (which usually is a hypertrophic scar).

Outline a Plan Early
It is important that a plan of action be outlined as quickly as possible, and this may include what seemingly is no action. By that I mean that if one must wait before corrective surgery, that is still a plan, and the patient will not feel forlorn or lost in ambiguity if it is so stated. Often I have told patients that the most difficult thing for us both is to wait. This requires restraint to avoid embarking precipitously on another operation that may compound the problem.

Marshal Support
The first task is to get the patient's support to help you to help him or her. For this to happen, the patient should be fully informed about his or her current status, what you intend to do, and what that will entail in terms of time, pain (if any), and cost. But one should also inform pertinent members of the patient's family, friends, and especially the referring physician or, if none, the family doctor. You and the patient need every ally possible.

As mentioned before, the plastic surgeon has to admit to the patient that there is a problem. When I first went into practice, one older plastic surgeon told me that whenever something did not turn out right, he never admitted it and instructed everyone in his office to do the same. In this way, he thought, the patient would not consider him negligent, and the hazard of a malpractice suit would be less. I cannot disagree more strongly with that precept. Although I would not advise beating our chests, wearing ashes and sackcloth, and crying "Mea culpa," I do not think that pretending the problem does not exist or attempting to cover one's tracks by lying will ever be justified from either a practical, moral, or even legal standpoint. Several patients have told me that what infuriated them the most was seeing their physician as a dishonest human being. No one wants his doctor to be the Artful Dodger. Unfortunately, this kind of person exists not only in Dickens' novels. It was Mark Twain who wrote, "The truth is what you tell when you can't think of anything else to say." Without sounding like an evangelist, I would state that the truth is not the last resort but the first approach; it clears the air and allows you to resume the task for which you have trained half a lifetime: caring for a patient without being encumbered by shoddy stratagems that ultimately fail.

Make Yourself Available

Another cardinal "do" is to make yourself available. Do not erect a barrier between you and the patient. The unfavorable result may actually be an opportunity to deepen the relationship and sometimes can be converted from a potentially miserable disaster into a satisfying experience. It is interesting that over the years several patients who have developed postoperative problems and were managed with a modicum of decency actually became enthusiastic supporters and subsequently referred other patients. Incidentally, giving the patient your home telephone number, for example, may make her or him more secure and may result in fewer telephone calls. The secretaries must be instructed that for this patient, the "hot line" is always open. If this is not done, the hard-to-reach doctor will soon be replaced by the easy-to-reach attorney. But, medicolegal considerations aside, it does not seem fair that you should make yourself scarce after you have contracted to do a job that might not have turned out as either you or the buyer wanted. We would certainly resent this attitude if a carpenter came to our home to perform a task and behaved in that fashion; surely we have more obligations to a patient whose face or life is at stake.

Using Your Consultant

Another aspect in managing the dissatisfied patient is the proper use of a consultant. Most patients want to remain with the original physician, but it can comfort the patient as well as the surgeon to have another opinion, especially if the case warrants it. You should sense when the patient wishes a consultation, and you should not make the patient jump hurdles to obtain one; however, the patient should not feel tossed off but directed to the other physician. I usually dictate a letter in the patient's presence stating what the problem is and that I would like his or her advice, which can be discussed freely with the patient. Occasionally, you may sense that a patient does not feel that he or she should pay for "your mistake." I would hope that we would consent to see patients for colleagues at no charge to maintain the delicate balance between the unhappy individual and the hard-pressed physician. If you, as the referring physician, believe that the patient should not be charged for the consultation, you should so inform the surgeon and offer to pay for the consultation yourself. Most of us, I am sure, would not allow a colleague to do so, but this practice has precedence. If a patient chooses to continue his or her care under another doctor, either the consultant or someone else, do not make the patient feel guilty. In similar situations, I have made sure that I knew when the patient was going into the hospital and have even called the patient in the hospital or at home afterward. The patient then realizes that you are truly interested in his or her well-being, and the doctor who has cared for the patient will also welcome your support and not feel that he or she has lost a professional friend.

Many patients have told me that when they have suggested to the doctor a "second opinion," the response has been hostile. A recent patient who had mild ectropion after eyelidplasty recalled that the surgeon "said that he never wanted to see me back if I went to someone else." That doctor's attitude was puerile and irrational since the patient was a reasonable person, justifiably concerned about her eyes, which fortunately improved simply by massage and waiting.

To illustrate some points in the management of the dissatisfied patient, let me give a few clinical examples. The patients are from my own practice. It is always easier to pontificate from the safe vantage point of someone else's patients, but what follows represents my own misadventures.

One problem situation involved a 58-year-old woman who, following a facelift, developed a moderate hematoma that was drained but left her with pathognomonic wrinkling. Over a few months this subsided, as did her feelings of hostility and anger, but it required twice weekly, then weekly visits, and also a consultation with another plastic surgeon—which I initiated. I took periodic photographs to document her progress, and I would show these to her. The patient, who had not prepaid her entire bill (my mistake), asked that a small amount remain unpaid because she said that she had not obtained the result she had expected and that she had endured considerable anxiety and stress in achieving what she got. Contrary to what the advice of some attorneys might be, I thought it reasonable to bend a little and our relations have been amicable since.

The second patient is the kind of woman about whom our residents ask, and very rightfully, "Why are you doing her?" She had a depressed air, and, indeed, she was depressed to a degree that I did not appreciate; she had not recovered sufficiently from her son's death several years before. When she requested a facelift, she said she wanted to get out more, to feel better about herself, and, even though she was in her early 60s, she wanted to look for a job. This seemed reasonable, but postoperatively she complained and still does, four years later, of vague discomfort, stiffness, and unusual sweating in her neck. She has seen a neurologist, a neurosurgeon, an orthopedic surgeon, a psychologist, and a psychiatrist—as well as another plastic surgeon. I have directed most of these referrals. She calls me from time to time and complains and then seems better after she has discussed it with me. The operation, with its unfortunate mysterious sequelae, has replaced her need to obtain employment. She represents an outstanding example of poor patient selection but also lingering distress of a patient, to whom the surgeon does have the obligation of "sticking with it." Fortunately, I have prevented her from seeking further surgery, which would prove even more deleterious to her well-being.

Mrs. W. is someone I remember well. She had an area of skin loss following a facelift. She was disappointed only to a minor degree, and with daily care the wound healed, so that in that area behind the ear, the scarring was not very noticeable; however, she returned a year or two later complaining that the scar hurt her severely. She seemed depressed and wondered how much the operation had really improved her appearance. Although the result may not have been outstanding, it certainly was more than acceptable. With this type of patient who is dissatisfied, it is necessary to probe, and indeed I found out that she had been very close to a married man who now was dying of cancer. She admitted that she wanted to speak to me again because she thought I might be sympathetic to her personal problems and probably this symptom of scar pain was really a pretext and a displacement. She wrote me later that her life was better; her friend had responded "remarkably well" to chemotherapy, and she no longer had pain behind the ear.

As physicians we know that pain is subjective, felt only by that individual who claims its presence. Since people vary widely in their pain tolerance, it is impossible to know precisely how much discomfort another person is truly having. Excessive pain after cosmetic surgery heralds complication: hematoma, infection, or, if after eyelidplasty, perhaps impending blindness. Chronic pain after esthetic procedures is also infrequent. It may signify a depressed or displeased patient. The busy plastic surgeon, if not vigilant, may prescribe diazepam, for example, in a "get off my back" response to a patient's complaining and listlessness. Without probing for an explanation of that patient's mood, the surgeon may perpetuate and aggravate the despondency by giving a tranquilizer. With patients after reconstruction, a persistent pain, requiring analgesics and allegedly preventing return to work, should make you suspect malingering for secondary gain to collect on workmen's compensation or to garner a large settlement in court. Depression is also a possibility. Make an effort to determine the dynamics of that patient's behavior.

Always record what you prescribe and check before giving more for pain or sleep. Count your prescriptions. I remember two patients in whom I noted a disquieting fondness for sleeping pills. After I told them of my concern, they agreed to stop what they thought was "just a habit." Indeed, it was. The physician is also susceptible to a habit: that of prescribing without thinking.

4 Types of Operations and Types of Patients

Another clinical memory concerns someone on whom I did a facelift—someone who seemed to be a very cheerful human being but who I now realize was in a manic or hypomanic phase. Her daughter had died in an auto accident two years before and so she had been seeing a psychiatrist who felt that she was handling her grief well and was out of the doldrums. About a year after the facelift, I was given an urgent message in the operating room to call her. She told me in no uncertain terms that she had the worst facelift of any of her friends. I remembered that she was given to bouts of excessive alcohol intake, although she sounded rational but obviously disturbed. I asked her to come to the office, and later, after a long discussion, I did a revision of her eyelidplasty—right upper lid. A few months after this, she returned—again hostile and complaining—could I do anything further? I told her frankly that since she felt the surgery had not been what she wanted, it would be risky for us both to participate in another operating room adventure. It is difficult to break off with a patient, but I think sometimes it is necessary or the downward trend will continue as a *folie à deux*.

Every so often we see a patient who has had surgery, such as a facelift, and at the time of follow-up visit we forget that we have already done her. She looks as if she is in the office for a facelift, and it is embarrassing to realize that the improvement you both had expected never materialized. Sometimes the patient says frankly that she is unhappy with the result, and you have to agree that her feeling is warranted. The remark may be, "It looks as if nothing had ever been done." There are some relationships that adversity cements, and I remember one particular patient for whom this was true. She wanted me to do the surgery again, and I did it, but even with a redo, the nature of her facial laxity was such that two years later she looked about the same as she had prior to ever having had the operation. At that point, I felt that my surgical intervention in her case was over.

A great advantage for the surgeon who has a private operating room is that the patient is not charged for subsequent touch-ups. This is not possible if one depends on the facilities of a hospital. Managing these financial obligations of the patient who has to have corrective surgery and has to pay for it personally can be "sticky." Perhaps it is wise to have in the original consent form a statement that the patient having cosmetic surgery is responsible not only for the bills at the time of the operation but also bills for the management of any complications that might result. As a matter of principle, I do not charge the patient, but the hospital certainly will.

In summary, the major errors in managing the dissatisfied patient are as follows: distorting reality, blaming the patient, inhibiting the patient's anger and fear and increasing guilt, remaining distant or unavailable, failing to consult, trying to jettison the patient, and not structuring a sound treatment plan that avoids premature corrective surgery.

It is perhaps too simple to state that we should treat the patient as we ourselves would want to be treated. In so doing, Emerson's words should be comforting: "Bad times . . . are occasions a good learner would not miss."

The Dissatisfied Patient and You as Consultant

So great is the ill-will among physicians that each denies honour and praise to the other. They would harm a patient and even kill him than grant a colleague his meed of praise.
Paracelsus
Die grosse Wundarznei (Book II)

The consultant who sees a patient with an unfavorable result arising from the work of another surgeon is in a singular position to do considerable good or irrevocable harm [108, 270]. Although in this situation, as in any other medical circumstance, the first obligation is to the patient, one can also help the other doctor.

The first step is to obtain as objective a history as possible. Exclamations of disbelief at the patient's story or the other surgeon's behavior should be assiduously avoided. Usually the patient who is angry and distraught gives too brief a history because he or she wishes something done immediately to correct the undesirable result. Since the operation the patient has relived the unfortunate surgical events thousands of times and may be impatient with the consultant for laboriously trying to fit together the sequence; however, securing a full account is crucial.

Typical statements from unhappy individuals are as follows:

> "I went to him because he is supposedly tops in his field. How could he have done this?"
>
> "She never told me this could happen. I was in and out of her office—one, two, three."
>
> "He was there to take my money before he operated. But afterward, I could never get near him. I'd call his office and his secretary would say, 'He is seeing patients now. He'll be in touch with you.' But he never called back."

As part of the history, it is advisable to ask patients about their general health and their professional and family life, as one would do if that person had come to you initially. What are his or her relations with spouse, parents, and employer? Is there a psychiatric history? Is the patient now abnormally depressed? How has he or she reacted to previous operations?

The physical examination is usually less of a problem than the history. The patient is almost eager to show the scars that "shouldn't be there," the breasts that "don't match," the nose that "looks awful," the tendon graft that "doesn't work." For the consultant, the pitfall is being so absorbed in the local problem that he or she neglects the patient in totality. The consultant might fail to notice, for example, how scars have healed from past trauma or other surgery; or he or she might not detect systemic disease, such as malfunctioning thyroid. During examination it is best, once again, to avoid comments, articulated or not, such as a low whistle, a stare of surprise, or an "Oh my" headshake. The patient will be alert to any sign of how bad the consultant feels the problem is or how badly he or she thinks the other surgeon performed.

The patient should be asked to return to the consulting room for a proper discussion with both of you seated. Most likely the patient resents the other doctor's not spending enough time with him or her and would not want another opinion on the fly, no matter how impressive the consultant's credentials.

Now comes the most difficult part of the consultation, literally "the moment of truth." My experience has been that it is best to give the patient as honest an appraisal of his or her problem as possible but to do so with warmth and empathy. It is helpful to begin simply, "Mrs. Palmer, as you know, you have had a breast reduction and your problem is that the scars are more noticeable than you want. It is true also, as you have said, that the breasts are not symmetric. I am sure that for you and Dr. _____ this has been very distressing since we both know that he would have wanted the best result for you." Having structured the problem, one can proceed to the treatment, which, for the patient, is the most important derivative of the consultation. "Now, Mrs. Palmer, we would all agree that we have to decide what to do. Looking backward is not productive and can be very upsetting." Although at times a consultant should defer his or her opinion because the other surgeon has requested it, generally it is wise to give a candid but not condemning evaluation at the time the patient is seen. Patients fear conspiracy among doctors; that we will protect the worst actions of the most incompetent to maintain the solidarity of our guild. Unfortunately, in some instances this is not mere paranoia.

It is important to ask the patient's permission before getting in touch with the other physician, unless the other physician has sent that patient specifically to the present consultant. We have no legal or ethical right to breach confidentiality without such consent. Aside from the legal implications, we will lose our credibility if the patient feels that there has been communication without his or her knowledge, and we will have rendered ourselves less effective in our helping role. Even if the patient gives permission but is in our office without the other surgeon's knowledge, there is significant strain on the consultant, especially if the other doctor is a close friend. The strain is even greater if the patient does not give permission for such contact. Usually, however, the patient will agree to it if you can make him or her realize that it is in his or her best interests to obtain as much information as possible about the entire medical course. If the patient is suspicious and has grudgingly consented, one may telephone the doctor in the patient's presence. This three-way discussion, besides allowing an exchange of facts and thoughts, does much to defuse an unpleasantly explosive situation.

Like the denouement in a well-constructed novel, the consultation should result in a plan of management. For all concerned, it is better to look forward in hope than backward in anger.

A practical matter must soon be resolved: Who is now responsible for the patient's future care? Sometimes the patient will settle the matter by refusing to return to the former doctor. Frequently the other surgeon has arranged the consultation and, of course, will continue to care.

I do not believe that it is wise medically or correct ethically to force patients to return to a doctor they no longer trust or like even though their attitudes might be justly founded. The plastic surgeon who consults, and we all do, must be willing to assume responsibility in these difficult situations, as we routinely do for the patient coming to us from surgeons not in our specialty. The fear of being unpopular or embroiled in a lawsuit should not lead us to avoid aiding the patient. As a practical matter, a patient whom you, as the second or third surgeon, refuse to treat, is more likely to seek redress by going to an attorney.

At some point in the consultation the truth should be reiterated: that in surgery, as in all of life, perfection is the aim, rarely the attainment; that in our own practice unfavorable results and frank complication have occurred and we can easily sympathize with both the patient and the other doctor. Some may call this being charitable; it is, in fact, being realistic. The patient must realize that our efforts will not magically rectify a difficult problem. In indicating the limitations of our own procedures, we must at the same time not make the patient feel that he or she has been so deformed as to be beyond help. This is the most delicate balance to achieve. Occasionally it does happen that nothing further can be done. The patient must understand this reality, but his or her comprehension and adaptation will be enhanced by a general explanation rather than a cold, preemptory presentation.

The consultant should be sufficiently mature not to use the patient's misery to denigrate a colleague or to plump his or her own ego. The golden rule is eminently pertinent here. Since all who operate are bound to have failures, rejoicing secretly in someone else's poor result is childish and short-sighted. Beware the boomerang!

A consultant who is able to help a patient in trouble also helps a family and a colleague. Few situations in medicine demand greater sense and sensibility but yield more satisfaction.

THE DIFFICULT PATIENT

The difficult patient is different from the dissatisfied patient, who is a step beyond. With the difficult patient, things are not going right, but they have not yet gone wrong, at least ultimately. You both have a chance.

When you are having increasing difficulty in relating to or in helping a patient with his or her problem, the direct approach is the best [146]. Tell the patient that you are concerned about the breakdown in communication. "You seem to be upset. Are you angry with me?" The patient's response will largely dictate the subsequent dialogue, which you should try to keep from becoming a petulant confrontation. After this airing, things generally improve. Occasionally a minor irritation has incited and perpetrated a patient's unhappiness and hostility. The complaint may be completely justified, or the patient may have misinterpreted your words or actions, or both. Frequently the issue is less important than the emotions it has aroused. The cause fades while the effect stays. However, that you have shown concern and have made an effort to be friendly and helpful may be all the evidence a patient needs to regain confidence in your commitment to his or her well-being. Sometimes the relationship that has been stunted may now grow into something vigorous and satisfying to you both. Crucial to recovery is the patient's cooperation, or better still, his or her participation. Some ideas of what an intelligent human being can do to help himself or herself may be found in Cousins' book, *The Anatomy of an Illness as Perceived by the Patient* [58]. Passive assent is preferable to active rebellion, but creative participation is the ideal. Although the last is rare, it is worth striving for, but it requires a skillful doctor with humility to recognize personal limitations and the potential of the patient.

I recall a patient who, two days after a parotid tumor (pleomorphic adenoma) was removed, was being "difficult," according to the nurses, although ostensibly everything was going very well. She complained about the nurses "never being around" when she wanted them. She said that the residents "didn't really care" about her and that I "just breezed in and breezed out" of her room. In actuality, her comment about me was probably true. As she became more testy, I became more distant—just the opposite of what I should have done. Finally, I asked her why she seemed to be always in a bad mood when things were going along very well with respect to her surgery. I did not have to probe deeply; her immediate response was, "It's my son. He told me before I came in for surgery that he was getting married and I can't stand the girl." After this catharsis, her mood in the hospital improved although the situation at home remained the same. Of course, the psychodynamics of all "difficult patients" are not that transparent. Moreover, in many instances, you are the cause of the problem—not something external to you such as a son's poor choice of your patient's daughter-in-law.

Recently I had to cancel a patient's facelift because I was ill for a day. She was furious. "Why me? In all my planning, I never considered the possibility that you would get sick," she moaned. She wanted me to cancel someone later in the week to get her on the schedule. I refused, despite numerous calls from her and her husband. We told her that she would be scheduled when the next opening was available—in a few weeks. On questioning the patient in more detail about why she was so distraught and so anxious to have the surgery as soon as possible, she told me that her father was dying in a nursing home and her mother was in the same condition at her house. She had hired a nurse for the week of her scheduled operation. Furthermore, her son was to be married in four weeks and she wanted to look "normal" for that occasion. I was more sympathetic with her plight and she was more reasonable, although I still detected smoldering resentment. Predictably, she was excessively conscious about each bruise and bump following the operation; that it went well was truly fortunate for us both.

Sometimes we consider a patient to be "difficult" when we think he or she should be grateful. Doctors, like most human beings, appreciate thanks for their efforts, and the human animal is not alone in this quest for gratification. A good retriever revels in the satisfaction of his or her owner. An occasional patient whom we have seen through severe illness not only appears ungrateful but hostile and distant after health is restored. This behavior may make the physician feel rejected, unloved, and even angry. The explanation may be that the patient not only has a disquieting memory of the illness and hospitalization but also is ashamed of having been exposed, mind and body, for all to see. The patient is like the person who under the ease of alcohol tells all the night before but then shies away from the confidant the next morning.

Few human beings can accept their vulnerability, and the patient who stalwartly refuses to look backward in gratitude may be asking you to reconsider her or him now as a normal human being in a normal setting. Frequently, these patients may thank you several months later, when they might admit that they had a difficult time in reintegrating. Some have said, "Sorry I was so difficult."

THE DISAPPEARING PATIENT: GET READY, GET SET—GONE!

About once a year, a patient comes to the operating room for an elective procedure, such as a breast reconstruction, a facelift, or an eyelidplasty, and will suddenly decide against it and ask to go home. Your response logically should be to determine why she has apparently changed her mind (in my experience, the patients who suddenly reverse their resolve have been women). Unless a specific incident, such as rudeness from a nurse or resident, has prompted her departure, you should support her decision and not try to dissuade her from it. Although you may be surprised by the suddenness of her action, you probably will have already observed signs of the patient's indecision even during the initial consultation: Perhaps she has asked you to tell her whether or not she should have the operation, or telephoned you frequently to pose innumerable questions more for assurance than for information. Characteristically, she may have changed her admission date several times, to the exasperation of your secretary. By leaving the hospital, the patient has done both of you a favor. If she was that much in conflict over her procedure, she would likely have been dissatisfied with her result.

Canceling an operation is not solely the patient's privilege. Obviously, you would do it for medical reasons, such as an upper respiratory infection or an electrocardiographic abnormality; however, occasionally you will have second thoughts on your preoperative visit about what you could accomplish for him or her.

Consequently the patient will expect more than you can deliver. It is better to part company.

THE PATIENT IN THE EMERGENCY ROOM

> *The patient dies while the physician sleeps.*
> William Shakespeare
> *The Rape of Lucrece*

Most agree with the principle that every physician should respond to an emergency with promptness, courtesy, and competence [50]. Yet, the reality is different. Herbert Spencer, the nineteenth-century English philosopher, believed that the course of most human lives in our society is absurd: As a youth, one is poor, and finally when enough money is accumulated, one is too old to enjoy it. Far better for the young to have it initially. Spencer would have seen his desideratum fulfilled in the procedure for staffing most emergency rooms. This is the realm of the under-40 generation. Surgeons just out of residency still revel in their accelerated pace and strain to be summoned in this initial phase of practice. Emergency room patients keep the young surgeon's skills sharpened and the rent paid. The new patient is a certain antidepressant for the beginning doctor. After a few years, elective surgery will increase and emergency calls decrease, for several reasons. Other younger doctors will have joined the staff; they have supplanted you in the "needy" category. Peers refer to peers; the distancing factor of aging is such that residents and nurses feel more comfortable in a medical interchange with those of their own age, provided, of course, that he or she is competent. Another reason for receiving fewer emergency calls as you get older is that you like them less and want them less. No longer do you respond with the same alacrity—instead of a whistle of delight, you emit a groan of reluctance. You may say something such as "O.K., I'll get there when I can."

With more years in practice, the type of work you do will also change. You may now be treating an occasional patient with a hand injury or a facial fracture. This is not the place to discuss how this evolution affects the image or influence of plastic and reconstructive surgery in your community, with your colleagues and the public, or the balance of power with other specialties, such as otolaryngology, oral surgery, and orthopedics.

At meetings, some surgeons in their late 60s state they still "cover" emergency rooms. If they are in a city, the reality is that although they may retain their place on the roster, someone younger is usually assuming call. A macho factor exists here, relating to their wanting not only to prove to themselves and others that they are energetic and as dedicated as before, but also to deny that they are doing esthetic rather than traumatic surgery, which is much like the medical student who does not want anyone to know that he or she is studying.

Whatever your decision about the emergency ward, your position must be unambiguous. If you are truly on call, then be available and gladly enter the fray.

In watching myself and others in the emergency room, I have noted some common errors in the care of patients:

1. *Being too brusque and abrupt.* Admittedly, any emergency call is unexpected and disrupts your schedule. Conveying your displeasure to patients increases their agony and guilt since they probably are blaming themselves for the accident. Most people are aware that some doctors "do not come out for emergencies"; they will greatly appreciate your efforts, and the image of our profession will get a needed boost. A kind word and a sympathetic attitude will help the relationship with the patient who is frightened and in pain and who may not have called you. In an emergency, the circumstances do not permit the gradual forging of a bond between patient and doctor. Yet, in plastic surgery, as one colleague commented, "The emergency room may be a nuisance but it makes you feel like a doctor." Imagine yourself or a loved one with facial injuries, and you may then realize that for the patient, the surgeon is the only agent of hope.

2. *Neglecting associated injuries.* This error arises from being too intent on the local problem to the exclusion of other sites of trauma, particularly the brain, spinal cord, chest, pelvis, or lower extremities. Facial lacerations are so compelling that even trained personnel may forego the usual workup to treat the obvious. You may be told that the patient is "fine except for the face." Examine the patient yourself before accepting anyone's appraisal.

Another mistake is the frequent omission in the chart of a statement concerning the patient's vision in the instance of facial injury. This basic evaluation should be made. Aside from the medical importance for the patient, it may have legal consequences for you.

3. *Giving excessive reassurance about the eventual scar.* During the repair of a facial laceration, it is tempting to overdo your reassurance of the patient with regard to the scarring that so concerns him or her. In more temperate moments, the plastic surgeon would be the first to state that wound healing is due only partly to the method of suturing. The patient may remember your prediction, and if the scar is worse than anticipated, you will receive the blame if you have been too optimistic. For documentation, photograph the patient before you begin your repair.

It is not your fault that the patient was injured; assume the responsibility only for careful care, not for the final result. Pare knew better: "I treat; God heals."

THE PATIENT WITH WHOM YOU ARE TERMINATING YOUR CARE BUT NOT YOUR CARING

At some point, a surgeon can do no more for a well patient with respect to treatment, operative or otherwise, although he or she may continue to be the patient's friend and medical advisor. Usually, the expectations and perceptions of the surgeon and the patient are similar, and terminating is natural and pleasurable; however, some finish under less favorable circumstances. In those situations, the patient is dissatisfied and angry, but, paradoxically, as Shakespeare wrote, "Parting is such sweet sorrow." "Sorrow" because you have not pleased the patient but "sweet" because his or her departure has freed you even though it has been a rejection. But you do have the obligation to tell the patient, preferably in your office and also by letter, that you are no longer responsible for his or her care. You might succeed in referring that person to another source of help. Or things may have deteriorated to the point that your every suggestion is an anathema. Certainly if the patient has a suspected or proven malignancy, these steps of proper termination are mandatory, not just for protecting yourself legally but for ensuring the patient's well-being.

Even the patient who thinks you have mismanaged his or her treatment will grudgingly recognize your attempts to do what a good physician should. And you will also be preserving the tradition of medicine, which is no mean objective.

Sometimes a patient will not want to leave. He or she may still want more to be done—more than you can do or wish to do. Reluctance on the part of the surgeon may not be due to technical limitations but rather to concern that the patient is becoming surgically dependent and cannot break away to get on with life. The patient should not base his or her future on the results of a minor scar revision, for example. Many surgeons during a long course of treating the patient may insist that the person resume work before the next stage, as a means of rehabilitation.

Occasionally, a patient is ready to quit, but the surgeon is relentless. Excessively perfectionistic, he or she subtly or openly coerces the patient into additional procedures to optimize the result. The patient's face has become an extension of the surgeon and his or her handiwork.

When to let well enough alone is a difficult judgment in all of life, not just within the realm of plastic and reconstructive surgery. As the surgeon, if you believe that the patient should be satisfied with what you consider an acceptable result that you cannot further improve, then gently suggest that someone else be consulted. Frequently, another surgeon will be able to offer a better solution, and, if not, his or her opinion will confirm yours and the patient may end the quest. If, however, the patient still has difficulty in living with the results, psychotherapy may be beneficial. The problem may be getting the patient to follow this advice. Family support may be crucial to convince the patient of its value.

There are other circumstances in which a patient may refuse to leave. For male surgeons, it is usually a female patient, perhaps of a hysterical personality type. She may not be the sole cause of the situation. Consciously or unconsciously, you may have been emitting signals that she has been eager to recognize. You must emphasize to the patient that you are happy she has done so well and seems satisfied with your care as a physician. Now she no longer needs your medical service, but others do. You must be strong enough to recognize that you have the power and the responsibility to terminate the relationship that has gone from the therapeutic to the amorous. Medicine is complicated enough and should be sufficiently challenging without these other ingredients, which serve not only to worsen the interaction between the doctor and the patient but ultimately to make the patient (and usually the doctor) more unhappy. Perhaps the ancient Indian practitioners were correct in their admonition: "A physician is forbidden to take anything but cooked rice from the hands of a woman."

Another danger is the Pygmalion complex [175, 176]. You recall the Greek legend about Pygmalion, a sculptor, who carved a beautiful ivory statue of a woman and then fell in love with it. In answer to his prayers, Aphrodite transformed his work of art into a living woman, whom Pygmalion married. Some female patients and some plastic surgeons have this primitive fantasy, which does not take much to nurture to a dangerous degree. With the entry of more women into medicine, one might postulate that the same problems will arise but that there will be sexual reversal of this classic theme.

Under certain circumstances, you may have little recourse but to unilaterally terminate your relationship with the patient. Among the situations that may justify the discharge of a patient are abusive treatment of you by the patient; continued refusal to pay bills when you have used all reasonable means to collect; when the disease from which the patient suffers is foreign to your expertise; repeated failure of the patient to follow your advice; excessive consultations by the patient with other physicians without your knowledge and consent; incompatibility of personalities; when you desire to limit your practice; and when you retire [49]. You have the obligation, however, to notify the patient in writing (registered mail) that you are discontinuing his or her treatment and to make an effort to supply an appropriate substitute. You should also try to communicate with the patient's family and friends to be sure they understand the reason for your action so that you cannot be accused of abandoning the patient.

THE DYING PATIENT

> *The noise of carriages and carts, the rattle of wheels, the cries of men and boys, all the busy sounds of a mighty multitude instinct with life and occupation, blended into one deep murmur, floated into the room . . . the breaking of the billows of the restless sea of life that rolled heavily on, without. Melancholy sounds to a quiet listener at any time; how melancholy to the watcher of the bed of death!*
> Charles Dickens
> Pickwick Papers (Chap. XLIV)

> *I was born to a lifetime of dying.*
> Henry de Montherlant
> Chaos and Night

> *We are but skin about a wind, with muscles clenched against mortality.*
> Djuna Barnes

The majority of patients in the care of most plastic surgeons are not in the end stage of disease [130]. Exceptions are those with advanced melanoma or malignancy of the head and neck. For the average plastic surgeon, the dying patient presents an unusual therapeutic situation. But no physician, even someone whose specialty is the terminal patient, should become so inured or detached that the demise of his or her patient is seen as a routine event, without significance and tragedy for someone.

This is not the place to present in detail observations such as those of Kübler-Ross [157, 158] and others [231] who have documented the sequence of dying: denial, isolation, anger, bargaining ("If only I can live until my grandson graduates"), depression, and finally acceptance. The point I wish to make is not to let the patient feel grotesque and isolated. Do not allow yourself to be fearful of contact with him or her. The issue is often not so much how a patient can accept the situation but how well the doctor does. For all of us, the clock is ticking; only when we are ill are we aware of its sound.

The fact that we do not have a cure does not render us useless [274]. This is the time to be a physician, not just a doctor [278]. No matter how many times you treat a dying patient, terminal illness never becomes easy, but why should we expect it to be? To help the patient and yourself and to make your efforts more effective, gather the support of the patient's family, good friends, the nurses, the oncologist, other patients, the radiotherapist, the family doctor, and the clergy, if appropriate for that person; however, with those others to help, resist the temptation to run away yourself. If the patient considers you to be his or her doctor for that particular time in life, do not disappoint him or her. Your ability to bring comfort to this person and his or her family will be good preparation for the next dying patient, perhaps ultimately for your own demise, unpleasant as it is to contemplate. The family also can benefit from support groups, which are increasingly available.

In *A Physician Faces Cancer in Himself*, Sanes [231], whose learning experience unfortunately came firsthand, offered advice about dealing with a presumably incurable patient, someone with disseminated cancer. He stressed the value of "competence, compassion, and communication"—desiderata for relating to any patient, not just the very ill. His advice was to be available; be punctual; take time ("One minute sitting down is worth five standing up when speaking to a patient or a member of his family"); be open but not casual, objective but not cold; be warm and concerned; avoid interruptions (e.g., telephone calls); be truthful and honest within the limits of available knowledge; use simple, understandable language, not medical terminology or jargon; avoid expressing your thoughts and emotions in nonverbal forms that may upset the patient or family; if the patient has cancer, say the word and specify the type of cancer; use a printed sheet or a diagram to help get the message across; do not try to give all the information at once; listen to the questions that family members ask and then answer them to the best of your ability; see that the family gets information and advice about nonmedical problems that may arise as a result of the patient's cancer; give the family your telephone number; assure them that you will not abandon the patient and them for the duration of the illness and beyond. Be prepared to repeat in the future some of what you have said during the first interview and to expand on it; acquaint the family about new developments, including changes in treatment and reasons for them; keep your promises to the patient and family; do not get angry if asked about a new proven or unproven treatment or procedure reported in the press or elsewhere and whether it could be applicable to the patient's case; do not get angry if a friend of the family intervenes; provide encouragement and support and preserve hope as far as possible.

Although cheerfulness is desirable, avoid humor that may be decidedly inappropriate and even cruel. Telling jokes to someone who has only a short ration of days improves neither their state of mind nor your image as a physician and friend. Occasionally, you may be using humor as a way of preventing the person from making you deal with the central, hard issues. Remember that the patient wants you to be there; whereas your desire may be to escape.

In discussing Tolstoi's classic *The Death of Ivan Ilych*, Trilling's [261] commentary is also memorable:

> Tolstoi does not reconcile us to the idea of our extinction and he does not mask the dreadfulness of dying. Quite the contrary—not only does he choose an instance of death that is long, drawn out and hideously painful . . . but he emphasizes the unmitigated aloneness of the dying man, the humiliation of his helplessness, and his abject terror at the prospect of his annihilation, as well as his bitter envy of those who still continue in existence while he is in the process of becoming nothing.

Although we physicians may be as helpless as the patient in thwarting death, we should be there to diminish the patient's loneliness and fear. Although we may not know always what to say, we certainly have our ears with which to listen.

THE PATIENT AND THE LAW

> *Law is not justice and a trial is not a scientific inquiry into truth. A trial is the resolution of a dispute.*
> Edison Hanes

> *Lawyers spend a great deal of time shoveling smoke.*
> Justice Oliver Wendell Holmes, Jr.

This heading could be the title of a text, which it deserves [224], but for purposes here, I wish to discuss only a few aspects.

Undoubtedly, malpractice suits would be rare if medical treatment met the expectations of every patient [125, 139]. The reality is cruelly different. The fact that most people in the United States believe that anyone can sue anyone else has resulted in the popularity of that indoor sport: going to court. A generation ago, a common saying was, "Go ahead, sue me! It's a free country." Today only a fool would utter such a statement. Since only one side usually wins, not all suits are victorious (or meritorious) and, in the case of physicians, more are acquitted than are found guilty. Presumably, the better the doctor-patient relationship, the less the likelihood of legal action [205]. Even with the best possible performance by a physician, however, an occasional patient will feel injured, wronged, overcharged, or undergratified. The only way to avoid a malpractice suit against you professionally is to relinquish being a doctor, a course so defensive and distasteful that few physicians, unless close to retirement or uncontrollably angry and almost self-destructive, will take. Just as cars have bumpers, so do doctors have malpractice insurance. No matter how carefully you select your patients and perform their operations, no one is immune from an occasional legal tussle with an unhappy patient and a willing attorney. Although it would be unwise to live in constant fear of a lawsuit, it is reasonable to take some measures to prevent a court action. Throughout this book I have tried to indicate those situations in which the behavior of a doctor can negatively affect his or her relationship with the patient. At any time, but especially at certain strategic junctures, the interaction can deteriorate. Unwise things can be done or said in the operating room or in a fit of irritability or fatigue. Proper patient selection, competent treatment, and careful record keeping are important practices in helping one avoid the halls of justice. The trick is to be careful, without becoming compulsive and paranoid, in dealing with patients. One would not wish to become a fretful physician, viewing each patient as potentially malevolent. Gone would be the pleasure of medicine and the delights of doctoring. However, hard hats are worn on construction jobs and precautions must be taken by every physician.

In the section on the dissatisfied patient, I have discussed specific measures to restore a crumbling alliance. Every human activity has its dangers and being a patient or a doctor is no exception. Even though the incidence of lawsuits has increased, it is still not an ordinary event for most physicians, although the concern with its possible occurrence is pervasive. Most doctors have a strong sense of its presence in the background—an unfailing source of disquiet.

I admit that when I open my mail and I note on the envelope the name of an attorney, I am aware of my well-functioning, sympathetic nervous system.

Gorney [121] has given ten commandments for minimizing risks of suits for malpractice.

1. Thou shalt attempt to understand thy patient.
2. Thou shalt listen to thy patient.
3. Thou shalt not "sell" thy trade.
4. Thou shalt treat thy patient as thyself.
5. Thou shalt own up to thy mistakes immediately.
6. Thou shalt not operate when in doubt.
7. Thou shalt not commit thyself to guarantees—stated or implied.
8. Thou shalt seek consultation when in doubt.
9. Thou shalt speak no evil of thy colleague.
10. Thou shalt eschew arrogance.

These dicta, which deserve not only to be remembered but to be followed, have been discussed in various contexts in this book, especially in relation to informing the patient and informed consent. To Gorney's rules should be added that of being cautious when attempting a new and unproven procedure and that of carefully reviewing the nursing notes daily as well as any report by a consultant [125].

Let us consider a few medical situations relating to the law.

Should You Treat Lawyers or Their Close Family in Elective Circumstances?

This question is not so absurd as it may at first seem since some plastic surgeons refuse to render therapy to attorneys or their spouses and children. The reason ostensibly is to avoid a lawsuit, but I believe that the major cause is generalized hostility toward the legal profession and its practitioners. This behavior on the part of physicians is puerile and is as unreasonable as what they consider the behavior of lawyers to be. Regarding all attorneys as enemies is paranoid and harmful thinking that will certainly create or reinforce their antipathy toward medicine. In my experience, lawyers and their families (perhaps they are conscious of the traditional antagonism between the professions) try to be exemplary patients. In fact, their understanding of the limitations of the operative procedure and the impossibility of guaranteeing results facilitates rapport. Of course, with any group—lawyers, teachers, manual laborers, plastic surgeons—some individuals will be difficult patients, and because of their personality traits, not their occupations, should be rejected for elective procedures. As physicians, we know that treating other doctors may not be an easy chore, although the risk of one doctor's suing another is much less than that of a patient outside the medical profession, but it is certainly not unknown.

Should You Treat a Patient Who Has Sued or May Sue a Physician?

Again, you must make your decision on the basis of the individual patient, and I have alluded to this kind of patient on page 256. Your first responsibility is toward the patient, who, in fact, may have been justified in instituting legal proceedings and you, the physician, should not add to his or her misery by abstaining from rendering proper care. But, just as that patient has a right to sue, so you have a right not to treat in circumstances other than an emergency.

Should You Assiduously Avoid Involvement in Any Malpractice Suit on Behalf of Any Defendant or Any Plaintiff?

The obvious answer is that you must decide according to the specific case. The reality is that testifying against another doctor will be an uncomfortable experience and may cause you considerable enmity. But you also have the responsibility of monitoring your profession. If the object of each attorney were to establish the truth, as is supposedly the aim of the judge and the courtroom, your position would be much easier. However, as one distinguished plaintiff attorney told me, "Most lawyers want to win their case and will do so in any way. They justify their actions by saying that it is for the good of their client. Truth is a happy by-product but do not be surprised if it gets lost in the scuffle." Some physicians refuse to go to court even to present testimony on behalf of a patient whom they have treated after facial trauma. They do not consider that presentation of their findings and management as part of their duty to the patient. Some doctors even request that the patient sign a form releasing them from court appearances. Although one might empathize with such an attitude, it does seem extreme. It may also not be legally binding. Furthermore I believe that a patient deserves my recounting his or her physical examination and treatment, either by letter (preferably) or in court should the need arise. Often this information can be obtained by a deposition in your office. It can also be subpoenaed.

Like most human beings, physicians will fight for some things and not for others. I do not like to wait in line at a restaurant but I will for a good movie. Some physicians will exert themselves in the legal arena whereas they will not exert themselves to write a paper or do research. One thing is certain: Whatever you decide, be prepared.

Sobering is the remark by Oscar Wilde to the effect that because "a man is willing to die for a cause, it does not make it right."

Cartwright has stated that the reasons for doctors getting sued are "prescribing the wrong medicines, performing the wrong procedures, misdiagnosing the patient's problem." [38]

Kahn, a plaintiff's attorney, has concluded that "the greatest clinical errors occur when doctors try to do something that's beyond their competence or experience. Surgeons in particular can fall into this trap [147]." To keep things in perspective with regard to our specialty, it is interesting that pregnancy and birth are the leading source of claims against anesthesiologists; but cardiac respiratory arrest is the most expensive. Fractures are a significant problem for emergency room physicians, with leg fractures among the most common causes of claim and spinal fractures the most expensive. Myocardial infarction is the most significant area of concern for lawsuits in family practice and general practice. For general surgeons the leading causes of suit are cholecystitis and other conditions relating to the gall bladder, breast and colon cancer, and inguinal hernia operations.

The internist has to be wary of misdiagnosis of myocardial infarction as well as lung, breast, and colon cancer [205]. Neurosurgeons and orthopedic surgeons enter the courtroom as a result of their operations on the spine. For obstetricians and gynecologists, as we know, pregnancy and delivery constitute the highest risk, followed by tubal ligations and hysterectomies. Failure in diagnosing meningitis will likely bring an attorney into the office of a pediatrician, and the urologist as well as his or her patients may have anguish after prostatectomy. For the otolaryngologist, the most expensive claims come from submucous resection. But not even the pathologist is free: Misdiagnosis of malignant melanoma may wrest him or her from the autopsy room to blink under the piercing lights of the courtroom. The leading area of malpractice suits for our specialty is esthetic surgery, the breasts being the legal minefield, especially reduction mammoplasty and subcutaneous mastectomy which, since fewer are now being done, have lost some of their malpractice potential.

From my experience in talking to other surgeons and in realizing how I could avoid, and probably did avoid, litigation the matter of finances is extremely important. It is the obvious fuse that can detonate with unwanted and catastrophic results for the surgeon.

IF YOU ARE SUED

To some lawyers, all facts are created equal.
Justice Felix Frankfurter

The stress of a law suit for doctors is now being recognized for what it is: A major negative element in one's life—approaching the stress of a divorce and almost that of a death. [283, 287] From interviews of sued physicians, about 40 percent viewed the process as the "single most stressful event in their lives."

We older physicians have had the pleasure of having our word relatively uncontested until quite recently [37]. Not only to be singled out publicly for presumed negligence but to be vilified in court and to stand in the docket being accused of character defects that we think we do not have—avarice, ignorance, indifference, selfishness—all this can easily prove too much for one's physical and mental equilibrium. As one colleague remarked, "If the charges are false, then one becomes almost insane from anger; if they are true, one almost dies of shame." There are some situations in which no doctor can ever win and the courtroom is one—even the physician who is judged the victor does not emerge from the arena unscathed. The worse consequence of the ordeal is to view every future patient not only with distrust but even hostility, sometimes poorly disguised. Even though this reaction is irrational, it does happen.

Studies have shown that those who have had to run the gauntlet of a malpractice claim tended to initiate practice changes such as ordering more diagnostic tests, using more outside consultants, and involuntarily excluding certain types of patients from treatment [44]. Not surprisingly, these physicians were also likely to discourage their own children from going into medicine. The once-sued physicians believe that the more time they spend with patients, the greater protection they have against litigation, and they tend to avoid high-risk procedures because of perceiving these as inducements to litigation. These are reasonable assumptions and courses of action.

From a practical point of view, the physician who is sued should seek support groups, consisting of other physicians who have gone through the same ordeal. Many insurance companies, hospitals, and medical societies have established this network. In addition, if the legal battle infringes into one's personal life, disrupting the family and even threatening to sever marriage bonds, psychotherapy, perhaps family therapy, should be sought. That we physicians are tardy to recognize our own medical problems needs no elaboration here. To recognize our emotional problems is even a greater task for us as a group. We tend to deny problems and to suddenly admit their existence and impulsively seek their correction. Unfortunately, some physicians who have been sued and who may have been somewhat unstable emotionally prior to the suit have chosen suicide as the way out—certainly not a course of treatment that they would have recommended to any patient in the same situation.

In short, being sued will undoubtedly alter one's perspective professionally and personally; hopefully the change and the disruption will be of manageable dimensions.

Having gone through a courtroom scene myself (and having described it fully and painfully elsewhere [95]), I can offer this advice: Try to think of yourself still as a worthwhile person and a needed physician—obviously easier to say and write than to do.

5
Stages in the Professional Life of the Plastic Surgeon

> *I observe the physician with the same diligence, as hee the disease.*
> John Donne
> *Devotions* (1603)

> *From inability to let well alone: from too much zeal for what is new and contempt for what is old; from putting knowledge before wisdom; science before art and cleverness before commonsense; from treating patients as cases and from making the cure of the disease more grievous than its endurance, Good Lord, deliver us.*
> Sir Robert Hutchinson
> (Cited in *Proc. R. Soc. Med.* 64 : 1038, 1971)

Throughout this book I have described and discussed the interaction between the patient and the plastic surgeon with numerous examples of when and how this bonding can be strengthened, weakened, or never achieved. In this chapter my purpose is to focus on the plastic surgeon and his or her professional life course [238, 262].

Shakespeare described seven ages of man. The reader will excuse my presenting only four ages of the plastic surgeon. The earliest encompasses the years of residency; the next, the period after residency, when new surgeons, to be successful, must *unlearn* part of their training; then comes the middle stage when the plastic surgeon is usually successful if ever he or she is to be successful; the final stage is when seniority comes, hopefully not senility, when other adaptive demands must be met. Always there is change, sometimes subtle, sometimes startling and ferociously demanding.

I would definitely suggest that every physician and surgeon whatever his or her specialty read Ward's [265] thoughts and recommendations about the earliest years as a consultant plastic surgeon. He describes the multiple roles and functions of a person who heads a unit, but, in truth, these are embodied to some degree in every plastic surgeon's professional life: the surgeon, the doctor (treating the patient as a totality), manager and administrator (office staff, residents, hospital personnel), advertiser and promoter (talking about one's work and that of associates in lectures, articles, even simple conversation), teaching and research (other members of the staff, perhaps residents and medical students), confidant and friends (not just patients but to other colleagues), visionary (going beyond one's predecessor's views), and the family and extracurricular man or woman.

The great French surgeon, Dupuytren, feared most "mediocrity." He lived in such a way personally and professionally to ensure that it never entrapped him. A century later another Frenchman, Marcel Proust, whose father and brother were physicians, made an observation that is at once sad and terrifying: "We end up doing whatever we do second best." There is a spectrum (perhaps even spectra) of personalities among plastic surgeons, as among all people, few of which, in my experience, will settle for second best. Most of us try energetically to resist it; however, what we think of ourselves and where we think we stand may be quite different from what others perceive.

My observation is that many residents, by the time they have finished their long years of training, have lost steam and want an existence that is materially adequate without being overly stressful. These are not by themselves unreasonable desires, but one would have expected them to have accomplished more. The choice is obviously each person's to make.

THE EARLIEST STAGE

A few pages cannot possibly do justice to that şingular period in a physician's life: his or her residency. For purposes here, I will focus on the residency in plastic surgery. Like the residency years that preceded it, usually in general surgery, training in plastic surgery places the resident in a half-slave, half-free status. If a word association game was conducted with "residency" as a stimulus, I expect that the most immediate responses would be "work," "work," "more work." The second would likely be "fatigue." If one were to probe below and beyond the work and fatigue inevitably associated with a residency, one would get to what Polk has written about in his ferociously cynical yet useful *The Medical Student's Survival Guide* [209]: "All physicians—in training—exhibit insecurity to one degree or another. What underlies this insecurity? Ignorance. The cure? Knowledge. . . ."

All of us who were residents can recall with ease, and with some humor admixed with a bit of pain, the many situations that have been impressed on our mind in which we acted perhaps appropriately or more often inappropriately, because we simply did not know what to do. Usually this occurred in an emergency when there was no time to consult with someone senior and more experienced. When residents get together, they usually talk less of their triumphs than of their defeats when the "chief" found them wanting and either granted them mercy or administered a verbal lashing. Now we recollect these events with the fondness that has replaced the fear that we felt at the time.

Obviously, residents are by definition inexperienced and ignorant. After residency ignorance may still prevail, but somehow with more experience, we are apt to forget how ignorant we really are. During residency, our deficiencies are brought home to us, if not by our observations, then by the willing comments of our mentors, our peers [31, 32], or others in the hospital where we trained, most particularly nurses.

That learning can be tiring and painful is well illustrated by the residency, but that it can also be pleasant, even joyous, is also true. Camaraderie is probably the strongest during residency when the "we are all in it together" feeling is mutually shared.

At the present time more people want to become plastic surgeons than there are residencies to make this wish possible. Whether or not the attraction of plastic surgery is due to the intrinsic value of our field or to the tangible rewards because much of plastic surgery will not be covered by insurance is hard to determine. I am not sure that those who enter a plastic surgical residency have a clear idea of how much the material advantages, if they truly exist, have affected their choice of this specialty.

Since many plastic surgical residencies still require four or five years of general surgical training before entry, those who make their way into a plastic surgical residency are very senior. Their adjustment is to put themselves in almost an intern–junior resident frame of mind to begin learning a new area of medicine and surgery. They have clawed their way up the ladder, only to find that they must work their way upward again, either during a two-year or three-year stint. Much of the training in general surgery, though applicable in certain situations and valuable with regard to concepts, is not particularly useful if the immediate operative challenge in plastic surgery is considered. For example, one now takes small, even bites of tissue when suturing, a disideratum that was not important in general surgery. One has to think small rather than big: How the incision heals becomes as important in plastic surgery to the patient and to the surgeon as survival after a cardiac transplantation becomes to the recipient and the cardiac surgeon. The end point is not survival in plastic surgery but utility, and in much of plastic surgery, not even that; it is appearance. This takes a shifting of mental gears, which many trainees find difficult, and a few, even impossible. If a resident in plastic surgery wishes to succeed, he or she must give as much importance to what colleagues in other fields consider "trivial" as he or she once did to what everyone considered major, e.g., a successful colectomy, a liver transplant, or acute management of a gunshot wound to the neck.

For the resident in plastic surgery, the swashbuckling days are over. Delicacy replaces machoism, whether the resident is male or female. The exhilaration felt after bringing the patient back from the brink of death is much less experienced in plastic surgery than it was when a resident was in general surgery. By the final year of training, the resident in plastic surgery chafes at the bit; it is time to go, to be free to live one's own life without the supervision and constraint of others. Yet, the resident, now secure in residency, begins to have anxiety about life after residency. Will I make a living? Where do I have to go to make a living? Are there too many plastic surgeons around? Is the Chief of Surgery who controls the whole surgical service going to be sympathetic with plastic surgery? If I go into private practice, will I become an anachronism? If I go into full-time plastic surgery within a university hospital, will I become a public servant, always under the thumb of the chief who sets my income and consequently my family's life-style? During residency, one usually wants more "cases" to do, more operations to perform, more patients of one's own; however, whatever happens during a residency, there is always someone more senior to provide support, to offer advice, and to protect when things go wrong. How one breaks out of residency with regard to establishing independence or dependence will determine much of what that person achieves professionally and within his or her own personal sphere. For the individual who is almost congenitally independent, going into a passive role would be akin to death. On the other hand, for someone who does best when directed, private practice, for example, could be disastrous. The Socratic injunction of "Know thyself," though always valuable, is certainly crucial when making the transition from residency.

The resident today, however, generally has a problem that we who are older did not have: For males, the cultural injunction was for our wives, if we were married, to follow us, to accede to our desires. This is not so today. The spouse may well be male, and there is more clamor for equality in the relationship and in the decision making than existed when I was a resident. Accommodating the desires and preferences of each other may place a significant strain on the relationship or the marriage. This is the time for strains, hopefully no breaks, but it may well entail professional advice (psychotherapy).

Suddenly, it seems, that final day in June arrives when the residency ends and the new stage of life begins. No matter how long the training, one wonders whether he or she is truly prepared for the new professional life. The resident, who has learned from those more experienced, then begins to compare himself or herself with the mentors, who are obviously more experienced but, when they left the residency, were probably relatively just as inexperienced. Now the former resident may actually have to pit himself or herself against his or her teacher, perhaps in the same institution, but, if not, perhaps in the same community. In this situation, the resident, soon to go into practice, receives no handicap.

THE SECOND STAGE: EARLY YEARS IN PRACTICE

Only a mediocre man is always at his best.
W. Somerset Maugham

During the first years after residency, new surgeons, to be successful, must *unlearn* part of their training. Not every facet of a residency is optimal for future performance [136]. The frenzied pace of most training programs forces residents to survive by rushing through tasks and by mastering shortcuts. For example, making rounds and not sitting down in a patient's room is standard procedure. In fact, a recognized ploy is to see patients so early in the morning that they will be too groggy to respond meaningfully to the routine question, "How are you today?" Rare is the surgeon who actually sits by the bedside and lets the patient talk without imparting an impression of having one foot already out the door. Most patients feel guilty about being a nuisance to their harried doctor. From guilt, it is an easy step to anger at the surgeon for not listening and not caring. These sentiments on the part of the patient are usually justified. We surgeons would do well to remember the advice of our great progenitor, Theodore Billroth [24]: "The patient longs for the doctor's daily visits; it is the event upon which all his thoughts and emotions turn. The physician can do all he has to do with speed and precision, but he must never appear to be in a hurry, and never absentminded." The dictum "Stop, look, and listen" has validity beyond the railroad crossing.

Another important difference after residency relates to responsibility. In most training programs, only the chief resident is truly responsible for his or her decisions, but even then, someone is available to share the grief: the head of the service or the staff member attending for that month. Big Brother or Big Sister may have been there to watch you but was also there to help you. Some chief residents, more than others, delegate to those junior members tasks and obligations that should be theirs, such as talking to the patient and the family about the coming operation. But on that final day in June, when school is out, when residents shed their student status and cross the Rubicon, it becomes necessary to adapt to the new circumstances of assuming more responsibility for their actions, unless they have chosen a protected environment as a subaltern. Not every young surgeon can accommodate easily to these new demands and expectations. Patients are now more likely to consider him or her as their principal physician during the course of their treatment. Although the young practitioner can get advice, he or she cannot hide in the shadows. An irate patient may forgive a resident who is learning but not a full-fledged surgeon who should know. This accountability has its benefits: The person who can be the target of blame can also receive praise. People will eventually recognize a job well done; the surgeon's status, material and otherwise, will improve. Having helped others, the young practitioner at the same time has helped himself or herself. The ancient Greeks recognized the importance of what psychologists today call positive reinforcement: "When there is no reward, there is no excellence."

The path of the young surgeon (or any doctor) includes pitfalls as well as pleasures [284]. Early in practice surgeons may extend their indications to operate in order to get experience, build a following, and pay the rent. ("A virgin surgeon needs no urgin'.") As residents, they were rewarded for scouting the wards for cases. "The more the better" could be their epithet. Those who supervise residents know that the problem is more to restrain them from the operating room than to urge them toward it. From June, when they finish their training, to a week later in July when they begin their practice, they predictably continue their accustomed behavior. Professional and financial pressures are greater now than during residency. A young surgeon who unwisely commits himself or herself to unwieldy fiscal burdens, such as a grand house with a grander mortgage, is liable to become more indiscriminate, consciously and unconsciously, in patient selection. As the feeling of entitlement increases, the sense of proportion decreases. For the young surgeon and spouse, luxuries become necessities. Perhaps they are following the advice of Oscar Wilde: "Take care of the luxuries; the necessities will take care of themselves." Unfortunately, the epigram may augur poorly for the patient, who may become grist for the prodigal surgeon's mill. Many human beings in other areas of life also have the problem of keeping their ambition and hedonism in moderation and their ideals in focus.

Although I have emphasized some negative aspects of the beginner in practice, strongly positive features of that stage in professional life exist. The most obvious is that new plastic surgeons are young enough to be energetic and enthusiastic. Furthermore, they probably have learned many things that an older plastic surgeon does not know: at the moment, for example, microsurgical techniques for free flap transfer and the many varieties and uses of musculocutaneous flaps. Another significant advantage is that they have more time to devote to being doctors. Because they have fewer patients, theoretically they can remain longer with each one. Since their total professional commitments are less onerous than those of someone who is established, they can engage in patient care with less fragmentation. In short, young plastic surgeons have tremendous potential, but unless they are careful, they may fall victim to what Alfred North Whitehead observed: "Youth is wasted on youth." They must remember that they have chosen a profession in which service is still expected. Helping others, patient by patient, is the most certain way of bringing success to themselves and, incidentally, favor to their profession. Just as a house is built brick by brick, so is a practice. There is no instant Osler or Halsted or Gillies. Overnight stardom is best left to athletics and the performing arts.

During this time, novice practitioners generally take whatever they can get, without precise regard to what eventually will become their pattern of practice. Obviously some plastic surgeons confine themselves from the outset to just microsurgery; others, to cranial facial surgery; but most do a variety of operations if only to pay the rent and feed the family. As mentioned earlier, a survey by the American Society of Plastic and Reconstructive Surgeons reported that the typical practice of its members is about 60 percent reconstructive and 40 percent esthetic, almost the same ratio as a survey four years earlier demonstrated. During this time, however, the young plastic surgeon who may be looking for patients and is not in a setting where he or she automatically gets patients, as in an established clinic or Health Maintenance Organization, may consider advertising as a way of stimulating the inflow. In a recent survey of the American Society for Aesthetic Plastic Surgery, about 30 percent of vendors displayed an ad in the yellow pages, something beyond the standard listings [3]. About 15 percent used direct mailing and another 20 percent used newspaper, magazine, radio, or television ads, or a combination to increase the number of patients. The decision regarding advertising is not simply a fiscal or professional one; it is a reflection of the plastic surgeon's personality and concept of what he or she would like to be or thinks he or she is. Once one advertises, another Rubicon is crossed. The advertiser has made a statement not only about himself or herself but about how he or she wishes to be in relation to colleagues [101]. In some communities, advertising is an anathema; in others, it is an expected routine; however, advertising is still an act that is noticed by one's associates, who are more likely to remember the ad than are the patients whom one wanted originally to notice it. Although a plastic surgeon who advertises may have similar skills and even a similar background as one who does not advertise, the subsequent professional image will differ, rightly or wrongly. It is quite possible through advertising to establish a bridge to patients but at the same time to burn a bridge to colleagues. That decision is obviously an individual one. What is legal is not always appropriate, as, for example, belching loudly at a banquet. As Wright [282] has noted, "Today, medicine encompasses far more than healing, saving, and serving. It has become a commodity, and consumer demands have grown beyond reasonable expectations. Furthermore, the current concept of medical care is beyond the physician-patient relationship; it now involves society and the community as a whole." All this must be kept in mind by every physician, every plastic surgeon.

THE MIDDLE STAGE

Heaven defend me from a busy doctor.
Welsh Proverb

After having been in practice 10 to 20 years, the plastic surgeon is probably in the full flush of his or her profession. Better known and more in demand, he or she now has the problem not of getting patients but of treating them properly. Great is the temptation to operate on more patients than would be wise because of a feeling of invincibility, that one's experience has been so extensive and one's skills so remarkable that nothing can possibly go wrong [92]. This type of thinking is an occupational disease associated with upward surgical mobility. To manage the large influx of patients, the surgeon may add systems and personnel that may hinder his or her connection with the patient. Enlarging the office and taking on one or more associates are part of the picture of growing bigger but not necessarily better. Where is that careful and considerate doctor of yore? As we rake in the money, we may also be raking in the patients, as if they were leaves. In some offices, for example, the receptionist may greet the patient, and a secretary may take information (address, age, occupation, insurance coverage) and obtain a history. A computer may even do the questioning or the patient may be asked to fill out a questionnaire. Later, a technician may take blood and ask for a urine sample or do an electrocardiogram. During this process, the patient may justifiably wonder, "Is there a doctor in the house?" In the name of efficiency, the system has been fabricated presumably so the doctor can treat more people more competently. The paradox is that although the doctor gains in time, the quality of his or her relationship with the patient may suffer. The patient is receiving adequate care but inadequate caring. Even in this age of acceleration, the interaction between the physician and patient, in order to be worthwhile, must take time. In the "olden days" (as my children refer to my youth, but actually, long before), the doctor-patient relationship was strong possibly because almost everything else was weak. Hospitals were nonexistent or primitive; nursing, pharmacology, and the knowledge of disease and the body mechanisms were comparatively rudimentary; surgery was the last resort and the most dangerous. The doctor, his skills, and his presence were the cornerstone of medicine. Now with more support, such as better nursing, better surgery, and better-trained colleagues, the individual doctor has become only part of the medical picture. He or she must fight to maintain position on the stage. Crowding but helping the doctor and patient are platoons of people—secretaries, receptionists, technicians, orderlies, other doctors, social workers, dietitians, respiratory-occupational-physical therapists—and this list is incomplete. The permeation of urban culture into almost every area of the United States and most Western societies has diluted the sense of mutual responsibility. Commitments of family members to each other are sadly tenuous and unenthusiastic. The young wish to live alone and leave the old to die alone. "Doing your own thing" and "taking care of numero uno" are trite phrases for a virulent disease that has infected medicine and has weakened the special bonding between doctor and patient. But nostalgia for what was is a futile indulgence since that era is gone forever. Even if we could have it back, would we want it? Would we wish to be once again without anesthesia, antibiotics, or vaccines?

Returning to the busy doctor's office of today, one might question whether taking the blood, obtaining an electrocardiogram, and removing sutures help the relationship between doctor and patient. Although it is impossible to designate a specific act as "the one" that a doctor should do, the reality of the therapeutic ambience exists. "The laying on of hands," ancient in traces, still is a potent emotional derivative for the patient and the physician. Physical contact with the patient—shaking hands, an arm around the shoulder, taking out stitches—brings the patient and doctor closer together. Consider the banal matter of dressings. For centuries, much has been written about their many functions and attributes; rarely mentioned, however, is that the act of applying, removing, or changing a dressing is an important focal point in the doctor-patient relationship and has ritualistic significance. The patient is usually more aware of the subtleties involved than is the physician. Respect for the dressing is respect for the patient and your craft.

Is the dressing neat, comfortable, and effective? Does it annoy the patient by repeatedly falling off? In the hospital, do you change the dressing initially or do you manage to avoid the task by relegating it to a nurse or resident? Do you give the impression to the patient and the staff that caring for the dressing is really beneath your position or beyond your time? If you do change the dressing, is it with gentleness and calmness? Or do you rush into the patient's room, abruptly turn on the lights, pull down the bedclothes, and rip off the dressing without a prelude of conversation or explanation? Are you careful about your aseptic technique when indicated? Do you then use sterile gloves? (It is interesting how many patients seem to remember more about Lister's precepts than do their doctors.) Do you have all your supplies ready or do you have to interrupt the procedure several times to get what you need? A disorganized, heavy-handed performance in changing a dressing would logically leave the patient wondering how carefully you did the operation.

Surgeons who see more patients than their skills and time can encompass will take the easy ways. Something has to go, and, unfortunately, it may be not just their dressings but their standards. The concern, compassion, and competence that brought them to the rung of the "successful" may soon be jettisoned. No longer are they what they were or what they should be. Because labels stick for a long time, a few years may have to pass before one's halo is noticeably faded. By then, the way back may be impossible because there is too much relearning to do.

Admittedly, some patients, comparatively few, do not mind that the doctor has spent minimal time with them. They are content to bathe in the reflected narcissism of their doctor—to delight in the physician's aura of success, as if his or her status will magically protect them against illness or guarantee the success of an operation. These patients find consolation in the elaborate "setup" of their doctor's office, which, for them, is evidence of favor with the gods.

For the discerning patient, however, the doctor has become a medical businessperson, marketing charm and competence without truly caring, still perhaps able to focus skills on the procedure but not capable of sustaining important medical duties. When a complication occurs, the doctor may instinctively hide behind secretaries, nurses, and assistants, who now become two-legged barriers to the patient. Now "all that glitters is not gold"; the parade, once resplendent, has turned into a dismal spectacle. Little wonder that with the scene soured, the patient may contemplate legal recourse.

The predicament of today's doctor in mid-career is the complexity and range of necessary activity—from office to home, and back and forth from one hospital to the next; the financial realities of maintaining a place of practice as well as a residence and family; the voraciousness of the paper tiger—unending forms and correspondence; the medicolegal specter; and the need to stay informed and to deal successfully and sympathetically, if possible, with thousands of patients, some on an emergency basis. Having more, doing more, but enjoying it less could be the slogan of our age. Busy doctors bolting from one commitment to another fit too well into today's tableau. In those air-conditioned cars, do they enjoy life as doctors or as human beings more than their predecessors did who visited their patients in horse-drawn buggies? Although individually we cannot do much to change our times, we can do something to modify our schedule. We must learn to protect ourselves from the superabundance of stimuli: noise, media, telephones, insurance forms, meaningless committee work. Henry David Thoreau's comment is pertinent: "It is not enough to be busy . . . the question is: what are we busy about?"

How many patients can we see and manage optimally? When the "successful" plastic surgeon begins to make mistakes or feels like a short-order cook, then it is time to pull back although it would have been better to have done so before [75]. The management of success is often more difficult than its acquisition [77].

Physicians have another problem. We are not like the painter who can discard a shoddy canvas. A mistake for us is also a mistake for somebody else, with possible lethal consequences. That Ted Williams once batted over .400 was astounding for a ballplayer, but not good enough for a physician and a patient.

Adding to the perplexity of maintaining the "human touch" with those who should be our intimates is the fact of specialization. Within the specialty of plastic surgery, there has been subspecialization. Fewer surgeons are doing a wide range of plastic and reconstructive surgery. Although many might complain about this trend, few can deny it. The phenomenon is related not only to the complexity of medicine and to the availability of more plastic surgeons, but also to the medicolegal climate in our country. Venturing beyond one's skills is not only dangerous for the patient but for ourselves from a malpractice standpoint.

A surgeon who repeats one procedure more often becomes increasingly adept at that procedure and less sure in other undertakings. This cycle reinforces the trend to doing more in a narrow range.

Furthermore, a conscious choice to treat what is more financially rewarding will provide another incentive to restrict one's focus. The longer a surgeon is in practice, the more limited his or her spectrum. The point soon comes when he or she can no longer do well or easily all the procedures that were familiar at the end of residency. In addition, new procedures will evolve for which he or she perhaps can never be trained, for example, microsurgical transfer of tissue and craniofacial surgery. The reality is that where one puts one's energies and maintains a high profile becomes the focal point of patient referral. Someone who gives numerous lectures on head and neck surgery is unlikely to receive referrals for hypospadias repair or for breast augmentation.

The danger of extreme specialization is the likelihood of our becoming technicians rather than remaining plastic surgeons or physicians, and there is the hazard—subtle at first, but pronounced later—of having arrested growth. By doing less and less more and more, doctors will only be able to do less later. They may be priming themselves for mental and spiritual obsolescence. If a physician has been so unwise and unlucky as to be known for only one procedure, which one does to the exclusion of others, what will happen if it should go out of style—like the mastoid operation of years ago? Will that surgeon have the will and the breadth to retread his or her cerebral hemispheres?

A few words about the operation itself are necessary, since the plastic surgeon in this mid-career stage will be doing the greatest number of procedures. As we know but like to forget, the operating room may be the arena for spectacular mistakes. A poorly planned or poorly performed operation can be devastating for the patient as well as for the surgeon. The young surgeon makes errors through ignorance and inexperience; the older surgeon errs from carelessness.

Although it is true that bad preoperative and postoperative management can ruin a good operation, rarely can a bad operation be transformed into a good one by bedside attention. This is particularly the case in plastic and reconstructive surgery, in which results depend directly on excellent technique. When the surgeon carries out the procedure in the operating room, it should not be for the first time. The operation should have been done in the mind's eye before, perhaps in the office but certainly in the 12 hours prior to operation, if the case is elective. The design of the flap, the type of immobilization, the availability of blood and proper equipment—considerations of this sort should not be left to happenstance. The ability to ad lib may lend a virtuoso quality to our field, but it should never replace tactical thinking. No operation is truly minor, but thinking that it may be is too common among busy, established surgeons, who have earned the treacherous label "successful."

If the patient is in satisfactory condition, no operation should be terminated until it has been done as well as possible. Boredom, fatigue, or the pressing schedule of an overcommitted surgeon should not compromise standards. A result that looks just fair at operation will generally look worse in the office. If a final glance discloses a remediable fault, we should not be reluctant to heed our assessment. A few more minutes can make a startling difference. Time spent then is more worthwhile than apologies and explanations later. Stitches are not sacred; they should be removed and replaced until the desired result is achieved. Michelangelo wisely commented, "Trivials make perfection but perfection is not trivial."

During the operation, the surgeon must never lapse into a cavalier and complacent attitude, but must be attentive to many things, including possible breaks in asepsis. You must check all solutions before using them, and communicate with the anesthesiologist about vital signs and changes in head and body position. At the end of the case, take the time to assess the result objectively; do not let your efforts and energies peter out and trust your reputation to gloss over imperfections. The great operation you might have done last week or two hours ago is irrelevant. It is what you are doing now that counts, for that patient presently in your care.

Concluding the case with the operation is a common folly, observed more among older surgeons than those just beginning practice [100]. In reality, the operation is not finished until the patient has been discharged from the surgeon's care. The hit-and-run technique has no place in surgery. Concern for the patient and his or her problems should not fade from consciousness as soon as the surgeon has applied the dressing (or is he or she too busy to do it or to supervise it?). Careful observation, detailed orders, and clear instructions are obviously critical. Those of us who are blessed with residents should not abrogate our responsibility. We should know, for example, when the patient has pain or some other complaint. We should also be fully aware of the patient's medications, vital signs, and laboratory data. Our standards should not go down with the setting sun. If a dressing or splint warrants removal, it should be done as quickly at night as during the day. The "wait for the morning" attitude may be effective for growing crocuses but not for managing patients.

Another frequent error, discussed earlier, is the attempt to be the bionic surgeon—know all, do all. If a situation presents problems beyond our usual ken, we should be quick to use consultants *before* the patient asks or a tragedy eventuates—not just to keep clean medicolegally but, more important, to ensure the patient the best treatment. Those who consult or refer early seldom need to repent later.

Another fault of many surgeons, particularly those with crowded schedules, is to follow up with a non–follow-up. Surgeons who fail to observe their patients long enough and carefully enough will lose a valuable chance to learn and to improve. In contrast, one who believes in extended, thorough observation will behold many things that are sometimes wondrous, occasionally painful, but always instructive. A year later the revised scar that initially looked so disappointing will have improved miraculously. In this hard world, the reverse is also true. The rhinoplasty that appeared "perfect" at six months can end up with many imperfections. It is always tempting to quit while ahead: to discharge the facelift patient, for example, when she is rejuvenated and grateful but only for a few months after surgery. If we truly wish to better our performance and to know our patients' reactions to their operations, we should follow them closely and objectively for a few years. During this time we must be genuinely committed to learning; we must not fit new facts into old impressions.

Every surgeon must beware of the sinister saboteur of good deeds: fatigue. An operation is a series of interdigitating sequential acts, whose quality depends on the soma and psyche of the surgeon, as well as those of the patient. This aspect of the doctor-patient relationship has been discussed before. The point for emphasis is that

5 Stages in the Professional Life of the Plastic Surgeon

the overworked, overstressed, or drug or alcohol dependent surgeon [124] does himself or herself little good and may do the patient considerable harm. It would seem logical for us to try to keep fit physically and emotionally for our daily performance. Athletes do, and their errors, though disappointing to spectators, rarely kill anyone. Patients, in fact, are very much aware of the health and habits of their doctors. Many patients in the hospital have said to me on afternoon rounds, "Get a good night's sleep, doctor." Or, even more explicit, "No partying tonight," with a nervous laugh. The statement that I am a teetotaler may provide reassurance if I am believed.

During the middle years—the most successful years—in practice, physicians, and plastic surgeons are no exception, undertake more than they should. Ottenberg [198] noted:

> A popular definition of executive is 'someone who has lost control of his/her time.' In this respect, many physicians qualify as executives. With their compliance, their secretaries have taken control of their time. The secretary divides the doctor's day, starting with the breakfast meetings; clinical appointments; teaching; conferences; possibly, a session with the community council or committee; a hasty snack, if there is time to eat anything at all; then more patients, well into early evening meeting or class. . . . Physicians who hold a number of occupational posts live on a treadmill. Moonlighting is an economic necessity early in their careers, but continuing to maintain two to four occupational positions, is common for doctors. . . . Treadmill living usually is rationalized early in the career, with periodic extensions of rationalization. This last, the doctor tells himself/herself, 'only until . . . (I feel secure in my private practice) (I am promoted in the department) (I obtain my own research grant).' The sad truth is that 'this' becomes a permanent way of life which escalates according to Parkinson's Law. Income rises, promotions occur, professional recognition is forthcoming—but demands on one's time keep expanding. What is the ultimate effect on the self-perception and on the attitude toward self-health of the physician who works 60–80 hours a week through the long years?

Ottenberg [198] again points out:

> Unscheduled time, especially quiet hours for creative efforts, time to be tolerant of crisis, and time for sociability, disappear in the production machine. The family receives only the tired father or mother—the overworked and often threatened physician who surfaces occasionally in the guise of 'successful' provider and careerist. . . . Too often the physician who is a parent is given recognition as the source of numerous 'advan-

tages.' In the family, there is decreasing satisfaction from providing more and more luxury that is devoid of meaningful personal participation. Many physicians subsidize trips abroad for their children when what may be needed is psychiatric evaluation and, possibly, psychotherapy. The grand tour sometimes precedes the grand emotional blowup. A circular process occurs, in which the professional parent works hard to pay for the luxury trip to take the emotional place of his/her absence, and succeeds only in increasing demand for more precocious spending.

This cycle is harder to get off for many plastic surgeons in the middle years than is the bicycle. More breeds more and the pace fails to slow. This is the time when plastic surgeons, if married and not careful, may forget their spouse for the near at hand, the available nurse or colleague or, unfortunately, patient, the last situation the most dangerous for the physician–plastic surgeon and, more importantly, the patient. The culmination in self-destruction reflects many things, not least of which is the loss of perspective. It is hard to get perspective when one is running all the time.

THE LAST STAGE

> *The young man knows the rules, but the old man knows the exceptions.*
> Oliver Wendell Holmes
> The Young Practitioner in *Medical Essays*

> *When I was young, patients were afraid of me; now that I am old, I am afraid of patients.*
> Johanna Peter Frank
> (Quoted by F. H. Garrison in *Bull. N.Y. Acad. Med.* 5 : 157, 1929)

> *Everyone has talent at 25. The difficulty is to have it at 50.*
> Edgar Degas

> *I have had just about all I can take of myself.*
> S. H. Behrman at 75

The surgeon who has attained seniority has privileges, for example, sitting in the front row at rounds, calling the heads of services by their first names, getting desirable operating time. Although not yet Dr. Chips, he or she may already be the topic of anecdotes among residents and nurses. He or she has become a parent and perhaps even a grandparent figure sooner than expected. Each July the senior plastic surgeons see others starting as they did 25 to 35 years ago. From an Olympian perch, he or she experiences a new calmness when viewing the hurly-burly below. Though grateful for no longer having to shove, nevertheless, he or she misses the scent and sweat of the fray. "This is for the young," is a consoling thought. With intellect more than emotions, the older physician tries to accept nature's cycle: youth replacing the elderly until they in turn must go. If the senior surgeon is wise, he or she will ease the way for youth or, at least, not try to impede its march. Fighting the inevitable will demean him or her, and colleagues will remember that person at the end rather than as he or she had been during the previous three decades. Most of us have seen or heard of older surgeons trying to keep someone from opening a practice in the same city or blocking referrals or denying operating room time. These acts are foolish and ultimately futile; they arise from the bitterness and insecurity of knowing that soon he or she must depart from the scene; the hard questions are when and how.

Buddha supposedly said, "Thousands of candles can be lighted from the single candle, and the life of the candle will not be shortened. Happiness never decreases by being shared."

A surgeon's manual skills are his or her professional and economic survival. For the older surgeon, these may have deteriorated to a noticeable degree—a fact that embarrasses him or her and endangers others. In a hospital operating room, he or she is under easy scrutiny. Lapses in performance are more obvious more quickly to more people than they would be in a private office or in one's own surgical facility where the surgeon controls the environment so that he or she cannot be so easily accountable. Furthermore, plastic surgeons cannot hide their handiwork, whereas errors of commission or omission are less obvious in other specialties such as psychiatry or neurology. A bad hand tremor appearing in a sexagenarian is a strong circumstantial evidence of aging as, in Thoreau's words, finding "a trout in the milk."

When an older surgeon makes an error in the operating room, colleagues, especially those younger, may wonder whether he or she is over the hill, forgetting that when they make errors, and younger people certainly do, great allowance is made for them—the promise of their competence is the reason for excusing mistakes by youth; whereas the expectation of deterioration becomes the cause for not making the same allowances when elders err. Many hospitals have a mandatory age for taking away operating room privileges. For an elderly surgeon who can no longer use the hospital facilities, an alternative is to build an outpatient unit, but this is a major financial and emotional commitment, especially at an advanced age. This dilemma may be resolved by joining an established "surgicenter" that is run usually by those younger whom hopefully he or she has not alienated. The essence of being a surgeon is performing operations. The older surgeon, like the old bull at mating time, may try to prove virility surgically and may undertake procedures that are beyond his or her capacity. How disastrous the consequences can be is exemplified by the life of the once-great German surgeon, Ferdinand Sauerbruch, who overstayed his time, to the detriment of himself and the death of others [259].

The older surgeon is usually not so creative as in the past. Older surgeons may have to settle for having their name appear at the end of a list of authors for whom they have provided money and laboratory space. Whereas once they had attracted attention because of their accomplishments, they may now maintain the center of the stage through intimidation. Adding to their problems may be the shameful ingratitude of younger surgeons, some of whom expect instant success, and when it is not forthcoming, they blame the senior surgeon.

The tradition of those older instructing those younger for the benefit of the patient has been one of the most important reasons for the survival of medicine. Competition in the marketplace should not absolve those older from sharing knowledge with those younger, or those younger from respecting their immediate predecessors. This is a lot to expect in our current society, which is notably deficient in its homage to the elderly. Witness the plight of aging parents. Realistically, also, the senior surgeon also has to contend with waning vigor. Nabokov described himself as follows: "Each man as he approaches his sixties, and sometimes even before, goes through a crisis not only of feeling old, but of being afraid of old age, afraid of seeing his powers decline. . . . Old age is a succession of renunciations. It's not so much the fear of the end, but the fear that the end comes in an unpleasant way" [185].

The older surgeon may dread retirement because during a busy professional career, he or she may not have accrued enough interests to be sustaining when not thinking or doing plastic surgery 18 hours a day (and dreaming of it the other 6). Watching the scramble around him or her, the older surgeon may think wistfully of the truth of the French proverb, "If youth knew; if old age could."

The last stage or any segment of a career does not exist by itself, independent of the vicissitudes of the personal life: family, friends (or lack of them), health, achievements, failures, joys, disappointments. Rare is a life that is uncomplicated, a straight, level line without unexpected peaks and troughs. As the ancient philosophers observed, the only constant is flux, a situation that relentlessly demands adaptation for survival. These processes and complexities of living need only acknowledgement here but not repetition since others have described them well already.

Adding to the problems of getting older in a medical career are obviously the problems of getting older. Chronological age sets the standard, even though people may say that it is "not so much how old you are but how old you feel." Inevitably, the two lines bisect. True to the point was Somerset Maugham's comment that "what makes old age hard to bear is not the failing of one's faculties, mental and physical, but the burden of one's memories." Less sanguine about the physical change that beset the elderly, Sir James Paget, whose name is indelibly linked with the diseases of the nipple and bone he described, remarked that "no man over 70 walks with the same pliant . . . step as he walked at 30 or 40; but many, over 70 . . . are not conscious of the change."

But finally the end must come to all plastic surgeons as it does to their patients. What others will say or think about us after we are gone, we will never know. Their thoughts about us now, while we are living, are by no means evident. No obituary can tell the whole story. In that regard, John Rowan Wilson's [280] obituary code, though humorous, is nevertheless sobering and instructive:

> "He did not suffer fools gladly"
>   He was the rudest bastard in miles
> "His surgery was charged with idealism"
>   He took outrageous risks with human life

"He generously encouraged his juniors who benefitted immensely from his sage guidance"
   His juniors did all his work and he took all the credit
"He was a man of Christian principles"
   He was a transparent hypocrite
"He was a connoisseur of fine wines"
   He drank
"He had personal problems"
   He drank secretly
"His wife remained an inspiration all his life"
   God knows how the poor woman stayed with him.

The only obituary that counts is what we write each day by what we do or do not do in every aspect of our life, not just in the operating room.

RUMINATIONS

After reading this book, one might ask the question that a visiting English surgeon put to me at the end of a day in my office and at the hospital, "Is all this patient care really necessary?" Compared to England, doctors in America, he thought, spend inordinate time with their patients (and did far too many tests). In his country, he observed that the patient expects less and probably gets less but likely does not appreciate the difference. The last part of the statement is yet to be documented, but studies have shown that nonoperative professional time expended per patient is less in the British Isles than in the United States [34]. Also in England as on the Continent, doctors are more likely to be authoritarian and the patient to be more compliant and, overtly, less questioning [61]. Few cross-cultural studies exist to supply the needed data on these matters, but with the clamor in America for us in the medical profession to become more like our colleagues in England, Canada, or Sweden, we are likely to be running these experiments in health care ourselves.

   An apparent paradox is that in those countries with some form of corporate or socialized medicine, the pendulum is swinging more to the private sector; whereas, in this country, we appear to be going the other way. Another paradox is that in the United States, where patients receive so much in comparison with other countries, they desire even more, and, more frequently than patients anywhere else, they will go to court if they believe that they have been abused. In the background is the lawyer, whose presence, though vexing and worrisome to the physician, has undoubtedly upgraded the rights of patients and the performance of doctors. It has also been a stimulus to give detailed explanations and explicit instructions to the patient, perhaps to a degree that is excessive and unnecessary, at least according to the standards of some other countries abroad.

Although differences exist in the doctor-patient relationship among technologically advanced countries, they may be insignificant in comparison with the universals, such as concern, compassion, and competence—qualities that positively affect most persons, be they sick or well. Admittedly, changes in the social and economic environment of medicine may create obstacles between patient and physician, but it is unlikely that there will be an interdiction against skill and empathy from the doctor and appreciation for the patient [277]. The importance of health and of those who help to ensure it guarantees that doctoring will not become humdrum and detached the routines in the post office. My optimism arises from the fact that the doctor-patient relationship has remained remarkably intact despite the buffetings of innumerable social changes through many centuries.

A colleague supposedly commented, "When patients go to a plastic surgeon, they want to know only two things: can he or she do it and how much will it cost?" The tenet of this book is that most patients want and deserve more, as we would if we were patients. Providing care without caring is like comparing food capsules to a gourmet meal; the former may provide the calories with a dull efficiency but without any enjoyment. The matter of pleasure and satisfaction is an important consideration. In the long run (and is not a medical career like a marathon?) we, the plastic surgeons, will continue to wither on our professional vine unless we extend ourselves to be more than vendors of services, dispensers of a narrow skill.

If, indeed, Dr. Francis Peabody's [206] dictum is correct, and I believe it is—that "the secret of the care of the patient is caring for the patient"—then how do we promote it or teach it? In fact, can we or should we [275]? That we should seems undeniable if we believe in the value of kindness in human relations and if we recognize that we live not by bread alone. The more difficult question is how to achieve "caring." I realize with temerity that I have strayed from my office to someone else's pulpit, but, at the risk of sermonizing, I wish to offer some thoughts that are not original. To foster concern in human beings for one another is still the primary challenge. The golden rule, honored by words, lies tarnished from disuse. If more noble reasons fail to spur humans to help each other, then perhaps a stimulus more base in the hierarchy of motivation may succeed. Forgive a surgeon's pragmatism, but we who walk upright and possess prehensile thumbs must be taught and must learn that it is in our best self-interest not to be totally selfish. Internalizing the precept is not synonymous with acting in accordance with it. The Italian proverb, "Between the saying and the doing lies the breadth of the sea," is apt here.

Now back to the office. After 12 harried hours of doctoring, when we look in the mirror, where is the concerned youth of yesteryear? In J. B. Priestley's [210] words, "Was the boy the better man?" Somewhere below the concretions of fatigue lies a vestige. Diversion and sleep will usually provide that crucial ingredient that enables us to reenter the medical arena; however, some doctors always place their convenience and needs before the plight of their patients. For those physicians, I recommend forced caring, i.e., consciously exerting oneself to care even though you and the patient may recognize the attempt is not spontaneous. With time, it might become so, but even if it never achieves that status, your efforts will be appreciated. If one cannot radiate warmth, one can at least try for incandescence.

The quality of trying, at least, even though the emotion or action is not automatic, has to do with what some have termed ego strength, courage, or grit. It is indispensable to win ball games, to save marriages, and to help patients.

In Camus's *The Stranger* [36], Meursault is condemned because he "does not play the game" and ultimately is judged guilty largely because of the damaging evidence that he had not wept at his mother's funeral. In Camus's words,

> A much more accurate idea of a character . . . will emerge if one asks just *how* Meursault doesn't play the game. The reply is a simple one: he

refuses to lie. To lie is not only to say what isn't true. It is also and above all, to say *more* than is true, and, as far as the human heart is concerned, to express more than one feels. This is what we all do, every day, to simplify life. He says what he is, he refuses to hide his feelings, and immediately society feels threatened.

In the instance of the doctor and the patient, each would *be* threatened if the other did not do some role playing: saying or acting according to each other's expectations. Camus' antihero ultimately loses his life because of his verbal reluctance and his unwillingness to "play the game." In the practice of medicine, the patient would become the casualty of our gratifying only our own needs and our own feelings all the time.

As physicians, though we may empathize with someone who is ill, the synchrony of our sentiments is only periodic, not continuous. Even then, we really do not experience what hurts and threatens a patient. The Portuguese say, "Only the one with the scar feels it." How rare the physician who named the condition "Christmas disease," in honor of the child first shown to lack clotting factor IX! This act on the part of the doctor is unique, since almost all eponyms glorify those who identify a malady rather than those who have to bear it.

In *The Patients,* Thorwald [260] presents recollections by individuals who underwent pioneering operations for failing organs, such as the heart, lung, and kidney. These were momentous surgical events with obvious heroes and heroines, yet the commonplace crises were epochs in the lives of any patient and his or her family: Ever present are risk, pain, fear, and uncertainty. Whenever I become ill, fortunately rarely, and then only with the "flu," I glimpse the dark world of patients. My uneasy sensations, even thousandfold, do not approximate those of the truly sick. Yet, from that brief episode, I am conscious of being a better physician; unfortunately, I confess, my uplifted state lasts just a few weeks; then I slide back into my usual patterns of doctoring, where I am on the comfortable outside looking in. This distance from the patient is not all bad; it allows us to be objective in our work and to continue without being engulfed by sorrow or revulsion. Yet, as Alan Alda [1], M.A.S.H.'s Hawkeye, said to the graduating class at

Columbia College of Physicians and Surgeons, "You've had to toughen yourself to death. From your first autopsy when you may have been sick, or cried, or just been numb, you've had to inure yourself to death in order to be useful to the living. But I hope in the process you haven't done too good a job of burying that part of you that hurts and is afraid."

As human beings, in our daily lives we usually place the "hows" before the "whys." We are not comfortable trying to resolve existential issues for ourselves. But a patient who is ill is forced to contemplate the monumental questions of death, purpose, meaning—while we, as physicians, at the bedside, or surgeons in the operating room, are busily fixing the body parts.

The Sacred Cow or Sleeping Dog Surgeon

This rather cryptic heading refers to the busy older physician–plastic surgeon who begins to think of himself or herself as too important to be disturbed for emergencies, especially those at night. He or she has caught the Great Man or Great Woman disease, which is dangerous not just for the patient, who has put his or her life in the plastic surgeon's hands, but for the plastic surgeon as well. When you begin to let residents do most of the work, when your nurses or secretaries screen *out* most of the calls, you are being blind to your duties. Soon residents and nurses will be fearful of calling you lest they get assaulted verbally. A problem that was once nascent, now becomes overgrown and perhaps impossible to resolve satisfactorily.

At this stage the plastic surgeon is on the way out when once he or she was on the way up. If an older plastic surgeon does not want to be available, he or she should retire and not remain in the game unless willing to play according to the rules—rules that once the plastic surgeon obeyed so well that it accounted for his or her achievement and present position. Retirement is a better alternative to complacent, shoddy care that results in injury to a patient.

RENEWAL

You, the plastic surgeon, probably came of age to care for patients independently when you were around 33. After another 33 years, your professional life would be nearing its end. In those three decades, you probably will have operated on at least 20,000 patients and will have consulted on at least two or three times that number—equal to a good-sized city's population. Your memory will be stronger for patients for whom things went spectacularly right or dramatically wrong. For the great majority of your patients, where you have given help where it was needed, few traces may remain in your mind; yet those patients likely will recall more about that encounter than you do. Although you intervene for a relatively brief period in the life of that person, you have the opportunity to do considerable harm or good. The impact of your treatment may resound throughout the remainder of that patient's life. In that interaction, you both have the opportunity to broaden your lives by at least one new relationship. Although it is true that like every human being, you may not remain static psychologically, physiologically, or chronologically, from where you sit you are the relatively constant feature in the tableau of patient and physician. The succession of patients is your reason professionally for being. Yet, most blessings on this planet are diluted and this is no exception. The need to turn out the work as well as the passage of years tends to erode enthusiasm. Recall the excitement of your first patient in practice: You tingled for involvement and felt the pleasure of exercising your skills, of helping someone, and of sensing gratitude in return. But after 20, 12, or even 2 years in practice, you experience satisfactions differently: The highs are not so high; however, it would be unfortunate if the pleasures of doctoring belonged only to the novitiate. Pleasures are there also for the seasoned clinician, the old campaigner. The problem, however, is to rekindle the dampened fires of enthusiasm. Ralph Waldo Emerson observed, "Nothing great was ever achieved without enthusiasm." But "great" need not describe only superachievements in medicine: the discovery of the circulation of blood, the importance of asepsis, or the existence of hormones. To be a good doctor to each patient is an important accomplishment. Let one who doubts the value of a good physician experience a bad one! To doctor daily requires renewal. How to "replenish the well," in Winston Churchill's terms, is the quiet challenge for each of us. To do again with joy what we have done many times before can be a task much harder than the medical problem itself. For some physicians, the next patient is a stimulant; for others, a stone. In the latter instance, the relationship between them will be mechanical and drab, perhaps without a scintilla of satisfaction for either. A pertinent story concerns three medieval workmen who were asked what they were doing. The first replied, "I toil from sunup to sundown and all I receive for my pains is a few francs a day." The second answered, "I am glad enough to wheel this wheelbarrow for I have been out of work for many months and I have a family to support." The third replied, "I am building Chartres Cathedral" [237].

Discussion of occupational tedium is usually in reference to factory workers or clerical personnel, but seldom physicians. The public may find it hard to believe that doctors, who have high incomes and still considerable respect (and are even subjects of television series), suffer as do all human beings from boredom and despondency. As a group, physicians are reluctant to express their frustrations. They have trained themselves in stoical tenacity and external imperturbability. *Aequanimitas* has become their byword not only at the bedside of patients but even at their own. Not unexpectedly, in comparison to the general population, physicians comprise a significant proportion of those who are alcohol and drug dependent. Whereas they are the first to suggest treatment for others, they are the last to seek it for themselves. The depressed physician would do well to heed the Biblical admonition: "Physician heal thyself," which is as pertinent today as it was two millennia ago. With most physicians, however, the problem is not illness but ennui. The paradox for doctors is that although they may think that their patients are wearing them down, they may not realize patients are also the means for buoying them up. The interaction between patient and doctor presents an opportunity not just for treatment but for personal growth. Your intervention hopefully has cured or improved the patient's illness or condition. His or her life is better because of you; is yours better because of the patient? In addition to vacations, athletics, hobbies, and religion, the relationship between the patient and the doctor can be a source of renewal, provided that the physician experiences it in a fuller dimension and with more imagination than the patterns of today's living seemingly require and allow. The physician has more than a ringside seat to the human condition. He or she is as much a participant as is the patient. Those who do not feel this communality will ultimately be the losers.

Pertinent to the life of a plastic surgeon is the couplet by Ellen Hooper:

> I slept and dreamed that life was beauty
> I woke—and found that life was duty.

One might say that the plastic surgeon should be able to unite beauty and duty since most of us perform both esthetic and reconstructive procedures. Yet, making somebody else "beautiful" can make us merely indifferent or irritable. How sad it is "when the vision lies in the dust of the marketplace." The trick is to acquire the vision first and then, equally or more difficult, to retain it. Far too many people have died long before they were buried. Life is too precious to be yawned at.

For physicians who have become plastic surgeons, the potential relationship between the patient and each of us offers an opportunity for personal and professional adventure [48]. Admittedly, the journey at first may seem less spectacular than what once faced Dr. Livingstone in Africa, but the terrain is equally uncharted and challenging and ever more mysterious.

REFERENCES

1. Alda, A. Commencement address to Columbia College, New York City, May 16, 1979.
2. Alexander, J. E. Challenges in esthetic plastic surgery. *Plast. Reconstr. Surg.* 52 : 237, 1973
3. American Society for Aesthetic Plastic Surgery membership survey. *Aesthetic Surgery,* Winter/Spring, 1989. Pp. 22–23.
4. American Society of Plastic and Reconstructive Surgeons. Fact sheet. Estimated number of cosmetic surgery procedures performed by American Society of Plastic and Reconstructive Surgeons members. Arlington Heights, Ill.: American Society of Plastic and Reconstructive Surgeons, 1989.
5. American Society of Plastic and Reconstructive Surgeons/Plastic Surgical Educational Foundation. Membership needs assessment and attitudinal survey. Summary and results. Arlington Heights, Ill.: American Society of Plastic and Reconstructive Surgeons, January 1988.

6. Aristotle. *Politics,* VII, II. In R. McKeon (ed.), *The Basic Works of Aristotle.* New York: Random House, 1941. P. 1280.
7. Aston, S. J. Preoperative patient evaluation. "What I tell my patients." *Aesthetic Surgery,* Winter/Spring, 1989. Pp. 6–7.
8. Baker, T. J. Computations of rhytidectomy. Presented at the 20th Annual Meeting of the New England Society of Plastic and Reconstructive Surgeons, Sturbridge, Mass., June 8, 1980.
9. Baker, T. J. Patient selection and psychological evaluation. *Clin. Plast. Surg.* 5 : 3, 1978.
10. Barber, B. *Informed Consent in Medical Therapy and Research.* New Brunswick, N.J.: Rutgers University Press, 1980.
11. Barsky, A. J. *Worried Sick. Our Troubled Quest for Wellness.* Boston: Little, Brown, 1988. Pp. 3–20.
12. Bartlett, E. E. What's Up Doc? The Patient and The Malpractice Suit. *Risk Management,* August 1987. Pp. 26–31.
13. Bass, L. W., and Wolfson, J. H. Professional courtesy is obsolete. *N. Engl. J. Med.* 299 : 772, 1978.
14. Beale, S., et al. Augmentation mammoplasty: the surgical and psychological effects of the operation and prediction of result. *Ann. Plast. Surg.* 13 : 279, 1984.
15. Beale, S., Lisper, H.-O., and Palm, B. A psychological study of patients seeking augmentation mammoplasty. *Br. J. Psychiatry* 136 : 133, 1980.
16. Belfer, M. L. Psychological Considerations of the Plastic Surgery Patient. In S. A. Sohn (ed.), *Fundamentals of Aesthetic Plastic Surgery.* Baltimore: Williams & Wilkins, 1987. Pp. 9–13.
17. Benet, S. V. No Visitors. In *Selected Works of Stephen Vincent Benet.* New York: Farrar & Rinehart, 1942. Vol. 2, p. 346.
18. Bennett, A. E. (ed.). *Communication Between Doctors and Patients.* London: Oxford University Press, 1976.
19. Bennett, G. *Patients and Their Doctors. The Journey Through Medical Care.* London: Baillière Tindall, 1979. Pp. 28–34.
20. Berenson, B. *Sketch for a Self-Portrait.* New York: Pantheon, 1949. P. 85.
21. Berger, K. J., and Bostwick, J., III. *A Woman's Decision: Breast Care, Treatment, and Reconstruction.* St. Louis: Mosby, 1984.
22. Bernstein, N. R. Oral communication, 1980.
23. Beth Israel Hospital. Your Rights as a Patient. (Brochure) Boston: Beth Israel Hospital.
24. Billroth, T. *The Medical Sciences in the German Universities. A Study in the History of Civilization.* New York: Macmillan, 1924. P. 154.
25. Bird, B. *Talking with Patients* (2nd ed.). Philadelphia: Lippincott, 1973.
26. Blacher, R. S. General Surgery and Anesthesia: The Emotional Experience. In R. S. Blacher (ed.), *The Psychological Experience of Surgery.* New York: Wiley, 1987. Pp. 1–25.

27. Bloom, A. A. Social work and the English language. *Social Casework* 61 : 332, 1980.
28. Bloom, S. W. *The Doctor and His Patient: A Sociological Interpretation.* New York: Russel Sage Foundation, 1963. Pp. 145–183.
29. Blumgart, H. L. Caring for the patient. *N. Engl. J. Med.* 270 : 449, 1964.
30. Bok, S. *Lying: Moral Choice in Public and Private Life.* New York: Pantheon, 1979.
31. Bosk, C. L. *Forgive and Remember. Managing Medical Failure.* Chicago: University of Chicago Press, 1979.
32. Bosk, C. L. Occupational rituals in patient management. *N. Engl. J. Med.* 303 : 71, 1980.
33. Bower, J. L. Oral communication, 1978.
34. Brewin, T. B. Not TLC but FPI. *J. R. Soc. Med.* 83 : 172, 1990.
35. Burk, J., Zelen, S. L., and Terino, E. O. More than skin deep: a self-consistency approach to the psychology of cosmetic surgery. *Plast. Reconstr. Surg.* 76 : 270, 1985.
36. Camus, A. Preface to *The Stranger.* In P. Thrody (ed.), *Lyrical and Critical Essays.* Translated from the French by E. C. Kennedy. New York: Knopf, 1968. Pp. 335–336.
37. Carrell, S. The physician-patient relationship. Perceptions and reality. The times they are a-changin'. *Facets,* March, 1990.
38. Cartwright, R. E. Cited by H. T. Paxton. Why doctors get sued. *Medical Economics,* April 18, 1988.
39. Cash, T. F., and Horton, C. E. Aesthetic surgery: effect of rhinoplasty on the social perception of patients by others. *Plast. Reconstr. Surg.* 73 : 543, 1983.
40. Cash, T. F., and Horton, C. E. A longitudinal study of the psychological effects of esthetic surgery. Unpublished data, 1990.
41. Cash, T. F., Winstead, B., and Janda, L. H. The great American shape-up. Body image survey report. *Psychology Today* 126 : 305, 1986.
42. Cassileth, B. R., et al. Informed consent—why are its goals imperfectly realized? *N. Engl. J. Med.* 302 : 896, 1980.
43. Chambliss, L., and Reier, S. How doctors have ruined health care. To hold down costs, we must first find out what we are paying for. *Financial World,* January 9, 1990.
44. Charles, S. C., et al. Sued and nonsued physicians. Satisfactions, dissatisfactions, and sources of stress. *Psychosomatics* 28 : 62, 1987.
45. Cheever, J. The Trouble of Marcie Flint. In *The Stories of John Cheever.* New York: Knopf, 1979. P. 289.
46. Cline, C. J. Is it a red or yellow light: a reexamination of traditional criteria for cosmetic surgery patient selection. Presented at the 58th Annual Scientific Meeting of the American Society of Plastic and Reconstructive Surgeons, Inc., San Francisco, October 29–November 3, 1989.

47. Cole, N. M. Informed consent: considerations in aesthetic and reconstructive surgery of the breast. *Clin. Plast. Surg.* 15 : 541, 1988.
48. Colfelt, R. H. *Together in the Dark. Mysteries of Healing.* Seattle: Madrona, 1987.
49. Committee of Ethics and Discipline. On terminating the physician-patient relationship. *Mass. Med. Soc. Newsl.* 19 : 3, 1979.
50. Committee on Trauma, American College of Surgeons. Guidelines for the patient-physician relationship in the emergency department. *Bull. Am. Coll. Surg.* 62 : 15, 1977.
51. Commonwealth of Massachusetts S1757. Chapter 214. An Act Providing Certain Rights to Patients and Residents in Hospitals, Clinics and Certain Other Facilities, 1979.
52. Conley, J. J. Introduction to *Complications of Head and Neck Surgery.* Philadelphia: Saunders, 1979. P. 12.
53. Copas, J. B., and Robin, A. A. The facial appearance sorting test (FAST): an aid to the selection of patients for rhinoplasty. *Br. J. Plast. Surg.* 42 : 65, 1989.
54. Courtiss, E. H., and Donelan, M. B. Skin sensation after suction liposuction: a prospective study of 50 consecutive patients. *Plast. Reconstr. Surg.* 81 : 550, 1988.
55. Courtiss, E. H., and Goldwyn, R. M. Breast sensation before and after plastic surgery. *Plast. Reconstr. Surg.* 58 : 1, 1976.
56. Courtiss, E. H., and Goldwyn, R. M. The Turbinates. In R. B. Stark (ed.), *Plastic Surgery of the Head and Neck.* New York: Churchill Livingstone, 1987. Pp. 624–627.
57. Courtiss, E. H., Goldwyn, R. M., and Anastasi, G. W. The fate of breast implants with infection around them. *Plast. Reconstr. Surg.* 63 : 812, 1979.
58. Cousins, N. *Anatomy of an Illness as Perceived by the Patient: Reflections on Healing and Regeneration.* New York: Norton, 1979.
59. Dicker, R. L., and Syracuse, V. R. *Consultation with a Plastic Surgeon.* Chicago: Nelson-Hall, 1975.
60. DiMatteo, M. R. A social-psychological analysis of physician-patient rapport: Toward a science of the art of medicine. *J. Soc. Issues* 35 : 12, 1979.
61. Doorey, A. J. The surgical work day in the British Isles. Some observations from a small sample studied in depth. *Arch. Surg.* 114 : 970, 1976.
62. Drane, J. F. *Becoming a Good Doctor: The Place of Virtue and Character in Medical Ethics.* Kansas City, MO: Sheen and Ward, The Catholic Association of the United States, 1988. Pp. 98–99.
63. Drinker, H., Knorr, N. J., and Edgerton, M. T., Jr. Factitious wounds. A psychiatric and surgical dilemma. *Plast. Reconstr. Surg.* 50 : 458, 1972.
64. du Gard, R. M. *The Thibaults.* New York: Viking, 1939.
65. Edgerton, M. T. Oral communication, 1979.
66. Edgerton, M. T., and Langman, M. L. Psychiatric Considerations.

In. E. H. Courtiss (ed.), *Male Aesthetic Surgery*. St. Louis: Mosby, 1982. Pp. 17–38.
67. Edgerton, M. T., Jacobson, W. E., and Meyer, E. Surgical-psychiatric study of patients seeking plastic (cosmetic) surgery: Ninety-eight consecutive patients with minimal deformity. *Br. J. Plast. Surg.* 13 : 136, 1961.
68. Edgerton, M. T., Meyer, E., and Jacobson, W. E. Augmentation mammaplasty. II: Further surgical and psychiatric evaluation. *Plast. Reconstr. Surg.* 27 : 279, 1961.
69. Entralgo, P. L. *Doctor and Patient*. New York: McGraw-Hill, 1969.
70. Ewalt, D. H., et al. Professional courtesy. *Ann. Plast. Surg.* 3 : 580, 1980.
71. Figueroa, C. Breast reduction—one woman's story. *Woman's Day*, February 20, 1979. P. 40.
72. Fili, W. J. *Face Lifts: Is There One in Your Future?* Broomall, Pa.: Filicon, 1977.
73. Filiberti, A., et al. Immediate versus delayed breast reconstruction. A psychological answer. *Eur. J. Plast. Surg.* 13 : 55, 1990.
74. Filiberti, A., Rimoldi, A., and Tamurini, M. Breast reconstruction: a psychological survey. *Eur. J. Plast. Surg.* 12 : 214, 1989.
75. Fischl, R. A. The busy physician or, why don't patients understand? *Ann. Plast. Surg.* 3 : 495, 1979.
76. Flanary, C. M., and Alexander, J. M. Patient responses to the orthognathic surgical experience: factors leading to dissatisfaction. *J. Oral Maxillofac. Surg.* 41 : 770, 1983.
77. Flowers, R. S. Blepharoplasty. In E. H. Courtiss (ed.), *Male Aesthetic Surgery*. St. Louis: Mosby, 1982. Pp. 207–239.
78. Fraser, C. On Analysis of Face-to-Face Communication. In A. E. Bennett (ed.), *Communication Between Doctors and Patients*. London: Oxford University Press, 1976. Pp. 7–28.
79. Fredrics, S. Oral communication, 1978.
80. Freedman, R. *Beauty Bound*. Lexington, Mass.: Heath, 1986. P. 9.
81. Freedman, R. *Bodylove*. New York: Harper & Row, 1990. Pp. 18–45.
82. Furnas, D. W. Operating room mirror for mammaplasty evaluation. *Ann. Plast. Surg.* 3 : 578, 1979.
83. Gallagher, E. G. The Doctor-Patient Relationship in the Changing Health Scene. Proceedings of an International Conference sponsored by the John E. Fogarty Center for Advanced Study in the Health Sciences, National Institutes of Health. Held at the National Institutes of Health, Bethesda, Md., April 26–28, 1976. Washington, D.C.: U.S. Government Printing Office.
84. Gamble, S. W. Changing roles in the '90's: Will RNs manage MDs? *Hospitals. The Management of Health Care Executives*. November 20, 1989. Pp. 42–44.

85. Gersuny, R. *Arzt und Patient. Winse fur Beide.* Stuttgart: Ferdinand Enke, 1904.
86. Gifford, S. Cosmetic Surgery and Personality Change: A Review and Some Clinical Observations. In R. M. Goldwyn (ed.), *The Unfavorable Result in Plastic Surgery: Avoidance and Treatment.* Boston: Little, Brown, 1972. Pp. 11–33.
87. Gifford, S. Emotional Attitudes Toward Cosmetic Breast Surgery: Loss and Restitution for the "Ideal Self." In R. M. Goldwyn (ed.), *Plastic and Reconstructive Surgery of the Breast.* Boston: Little, Brown, 1976. Pp. 103–121.
88. Goffman, E. *The Presentation of Self in Everyday Life.* Garden City, N.Y.: Doubleday, 1959.
89. Goin, M. K. Psychiatric Considerations. In E. H. Courtiss (ed.), *Aesthetic Surgery Trouble: How to Avoid It and How to Treat It.* St. Louis: Mosby, 1978. Pp. 17–24.
90. Goin, M. K. Psychological reactions to surgery of the breast. *Clin. Plast. Surg.* 9 : 347, 1982.
91. Goin, J. M., and Goin, M. K. *Changing the Body. Psychological Effects of Plastic Surgery.* Baltimore: Williams & Wilkins, 1981.
92. Goin, J. M., and Goin, M. K. Psychological Aspects of Aesthetic Plastic Surgery. In J. L. Lewis, Jr. (ed.), *The Art of Aesthetic Plastic Surgery.* Boston: Little, Brown, 1989. Pp. 39–47.
93. Goin, J. M., and Goin, M. K. Psychological Understanding and Management of the Plastic Surgery Patient. In N. G. Georgiade et al. (eds.), *Essentials of Plastic, Maxillofacial and Reconstructive Surgery.* Baltimore: Williams & Wilkins, 1987. Pp. 1127–1143.
94. Goin, M. K., Burgoyne, R. W., and Goin, J. M. Face-lift operations: the patient's secret motivations and reactions to "informed consent." *Plast. Reconstr. Surg.* 58 : 273, 1976.
95. Goldwyn, R. M. *Beyond Appearance: Reflections of a Plastic Surgeon.* New York: Dodd, Mead, 1986. Pp. 220–226.
96. Goldwyn, R. M. Breast reconstruction after mastectomy. *N. Engl. J. Med.* 317 : 1711, 1987.
97. Goldwyn, R. M. Disease is a family affair. *Arch. Surg.* 106 : 610, 1973.
98. Goldwyn, R. M. Fees. A perspective. *Arch. Surg.* 107 : 127, 1973.
99. Goldwyn, R. M. High hopes and malpractice. *Arch. Surg.* 111 : 1042, 1976.
100. Goldwyn, R. M. Ingredients for Failure. In R. M. Goldwyn (ed.), *The Unfavorable Result in Plastic Surgery: Avoidance and Treatment.* Boston: Little, Brown, 1972. Pp. 2–4.
101. Goldwyn, R. M. Marketing the sure way. *Plast. Reconstr. Surg.* 85 : 105, 1990.
102. Goldwyn, R. M. Operating for the aging face. *Psychol. Med.* 3 : 187, 1972.
103. Goldwyn, R. M. Patient Selection: The Importance of Being Cau-

tious. In E. H. Courtiss (ed.), *Aesthetic Surgery Trouble: How to Avoid It and How to Treat It.* St. Louis: Mosby, 1978. Pp. 14–16.
104. Goldwyn, R. M. Plastic surgeons on the make. *Plast. Reconstr. Surg.* 72 : 251, 1985.
105. Goldwyn, R. M. Reality in plastic surgery: a plea for complete disclosure of results. *Plast. Reconstr. Surg.* 80 : 713, 1987.
106. Goldwyn, R. M. Reporting or hiding a complication. *Plast. Reconstr. Surg.* 71 : 843, 1983.
107. Goldwyn, R. M. The advent of liposuction. *Plast. Reconstr. Surg.* 72 : 705, 1983.
108. Goldwyn, R. M. The Consultant and the Unfavorable Result. In R. M. Goldwyn (ed.), *The Unfavorable Result in Plastic Surgery: Avoidance and Treatment.* Boston: Little, Brown, 1972. Pp. 5–7.
109. Goldwyn, R. M. The Dissatisfied Patient. In D. Gowlian and E. H. Courtiss (eds.), *Symposium on Surgery of the Aging Face.* St. Louis: Mosby, 1978. Vol. 19, pp. 81–84.
110. Goldwyn, R. M. The Factitious Skin Wound. In R. Rudolph and J. M. Noe (eds.), *Chronic Problem Wounds.* Boston: Little, Brown, 1983. Pp. 159–164.
111. Goldwyn, R. M. The plastic surgeon: doctor or physician. *Ann. Plast. Surg.* 8 : 189, 1982.
112. Goldwyn, R. M. The Unfavorable Result in Aesthetic Plastic Surgery. In J. R. Lewis, Jr. (ed.), *The Art of Aesthetic Plastic Surgery.* Boston: Little, Brown, 1989. Pp. 55–58.
113. Goldwyn, R. M. The Woman and Esthetic Surgery. In M. T. Notman and C. C. Nadelson (eds.), *The Woman Patient. Medical and Psychological Interfaces. I: Sexual and Reproductive Aspects of Women's Health Care.* New York: Plenum, 1978. Pp. 271–280.
114. Goldwyn, R. M. Unexpected bleeding after elective nasal surgery. *Ann. Plast. Surg.* 2 : 201, 1979.
115. Goldwyn, R. M. (ed.). *Long-Term Results in Plastic and Reconstructive Surgery.* Boston: Little, Brown, 1980, Vols. 1 and 2.
116. Goldwyn, R. M. (ed.). *Reduction Mammaplasty.* Boston: Little, Brown, 1990.
117. Goldwyn, R. M. (ed.). *The Unfavorable Result in Plastic Surgery: Avoidance and Treatment* (2nd ed.). Boston: Little, Brown, 1984.
118. Goldwyn, R. M., and Kasdon, E. J. The "disappearance" of residual basal cell carcinoma of the skin. *Ann. Plast. Surg.* 1 : 286, 1978.
119. Goldwyn, R. M., and Strome, M. Unsuspected adenoid cystic carcinoma in secondary rhinoplasty. *Ann. Plast. Surg.* 2 : 338, 1979.
120. Gorney, M. AIDS and the aesthetic surgeon. *Aesthetic Surgery,* Winter/Spring, 1989. Pp. 10–11.
121. Gorney, M. Malpractice. In E. H. Courtiss (ed.), *Aesthetic Surgery Trouble: How to Avoid It and How to Treat It.* St. Louis Mosby, 1978. Pp. 1–13.
122. Grazer, F. M., and Goldwyn, R. M. Abdominoplasty: Assessed by

survey with emphasis on complications. *Plast. Reconstr. Surg.* 59 : 513, 1977.
123. Grazer, F. M., and Klingbeil, J. R. *Body Image: A Surgical Perspective.* St. Louis: Mosby, 1980.
124. Green, R. C., Jr., Carroll, G. J., and Buxton, W. D. *The Care and Management of the Sick and Incompetent Physician.* Springfield, Ill.: Thomas, 1978.
125. Griggs, J. Avoiding malpractice suits. *Surg. Rounds* 3(5) : 64, May 1980.
126. Grundner, T. M. On the readability of surgical consent forms. *N. Engl. J. Med.* 302 : 900, 1980.
127. Gurdin, M. D. Oral communication, 1977.
128. Harris, D. L. Self-consciousness of disproportionate breast size: a survey of psychological reactions to abnormal appearance. *Br. J. Plast. Surg.* 36 : 191, 1983.
129. Harris, D. L. The symptomatology of abnormal appearance: an anecdotal survey. *Br. J. Plast. Surg.* 35 : 312, 1982.
130. Haug, M. Doctor patient relationships and the older patient. *J. Gerontol.* 34 : 852, 1979.
131. Hawtof, D. B., and Smith, D. Language in the operating room. *Ann. Plast. Surg.* 18 : 186, 1987.
132. Hay, G. G., and Heather, B. B. Changes in psychometric test results following cosmetic nasal operations. *Br. J. Psychiatry* 122 : 89, 1973.
133. Henderson, L. J. Physician and Patient as a Social System. In J. D. Stoerkle (ed.), *Encounters Between Patients and Doctors: An Anthology.* Cambridge: MIT Press, 1987. Pp. 137–146.
134. Herzlich, C., and Pierret, D. *Illness and Self in Society.* Baltimore: Johns Hopkins University Press, 1987. P. 183.
135. Hetter, G. P. Satisfactions and dissatisfactions of patients with augmentation mammaplasty. *Plast. Reconstr. Surg.* 64 : 151, 1979.
136. Hoffmeir, P. A., and Bohner, J. A. *From Residency to Reality.* New York: McGraw-Hill, 1988.
137. Hollyman, J. A., et al. Surgery for the psyche: a longitudinal study of women undergoing reduction mammoplasty. *Br. J. Plast. Surg.* 39 : 222, 1986.
138. Hsiao, W. C., et al. Resource-based relative values from eight surgical specialties. *J.A.M.A.* 260 : 2418, 1988.
139. Jacobson, P. D. Medical malpractice and the tort system. *J.A.M.A.* 262 : 3320, 1989.
140. Jacobson, W. E., Edgerton, M. T., and Meyer, E. Psychiatric evaluation of male patients seeking cosmetic surgery. *Plast. Reconstr. Surg.* 26 : 356, 1960.
141. Jamison, K. R., Wellisch, D. K., and Pasnau, R. O. Psychosocial aspects of mastectomy I. The woman's perspective. *Am. J. Psychiatry.* 135 : 432, 1978.
142. Jaspars, J., King, J., and Pendleton, D. The Consultation: A Social

Psychological Analysis. In D. Pendleton and J. Hasler (eds.), *Doctor-Patient Communication*. London: Academic, 1983. Pp. 139–157.
143. Jobe, R. *The Sophisticated Shopper's Guide to Plastic Surgery*. Rolling Hills Estates, Calif.: Erdmann, 1990. Pp. 20–22.
144. Johnson, D. Doctor talk. *New Republic,* August 18, 1979. Pp. 25–27.
145. Joseph, J. Motivation for reduction rhinoplasty and the practical significance of the operation in life. Translated from the German by S. Milstein. *Plast. Reconstr. Surg.* 73 : 692, 1984.
146. Kahan, E. B., and Gaskill, E. G. The "Difficult" Patient: Observations on the Staff-Patient Interaction. In M. T. Notman and C. C. Nadelson (eds.), *The Woman Patient. Medical and Psychological Interfaces. I: Sexual and Reproductive Aspects of Women's Health Care.* New York: Plenum, 1978. Pp. 257–269.
147. Kahn, E. Cited by H. T. Paxton. Why doctors get sued. *Medical Economics,* April 18, 1988.
148. Kalick, S. M. Aesthetic surgery: How it affects the way patients are perceived by others. *Ann. Plast. Surg.* 2 : 128, 1979.
149. Kalick, S. M. Written communication, 1980.
150. Karsh, E. The Doctor-Patient Relationship Through the Ages. In W. E. Preece (ed.), *Medical and Health Annual*. New York: Encyclopaedia Britannica, 1977.
151. Kaye, B. L. *Facial Rejuvenation Surgery. A Colorphotographic Atlas.* Philadelphia: Gower Medical-Lippincott, 1987. P. 130.
152. Kiyak, H. A., and Zeitler, D. L. Self-assessment of profile and body image among orthognathic surgery patients before and two years after surgery. *J. Oral Maxillofac. Surg.* 46 : 365–371, 1988.
153. Knorr, N. J., Edgerton, M. T., and Hoopes, J. E. The insatiable cosmetic surgery patient. *Plast. Reconstr. Surg.* 40 : 285, 1967.
154. Knorr, J. J., Hoopes, J. E., and Edgerton, M. T. Psychiatric surgical approach to adolescent disturbances in self image. *Plast. Reconstr. Surg.* 41 : 248, 1968.
155. Knox, R. A. What's ailing doctors? *Boston Globe Magazine,* March 18, 1990.
156. Kolata, G. Wariness is replacing trust between healer and patient. *The New York Times,* February 20, 1990.
157. Kübler-Ross, E. *On Death and Dying*. New York: Macmillan, 1969.
158. Kübler-Ross, E. *Questions and Answers on Death and Dying*. New York: Macmillan, 1974.
159. Kunstler, W. E. Aesthetic considerations in surgical operations from antiquity to recent times. *Bull. Hist. Med.* 12 : 27, 1942.
160. Lavell, S., and Lewis, C. M. SAFE: A practical guide to psychological factors in selecting patients for facial cosmetic surgery. *Ann. Plast. Surg.* 12 : 256, 1984.
161. Lederer, H. D. How the Sick View Their World. In E. G. Jaco (ed.), *Patients, Physicians, and Illness. Sourcebook in Behavioral Science and Medicine.* New York: Free Press, 1958. Pp. 247–256.

162. Leff, L. A Secret of Success: Be Good at Getting Wrinkles Ironed Out. *Wall Street Journal,* November 15, 1979.
163. Leigh, H., and Reiser, M. F. *The Patient. Biological, Psychological, and Social Dimensions of Medical Practice.* New York: Plenum, 1980. Pp. 3–90.
164. Lepore, M. J. *Death of the Clinician. Requiem or Reveille?* Springfield, Ill.: Thomas, 1982.
165. Levinson, J. Breast reconstruction: a patient's view (Letter to Editor), *Plast. Reconstr. Surg.* 73 : 703, 1984.
166. Ley, P. Towards Better Doctor-Patient Communications. In A. E. Bennett (ed.), *Communication Between Doctors and Patients.* London: Oxford University Press, 1976. Pp. 77–98.
167. Linn, L. Cosmetic Surgery, with Particular Reference to Rhinoplasty. In R. S. Blacher (ed.), *The Psychological Experience of Surgery.* New York: Wiley, 1987. Pp. 194–206.
168. Lipkin, M. *The Care of Patients: Concepts and Tactics.* New York: Oxford University Press, 1974. Pp. 171–175.
169. Lipp, M. R. *Respectful Treatment. The Human Side of Medical Care.* Hagerstown, Md.: Harper & Row, 1977. Pp. 124–130.
170. MacGregor, F. C. Social, psychological and cultural dimensions of cosmetic and reconstructive plastic surgery. *Aesthetic Plast. Surg.* 13 : 1, 1989.
171. MacGregor, F. C. *Transformation and Identity. The Face and Plastic Surgery.* New York: Quadrangle/Times Books, 1974.
172. MacGregor, F. C., et al. *Facial Deformities and Plastic Surgery. A Psychosocial Study.* Springfield, Ill.: Thomas, 1953.
173. Magraw, R. M. Social and Medical Contracts: Explicit and Implicit. In R. J. Bulger (ed.), *Hippocrates Revisited.* New York: Med-Com, 1973. Pp. 148–157.
174. Magraw, R. M., and Magraw, D. B. *Ferment in Medicine. A Study of the Essence of Medical Practice and of its New Dilemmas.* Philadelphia: Saunders, 1966. Pp. 104–123.
175. Maltz, M. *Doctor Pygmalion. The Autobiography of a Plastic Surgeon.* London: Museum, 1954.
176. Maltz, M. *New Faces—New Futures: Rebuilding Character with Plastic Surgery.* New York: Smith, 1936.
177. Manning, P. R., and DeBakey, L. *Medicine: Preserving the Passion.* New York: Springer-Verlag, 1987.
178. Marcus, P. Psychological aspects of cosmetic rhinoplasty. *Br. J. Plast. Surg.* 37 : 313, 1984.
179. Matheson, G., and Drever, J. M. Psychological preparation of the patient for breast reconstruction. *Ann. Plast. Surg.* 24 : 238, 1990.
180. Melick, D. W. Cited by R. M. Magraw and D. B. Magraw. *Ferment in Medicine. A Study of the Essence of Medical Practice and of its New Dilemmas.* Philadephia: Saunders, 1966. P. 104.
181. Meyer, E. Psychiatric Aspects of Plastic Surgery. In J. M. Converse

(ed.), *Reconstructive Plastic Surgery* (1st ed.). New York: Saunders, 1964. Vol. 1, pp. 365–383.
182. Morini, S. Sculpture. What plastic surgery can do to give you a beautiful bosom. *Vogue,* January 15, 1971. P. 83.
183. Murray, J. A. M., et al. Open v. closed reduction of the fractured nose. *Arch. Otolaryngol. Head Neck Surg.* 110 : 797, 1984.
184. Musgrave, R. H., and Garrett, W. S., Jr. Preoperative Consultation: A Different Concept. In D. R. Millard, Jr. (ed.), *Symposium on Corrective Rhinoplasty.* St. Louis: Mosby, 1976. Pp. 50–55.
185. Nabokov, V. Quoted in *The New York Times Book Review,* October 24, 1971. P. 22.
186. Nadelson, T. Oral communication, 1990.
187. Nadelson, T. The Münchausen syndrome. Borderline character features. *Gen. Hosp. Psychiatry.* 1 : 11, 1979.
188. Napoleon, A., and Lewis, C. M. Psychological considerations in lipoplasty: the problematic or "special care" patient. *Ann. Plast. Surg.* 23 : 430, 1989.
189. Napoleon, A., and Lewis, C. M. Psychological considerations in the elderly cosmetic surgery candidate. *Ann. Plast. Surg.* 24 : 165, 1990.
190. National Blood Resource Education Program Expert Panel. The use of autologous blood. *J.A.M.A.* 264 : 414, 1990.
191. Noe, J. M., and Kalish, S. A New Approach to Wound Dressings. In *Wound Care.* Greenwich, Conn.: Chesebrough-Ponds. Pp. 1–18.
192. Norman, J. Are you giving away too much care? *Medical Economics for Surgeons,* March 1990. Pp. 47–53.
193. Notman, M. T. A Psychological Consideration of Mastectomy. In M. T. Notman and C. C. Nadelson (eds.), *The Woman Patient. Medical and Psychological Interfaces. I: Sexual and Reproductive Aspects of Women's Health Care.* New York: Plenum, 1978. Pp. 247–255.
194. Novak, M. Psychocutaneous medicine: The distrustful patient. *Cutis* 19 : 362, 197.
195. Offer, D., Ostrow, E., and Howard, K. *The Adolescent: A Psychological Self-Portrait.* New York: Basic, 1981.
196. Ohlsen, L., Ponten, B., and Hambert, G. Augmentation mammoplasty: A surgical and psychiatric evaluation of the results. *Ann. Plast. Surg.* 2 : 42, 1979.
197. Osmond, H. God and the doctor. *N. Engl. J. Med.* 302 : 555, 1980.
198. Ottenberg, P. The physician disease: success and work addiction. *Psychiatric Opinion,* April, 1975.
199. Ousterhout, D. K. *Aesthetic Applications of Craniofacial Techniques.* Boston: Little, Brown, 1990.
200. Ousterhout, D. K. Feminization of the forehead: contour changes to improve female aesthetics. *Plast. Reconstr. Surg.* 79 : 701, 1987.
201. Parsons, T. Definitions of Health and Illness in the Light of American Values and Social Structure. In E. G. Jaco (ed.), *Patients, Physicians and Illness. Sourcebook in Behavioral Science and Medicine.* New York: Free Press, 1958. Pp. 165–187.

202. Parsons, T. Social Structure and Dynamic Process: The Case of Modern Medical Practice. In T. Parsons (ed.), *The Social System*. New York: Free Press, 1951. Pp. 428–479.
203. Parsons, T. The sick role and the role of the physician reconsidered. *Milbank Mem. Fund Q.* 53 : 257, 1975.
204. Patzer, G. L. *The Physical Attractiveness Phenomenon*. New York: Plenum, 1985. P. 142.
205. Paxton, T. C. Why Doctors Get Sued. *Medical Economics*, April 18, 1988. Pp. 42–50.
206. Peabody, F. W. Care of patient. *J.A.M.A.* 88 : 877, 1927.
207. Penn, J. G., and Baker, J. L., Jr. An office-based elective surgical center. *Ann. Plast. Surg.* 4 : 94, 1980.
208. Phelps, D. B., Buchler, W., and Bostwick, J. A., Jr. The diagnosis of facititious ulcer of the hand: a case report. *J. Hand Surg.* 2 : 105, 1977.
209. Polk, S. R. *The Medical Student's Survival Guide* (2nd ed.). Myrtle Beach, SC: Trentland, 1988. P. 201.
210. Priestley, J. B. *Margin Released. A Writer's Reminiscences and Reflections*. New York: Harper & Row, 1962. P. 38.
211. Pruzinsky, T. Collaboration of plastic surgeon and medical psychotherapist: elective cosmetic surgery. *Med. Psychother. An Int. J.* 1 : 1–13, 1988.
212. Pruzinsky, T. The changing face of plastic surgery: developments and trends in requests for elective cosmetic surgery. *Med. Psychother. An Int. J.* 2 : 137, 1988.
213. Pruzinsky, T., and Cash, T. F. Medical Interventions for the Enhancement of Adolescents' Physical Appearance: Implications for Social Competence. In T. F. Cash and T. Pruzinsky (eds.), *Body Images: Development, Deviance, and Change*. New York: Guilford, 1990.
214. Pruzinsky, T., and Edgerton, M. T. Body Image Change in Cosmetic Plastic Surgery. In T. F. Cash and T. Pruzinsky (eds.), *Body, Images: Development, Deviance, and Change*. New York: Guilford, 1990.
215. Pruzinsky, T., and Persing, J. A. Psychological Perspectives and Aesthetic Applications of Reconstructive Surgery Techniques. In D. K. Ousterhout (ed.), *Aesthetic Applications of Craniofacial Techniques*. Boston: Little, Brown, 1990.
216. Rees, T. D. *Aesthetic Plastic Surgery*. Philadelphia: Saunders, 1980.
217. Rees, T. D. Selection of Patients. In T. D. Rees and D. Wood-Smith (eds.), *Cosmetic Facial Surgery*. Philadelphia: Saunders, 1973. Pp. 17–26.
218. Rees, T. D. The Initial Office Consultation. Teaching course of the American Society of Aesthetic Plastic Surgeons, 13th Annual Meeting, Orlando, Fla., May 21, 1980.
219. Rees, T. D. Written communication, 1980.

220. Reich, J. Factors influencing patient satisfaction with the results of esthetic plastic surgery. *Plast. Reconstr. Surg.* 55 : 5, 1975.
221. Reich, J. The surgery of appearance. Psychological and related aspects. *Med. J. Aust.* 2 : 5, 1969.
222. Robbe-Grillet, A. *Jealousy*. In two novels: *Jealousy* and *In the Labyrinth*. Translated from the French by R. Howard. New York: Grove, 1965. Pp. 41–42.
223. Roberts, C. M. *Doctor and Patient in the Teaching Hospital. A Tale of Two Life-Worlds.* Lexington, MA: Lexington, 1977.
224. Robertson, J. D., and Keavy, W. T. *Plastic Surgery Malpractice and Damages.* New York: Wiley, 1990.
225. Robin, A. A., et al. Reshaping the psyche. The concurrent improvement in appearance and mental state after rhinoplasty. *Br. J. Psychiatry,* 152 : 539–543, 1988.
226. Rogers, B. O. The development of aesthetic plastic surgery: A history. *Aesthetic Plast. Surg.* 1 : 3, 1976.
227. Rollin, B. The Best Years of My Life. *New York Times Magazine,* April 6, 1980. P. 36.
228. Rosenberg, M. L. *Patients: The Experience of Illness.* Philadelphia: Saunders, 1980.
229. Rudofsky, B. *The Unfashionable Human Body.* New York: Anchor, 1974.
230. Sanes, S. *A Physician Faces Cancer in Himself.* Albany: State University of New York Press, 1979. Pp. 40–50, 188–197.
231. Schedler, T. R. Written communication, December 28, 1989.
232. Schlebusch, L., and Levin, A. A psychological profile of women selected for augmentation mammaplasty. *S. A. Med. J.* 64 : 481, 1983.
233. Schonfeld, W. A. Gynecomastia in adolescence: Effect on body image and personality adaptation. *Psychosom. Med.* 24 : 379, 1962.
234. Schultz, R. C. *Outpatient Surgery*. Philadelphia: Lea & Febiger, 1979.
235. Schweitzer, I., and Hirschfield, J. J. Postrhytidectomy psychosis: a rare complication. *Plast. Reconstr. Surg.* 74 : 419, 1984.
236. Seneca de Beneficiis, VI, 16. Cited by P. L. Entralgo, *Doctor and Patient.* New York: McGraw-Hill, 1969. P. 7.
237. Shahn, B. *The Shape of Content.* Cambridge: Harvard University Press, 1978. P. 91.
238. Sheehy, G. *Passages.* New York: Dutton, 1976.
239. Sheen, J. H., and Sheen, A. P. *Aesthetic Rhinoplasty* (2nd ed.). St. Louis: Mosby, 1987. Pp. 652–653.
240. Shipley, R. H., O'Donnel, J. M., and Bader, K. F. Psychosocial effects of cosmetic augmentation mammaplasty. *Aesthetic Plast. Surg.* 2 : 429, 1978.
241. Siegler, M., and Osmond, H. *Patienthood. The Art of being a Responsible Patient.* New York: Macmillan, 1979. Pp. 51–52, 80.
242. Sigerist, H. E. *A History of Medicine. II: Early Greek, Hindu, and*

Persian Medicine. New York: Oxford University Press, 1961. Pp. 309–310.
243. Sihm, F., Jagd, M., and Pers, M. Psychological assessment before and after augmentation mammaplasty. Scand. J. Plast. Reconstr Surg. 12 : 296, 1978.
244. Slavin, S. A., and Goldwyn, R. M. The cocaine user: The potential problem patient for rhinoplasty. Plast. Reconstr. Surg. 86 : 436, 1990.
245. Smith, J. W., and Baker, S. S. "Doctor, Make Me Beautiful." New York: McKay, 1973.
246. Snyder, M. The many me's of the self-monitor. Psychology Today 13(10) : 32, March 1980.
247. Sontag, S. Illness as Metaphor. New York: Farrar, Straus, & Giroux, 1978.
248. Sontag, S. The double standard of aging. Saturday Review, September 23, 1972. Pp. 29–38.
249. Spencer, F. C. The Gibbon Lecture. Competence and compassion: Two qualities of surgical excellence. Bull. Am. Coll. Surg. 64 : 15, 1979.
250. Stallings, J. O., with Moss, T. A New You. How Plastic Surgery Can Change Your Life. New York: Van Nostrand Reinhold, 1977.
251. Stein, L. I., Watts, D. T., and Howell, T. The doctor-nurse game revisited. New Engl. J. Med. 322 : 546, 1990.
252. Stevens, L. A. The Psychological Aspects of Breast Surgery. In R. S. Blacher (ed.), The Psychological Experience of Surgery. New York: Wiley, 1987. Pp. 87–98.
253. Stoeckle, J. D. (ed.). Encounters Between Patients and Doctors: An Anthology. Cambridge: MIT Press. Pp. 1–129.
254. Tardy, M. E. Rhinoplasty in midlife. Otolaryngol. Clin. North Am. 13 : 289, 1980.
255. Teimourian,, B. Suction Lipectomy and Body Sculpting. St. Louis: Mosby, 1986. Pp. 685–768.
256. Teimourian, B., and Adhan, M. N. Survey of patients' responses to breast reconstruction. Ann. Plast. Surg. 9 : 321, 1982.
257. Teimourian, B., and Rogers, W. B., III. A national survey of complications associated with suction lipectomy: a comparative study. Plast. Reconstr. Surg. 84 : 628, 1989.
258. Thomson, J. A., Jr., Knorr, N. J., and Edgerton, M. T., Jr. Cosmetic surgery: The psychiatric perspective. Psychosomatics 19 : 7, 1978.
259. Thorwald, J. The Dismissal: The Last Days of Ferdinand Sauerbruch. New York: Pantheon, 1961.
260. Thorwald, J. The Patients. New York: Harcourt Brace Jovanovich, 1971.
261. Trilling, L. Commentary on L. Tolstoi's The Death of Ivan Ilych. In L. Trilling (ed.), The Experience of Literature. A Reader with Commentaries. Garden City, N.Y.: Doubleday, 1967. P. 525.
262. Vaillant, G. E. Adaptation to Life. Boston: Little, Brown, 1977.
263. Vistnes, L. M., and Jobe, R. Rhytidectomy with Emphasis on the

Differences Between Males and Females. In E. H. Courtiss (ed.), *Male Aesthetic Surgery*. St. Louis: Mosby, 1982. Pp. 253–262.
264. Walster, E., et al. Importance of physical attractiveness in dating behavior. *J. Pers. Soc. Psychol.* 4 : 508, 1966.
265. Ward, C. M. First steps of a consultant in plastic surgery: A personal experience. *B. J. Plast. Surg.* 38 : 84, 1985.
266. Webster, R. C., and Smith, R. C. (eds.). *The Aging Face and Neck. Consultations with Richard Webster, M.D. and Associates*. New York: Field, Rich, 1985. P. 203.
267. Weiss, T. E. What is hostility? *Phys. East* 1 : 20, 1979.
268. Wellisch, D. K., et al. The psychological contribution of nipple addition in breast reconstruction. *Plast. Reconstr. Surg.* 80 : 699, 1987.
269. Wellisch, D. K., Jamison, K. R., and Pasnau, R. O. Psychosocial aspects of mastectomy. II. The man's perspective. *Am. J. Psychiatry* 135 : 543, 1978.
270. Wengle, H-P. The psychology of cosmetic surgery: A critical overview of the literature 1960–1982—Part I. *Ann. Plast. Surg.* 16 : 435, 1986.
271. Wengle, H-P. The psychology of cosmetic surgery: Old problems in patient selection seen in a new way—Part II. *Ann. Plast. Surg.* 16 : 487, 1986.
272. Whitaker, L. Skeletal Foundation of Aesthetic Cranial and Facial Surgery. In E. H. Courtiss (ed.), *Male Aesthetic Surgery*. St. Louis: Mosby, 1982. Pp. 145–160.
273. White, A. G. The patient sits down: A clinical note. *Psychosom. Med.* 15 : 256, 1953.
274. White, L. P. (ed.). Care of patient with fatal illness. *Ann. N.Y. Acad. Sci.* 164 : 635, 1969.
275. White, R. Quoted in "Honorable Intentions. Six ways of looking at a primary care residency." *Harvard Med. Alumni Bull.* 54 : 11, 1980.
276. Williams, J. The Initial Office Consultation. Teaching course. The 13th Annual Meeting of the American Society for Aesthetic Plastic Surgery, Orlando, Fla., May 21, 1980.
277. Williams, P., and Harrison, T. *McIndoe's Army. The Injured Armies Who Faced the World*. London: Pelham, 1979. P. 31.
278. Williams, R. H. Management of the Sick with Kindness, Compassion, Wisdom, and Efficiency. In R. H. Williams (ed.), *To Live and to Die: When, Why, How*. New York: Springer-Verlag, 1974. Pp. 134–149.
279. Williams, W. C. Le Médecin Malgré Lui. In *The Complete Collected Poems of William Carlos Williams, 1906–1938*. Norfolk Conn.: New Directions, 1938. P. 19.
280. Wilson, J. R., cited by Ward, C. M. First steps of a consultant in plastic surgery: A personal experience. *Br. J. Plast. Surg.* 38 : 84, 1985.
281. Wright, M. R. Management of patient dissatisfaction with results of cosmetic procedures. *Arch. Otolaryngol.* 106 : 466, 1980.

282. Wright, M. R. Self-perception of the elective surgeon and some patient perception correlates. *Arch. Otolaryngol.* 106 : 460, 1980.
283. Wright, M. R. Surgical addictions. A complication of modern surgery? *Arch. Otolaryngol.* 12 : 870, 1986.
284. Wright, M. R. The elective surgeon's reaction to change and conflict. *Arch. Otolaryngol.* 110 : 318, 1984.
285. Wright, M. R. The male aesthetic patient. *Arch. Otolaryngol.* 113 : 724, 1987.
286. Wright, M. R. The psychology of rhinoplasty. *Fac. Plast. Surg.* 5 : 109, 1988.
287. Wright, R. H. What to do until the malpractice lawyer comes. A survivor's manual. *Am. Psychol.* 12 : 1535, 1981.
288. Zalon, J., with Block, J. L. *I Am Whole Again. The Case for Breast Reconstruction After Mastectomy.* New York: Random House, 1978.
289. Zerubavel, E. *Patterns of Time in Hospital Life. A Sociological Perspective.* Chicago: University of Chicago Press, 1979.

APPENDIX

Personal Authorization Forms

Excision of Lesions

Eyelidplasty

Rhytidectomy (Facelift)

Brow (Forehead) Lift

Rhinoplasty

Dermabrasion

Chemical Face Peel

Abdominal Lipectomy

Liposuctioning

Augmentation Mammoplasty

Mastopexy (Correction of Breast Ptosis)

Reduction Mammoplasty

Breast Reconstruction

Stipulation that patient is responsible for hospital costs associated with any surgery undertaken to improve result or to treat complication

I use the following forms for my patients. They have been partly derived from what some of my colleagues have found helpful. I offer them here with the hope that they will aid or guide readers, who should not copy them slavishly with the expectation that they will satisfy their own needs or those of their patients or the legal requirements where they live. Even if these forms were adequate now, they might not be later.

Robert M. Goldwyn, M.D., Inc.

Authorization for Excision of Lesions

_____
Patient's Name

1. I authorize Robert M. Goldwyn, M.D. (the "Doctor") to perform an operation on me (or my _____) to: (description of procedure) _____
   _____
   _____
   _____
   _____
   _____
2. The nature and effects of the operation, the risks and complications involved, as well as alternate methods of treatment, have been fully explained to me by the Doctor and I understand them.
3. I authorize the Doctor to perform any other procedure that he may deem desirable in attempting to improve the condition stated in Paragraph 1 or any unhealthy or unforeseen condition that may be encountered during the operation.
4. I consent to the administration of anesthetics by the Doctor or under the direction of the physician responsible for this service.
5. I understand that the practice of medicine and surgery is not an exact science and that reputable practitioners cannot guarantee results. No guarantee or assurance has been given by the Doctor or anyone else as to the results that may be obtained.
6. I understand that the two sides of the human body are not the same and can never be made the same.
7. For the purpose of advancing medical education, I consent to the admittance of authorized observers to the operating room.
8. I give permission to Robert M. Goldwyn, M.D., Inc. to take still or motion clinical photographs with the understanding that such photographs remain the property of the corporation.

I certify that I have read the above authorization, that the explanations referred to therein were made to my satisfaction, and that I fully understand such explanations and the above authorization.

Signed _____
(Patient or person authorized to consent for patient)

Witness _____   Date _____

Robert M. Goldwyn, M.D., Inc.

Authorization for Eyelidplasty

Patient's Name

1. I authorize Robert M. Goldwyn, M.D. (the "Doctor") and his assistants to perform on me the operation known as eyelidplasty or blepharoplasty (a plastic surgical operation on the eyelids and surrounding structures).
2. The nature and effects of the operation, the risks and complications involved, as well as alternative methods of treatment, have been fully explained to me by the Doctor and I understand them.

    The following points, among others, have been specifically made clear:
    a. Incisions are used in and about the eyelids, and the incisions heal with scar tissue.
    b. The incision lines usually are conspicuous early postoperatively and for an indefinite period of time.
    c. There will be discoloration about the eyes for several days, and in some cases this can persist for considerably longer periods.
    d. There is the possibility of ectropion (a turning out of the eyelid).
    e. There is the rare possibility of blindness.
    f. The procedure is subject to the same postoperative complications as with other surgical procedures.
    g. Because of the nature of the procedure, an exact end-result cannot be predicted, and I have not been given any guarantee of specific results.
3. I authorize the Doctor to perform any other procedure that he may deem desirable in attempting to improve the condition stated in Paragraph 1 or any unhealthy or unforeseen condition that may be encountered during the operation.
4. I consent to the administration of anesthetics by the Doctor or under the direction of the physician responsible for this service.
5. I understand that the practice of medicine and surgery is not an exact science and that reputable practitioners cannot guarantee results. No guarantee or assurance has been given by the Doctor or anyone else as to the results that may be obtained.
6. I understand that the two sides of the human body are not the same and can never be made the same.
7. For the purpose of advancing medical education, I consent to the admittance of authorized observers to the operating room.

8. I give permission to Robert M. Goldwyn, M.D., Inc. to take still or motion clinical photographs with the understanding that such photographs remain the property of the corporation.
9. I am not known to be allergic to anything except: (list) ____

I certify that I have read the above authorization, that the explanations referred to therein were made to my satisfaction, and that I fully understand such explanations and the above authorization.

Signed _____
(Patient or person authorized to consent for patient)

Witness _____ Date _____

Robert M. Goldwyn, M.D., Inc.

Authorization for Rhytidectomy (Facelift)

Patient's Name

1. I authorize Robert M. Goldwyn, M.D. (the "Doctor") and his assistants to perform on me the operation known as rhytidectomy or facelift.
2. The nature and effects of the operation, the risks and complications involved, as well as alternative methods of treatment, have been fully explained to me by the Doctor and I understand them.

    The following points, among others, have been specifically made clear:
    a. Scars result from this operation. Every effort will be made to conceal or to make them as inconspicuous as possible.
    b. There may be facial swelling that may persist for several weeks.
    c. There may be discoloration (black and blue marks) that may persist for several weeks.
    d. There may be scattered areas of numbness over the face and neck following the surgery that may persist for an indefinite period of time.
    e. No guarantee has been made regarding the amount or percentage of improvement in terms of apparent age or the permanency of the results.
    f. At times fluid or blood may accumulate in the operative sites and these may require aspiration or drainage.
    g. There may be hair loss bilaterally.
    h. There is a possibility of injury to the facial nerves that could result in temporary or permanent weakness of some of the facial muscles.
    i. Part of the undermined skin could be lost, which could result in wide scars or necessitate a skin graft.
    j. Infection is possible in any type of surgery, including rhytidectomy.
3. I authorize the Doctor to perform any other procedure that he may deem desirable in attempting to improve the condition stated in Paragraph 1 or any unhealthy or unforeseen condition that may be encountered during the operation.
4. I consent to the administration of anesthetics by the Doctor or under the direction of the physician responsible for this service.

5. I understand that the practice of medicine and surgery is not an exact science and that reputable practitioners cannot guarantee results. No guarantee or assurance has been given by the Doctor or anyone else as to the results that may be obtained.
6. I understand that the two sides of the human body are not the same and can never be made the same.
7. For the purpose of advancing medical education, I consent to the admittance of authorized observers to the operating room.
8. I give permission to Robert M. Goldwyn, M.D., Inc. to take still or motion clinical photographs with the understanding that such photographs remain the property of the corporation.
9. I am not known to be allergic to anything except: (list) _____

I certify that I have read the above authorization, that the explanations referred to therein were made to my satisfaction, and that I fully understand such explanations and the above authorization.

Signed _____
(Patient or person authorized to consent for patient)

Witness _____   Date _____

Robert M. Goldwyn, M.D., Inc.

Authorization for Brow (Forehead) Lift

Patient's Name

1. I authorize Robert M. Goldwyn, M.D. (the "Doctor") and his assistants to perform on me (or my _____) the operation known as brow (forehead) lift.
2. The nature and effects of the operation, the risks and complications involved, as well as the alternative methods of treatment, have been fully explained to me by the doctor and I understand them.

   The following points, among others, have been specifically made clear:
   a. There will be early pain after operation, usually for 24 to 48 hours, but it could be longer.
   b. Numbness of the scalp and forehead can occur and is usually temporary but can be permanent.
   c. Itching of the scalp or forehead is also common.
   d. The hairline will be raised.
   e. It is possible to lose from lack of blood supply (necrosis) areas of the scalp and have the wounds heal over a period of weeks.
   f. There can be temporary or permanent loss of some hair.
   g. Scars can be wide.
   h. Bleeding can occur.
   i. Infection is possible.
   j. There may be temporary or permanent injury to nerves so that the eyebrow on one or both sides will not move and/or cannot be raised.
   k. It is possible that it will be difficult to close the eyes. This is usually a temporary condition but may be permanent.
3. I authorize the Doctor to perform any other procedure that he may deem desirable in attempting to improve the condition stated in Paragraph 1 or any unhealthy or unforeseen condition that may be encountered during the operation.
4. I consent to the administration of anesthetics by the Doctor or under the direction of the physician responsible for this service.
5. I understand that the practice of medicine and surgery is not an exact science and that reputable practitioners cannot guarantee results. No guarantee or assurance has been given by the Doctor or anyone else as to the results that may be obtained.
6. I understand that the two sides of the human body are not the same and can never be made the same.

7. For the purpose of advancing medical education, I consent to the admittance of authorized observers to the operating room.
8. I give permission to Robert M. Goldwyn, M.D., Inc. to take still or motion clinical photographs with the understanding that such photographs remain the property of the corporation.
9. I am not known to be allergic to anything except: (list) _____

I certify that I have read the above authorization, that the explanations referred to therein were made to my satisfaction, and that I fully understand such explanations and the above authorization.

Signed _____
(Patient or person authorized to consent for patient)

Witness _____ Date _____

Robert M. Goldwyn, M.D., Inc.

Authorization for Rhinoplasty

Patient's Name

1. I authorize Robert M. Goldwyn, M.D. (the "Doctor") and his assistants to perform on me (or my _____) the operation known as rhinoplasty, or commonly called cosmetic surgery to the nose. This may also include a procedure on the nasal septum for changing its size, configuration, or alignment in order to alter the breathing pattern.
2. The nature and effects of the operation, the risks and complications involved, as well as alternative methods of treatment, have been fully explained to me by the Doctor and I understand them.

    The following points, among others, have been specifically made clear:
    a. There will be swelling for an indeterminate period. Much of the swelling will normally disappear in a few days but the remainder may require several weeks, or even months to disappear completely.
    b. There will be discoloration (black and blue marks) on and about the face, principally around the eyes, for several days. In some cases the discoloration persists for considerably longer periods.
    c. Infrequently a permanent perforation may result from operation on the septum.
    d. Because of the nature of the procedure, it is stressed that no exact end-result can be predicted. No exact end-result has been promised.
    e. The procedure is subject to the same postoperative complications as other surgical procedures, e.g., infection, bleeding, pain.
3. I authorize the Doctor to perform any other procedure that he may deem desirable in attempting to improve the condition stated in Paragraph 1 or any unhealthy or unforeseen condition that may be encountered during the operation.
4. I consent to the administration of anesthetics by the Doctor or under the direction of the physician responsible for this service.
5. I understand that the practice of medicine and surgery is not an exact science and that reputable practitioners cannot guarantee results. No guarantee or assurance has been given by the Doctor or anyone else as to the results that may be obtained.
6. I understand that the two sides of the human body are not the same and can never be made the same.

7. For the purpose of advancing medical education, I consent to the admittance of authorized observers to the operating room.
8. I give permission to Robert M. Goldwyn, M.D., Inc. to take still or motion clinical photographs with the understanding that such photographs remain the property of the corporation.
9. I am not known to be allergic to anything except: (list) ____

_____

I certify that I have read the above authorization, that the explanations referred to therein were made to my satisfaction, and that I fully understand such explanations and the above authorization.

Signed _____
(Patient or person authorized to consent for patient)

Witness _____ Date _____

Robert M. Goldwyn, M.D., Inc.

Authorization for Dermabrasion

Patient's Name

1. I authorize Robert M. Goldwyn, M.D. (the "Doctor") and his assistants to perform on me an operation known as dermabrasion or commonly referred to as sanding or planing.
2. The nature and effects of the operation, the risks and complications involved, as well as alternative methods of treatment, have been fully explained to me by the Doctor and I understand them.

    The following points, among others, have been specifically made clear:
    a. During the dermabrasion process, I will experience discomfort and swelling, and my face will be covered with a crust, which will usually separate within 5 to 10 days.
    b. The skin will have a reddish appearance that could persist for an indefinite period.
    c. At the junction of the treated and untreated areas, there may be a difference in color, pigmentation, and texture of the skin.
    d. In some cases there may be alteration of pigmentation or the appearance of small cysts in the treated areas.
    e. Scarring is rare but may result from the procedure.
    f. Although a certain amount of improvement is anticipated, the exact amount of change in the appearance of the skin cannot be accurately predicted.
    g. The procedure will not prevent recurrence of the original problem, i.e., acne.
3. I authorize the Doctor to perform any other procedure that he may deem desirable in attempting to improve the condition stated in Paragraph 1 or any unhealthy or unforeseen condition that may be encountered during the operation.
4. I consent to the administration of anesthetics by the Doctor or under the direction of the physician responsible for this service.
5. I understand that the practice of medicine and surgery is not an exact science and that reputable practitioners cannot guarantee results. No guarantee or assurance has been given by the Doctor or anyone else as to the results that may be obtained.
6. I understand that the two sides of the human body are not the same and can never be made the same.
7. For the purpose of advancing medical education, I consent to the admittance of authorized observers to the operating room.

8. I give permission to Robert M. Goldwyn, M.D., Inc. to take still or motion clinical photographs with the understanding that such photographs remain the property of the corporation.
9. I am not known to be allergic to anything except: (list) ____

I certify that I have read the above authorization, that the explanations referred to therein were made to my satisfaction, and that I fully understand such explanations and the above authorization.

Signed _____
(Patient or person authorized to consent for patient)

Witness _____ Date _____

Appendix

Chemical Face Peel

Special Consent to Operation or Other Procedure

Patient: _____
Date: _____ Time: _____

1. I hereby authorize _____ and/or associates to perform a surgical procedure known as a chemical face peel on

   _____
   (Name of Patient) or (Myself)

2. The procedure listed in Paragraph 1 has been personally explained to me by the above doctor(s), and I completely understand the nature and consequences of the procedure. The following points, among others, have been specifically made clear:
   a. The process involves the application of chemicals to the face and this may require the use of a face mask for several days afterward.
   b. During the face-peeling process, I will experience discomfort and swelling, and my face will be covered with a crust, which will usually separate within 5 to 10 days.
   c. The skin will have a reddish appearance that may persist for an indefinite period; at the junction of the treated and untreated areas there may be a difference in color and texture of the skin.
   d. Scarring is rare but may result from the procedure.
   e. Although a certain amount of improvement is anticipated, the exact amount of change in the appearance of the skin cannot be accurately predicted.

3. I recognize that, during the course of the operation, unforeseen conditions may necessitate additional or different procedures than those set forth above. I therefore further authorize and request that the above-named surgeon, his assistants, or his designees perform such procedures as are, in his professional judgment, necessary and desirable, including, but not limited to, procedures involving pathology and radiology. The authority granted under this Paragraph 3 shall extend to remedying conditions that are not known to the above doctors at the time the operation is commenced.

4. I consent to the administration of local anesthesia to be applied by or under the direction and supervision of the above doctors, with the exception of

   _____
   (None or a Particular One)

5. I recognize that when general anesthesia is used, it presents additional risks over which the above doctors have no control, and I agree to discuss the risks of general anesthesia with the anesthesiologist before surgery is performed.
6. I am aware that the practice of medicine and surgery is not an exact science, and I acknowledge that no guarantees have been made to me as to the results of the operation or procedure.
7. I consent to be photographed before, during, and after the treatment and understand that these photographs will be the property of the above doctors and may be published in scientific journals and/or shown for scientific reasons.
8. I agree to keep the above doctors informed of any change of address so that they can notify me of any late findings, and I agree to cooperate with the above doctors in my care after surgery until completely discharged.
9. I am not known to be allergic to anything except: (list) ____

I have read the above consent and received a copy of it. I fully understand the contents of the consent and authorize and request the above doctors to perform this surgical procedure on me.

_____ _____
Witness   Patient

IF PATIENT IS A MINOR, COMPLETE THE FOLLOWING:
Patient is a minor ____ years of age, and we, the undersigned, are the parents, guardians, or legal representatives of the patient.

I have read the above consent and received a copy of it. I fully understand the contents of the consent and authorize and request the above doctors to perform this surgical procedure on me.

_____ _____
Witness   Parent or Legal Guardian

_____ _____
Witness   Parent or Legal Guardian

Robert M. Goldwyn, M.D., Inc.

Authorization for Abdominal Lipectomy

Patient's Name

1. I authorize Robert M. Goldwyn, M.D. (the "Doctor") and his assistants to perform on me an operation known as abdominal lipectomy or commonly called abdominoplasty.
2. The nature and effects of the operation, the risks and complications involved, as well as alternative methods of treatment, have been fully explained to me by the Doctor and I understand them.

    The following points, among others, have been specifically made clear:
    a. There will be a long transverse scar across the lower abdomen. The exact quality of this scar and its width cannot be determined before operation since different individuals scar differently.
    b. Areas of the abdomen may be numb after operation. This is often temporary but could be permanent.
    c. There may be accumulations of fluid beneath the skin that may require drainage or aspiration, and it may be necessary to repeat this procedure several times.
    d. There is a possibility that blood may collect beneath the skin flaps during the postoperative period. If this happens, it may be necessary to open the incision under general anesthesia and remove this accumulation of blood.
    e. Blood transfusion is not required in the majority of instances; however, occasionally blood transfusion may be necessary. If a blood transfusion is given, it carries the risk of hepatitis and/or a transfusion reaction.
    f. There is a possibility of some skin loss, and this may require skin grafting or another secondary surgical procedure.
    g. Swelling and discoloration around the operative area may persist for several weeks.
    h. There will be a circular elliptical scar around the umbilicus, and the umbilicus may have a different appearance following operation.
    i. In association with abdominoplasty, complications such as infection, phlebitis in the legs and pelvis, pulmonary embolism, and even death have been reported.
3. I authorize the Doctor to perform any other procedure that he may deem desirable in attempting to improve the condition stated in Paragraph 1 or any unhealthy or unforeseen condition that may be encountered during the operation.

4. I consent to the administration of anesthetics by the Doctor or under the direction of the physician responsible for this service.
5. I understand that the practice of medicine and surgery is not an exact science and that reputable practitioners cannot guarantee results. No guarantee or assurance has been given by the Doctor or anyone else as to the results that may be obtained.
6. I understand that the two sides of the human body are not the same and can never be made the same.
7. For the purpose of advancing medical education, I consent to the admittance of authorized observers to the operating room.
8. I give permission to Robert M. Goldwyn, M.D., Inc. to take still or motion clinical photographs with the understanding that such photographs remain the property of the corporation.
9. I am not known to be allergic to anything except: (list) ‾‾‾‾

I certify that I have read the above authorization, that the explanations referred to therein were made to my satisfaction, and that I fully understand such explanations and the above authorization.

Signed ‾‾‾‾‾‾‾‾‾‾‾‾‾‾‾‾‾‾‾‾‾‾‾‾‾‾
(Patient or person authorized to consent for patient)

Witness ‾‾‾‾‾‾‾‾‾‾‾‾‾‾‾‾‾‾‾‾‾‾ Date ‾‾‾‾‾‾‾‾‾‾

Robert M. Goldwyn, M.D., Inc.

Authorization for Liposuctioning

Patient's Name

1. I authorize Robert M. Goldwyn, M.D. (the "Doctor") and his assistants to perform on me (or my _____) the operation known as liposuctioning.
2. The nature and effects of the operation, the risks and complications involved, as well as alternative methods of treatment, have been fully explained to me by the Doctor and I understand them.

    The following points, among others, have been specifically made clear:
    a. Uneven contour, surface irregularities, and lumpiness may result. These problems may occur after liposuction and normally resolve or greatly improve in six months with just time and with massage by the patient. Frequently, the skin will have a rippled texture prior to operation and this usually lasts following liposuction.
    b. Numbness may be present in areas treated by liposuction, but it normally disappears in three or four months.
    c. Infection can occur with any operation. Its incidence after liposuction is low.
    d. Pain may be felt in the lateral thighs and ankle area, even several months after operation. It may be aggravated by jogging or exercise. This discomfort usually disappears.
    e. Because the liposuction requires dissection and leaves empty spaces, blood and serum may collect but usually disappear within a few weeks. Bruising is common and can last for two weeks and occasionally longer.
    f. Areas of skin loss can occur but are infrequent.
    g. Scars from liposuction are usually minimal, and they are usually hidden, whenever possible; however, no one can precisely predict wound healing.
    h. Diffuse or irregular swelling can last for as long as six months after operation. The ankles and the feet tend to stay swollen the longest (from four to six months) after liposuction of the knees, calves, or ankles.
3. I authorize the Doctor to perform any other procedure that he may deem desirable in attempting to improve the condition stated in Paragraph 1 or any unhealthy or unforeseen condition that may be encountered during the operation.
4. I consent to the administration of anesthetics by the Doctor or under the direction of the physician responsible for this service.

Appendix

5. I understand that the practice of medicine and surgery is not an exact science and that reputable practitioners cannot guarantee results. No guarantee or assurance has been given by the Doctor or anyone else as to the results that may be obtained.
6. I understand that the two sides of the human body are not the same and can never be made the same.
7. For the purpose of advancing medical education, I consent to the admittance of authorized observers to the operating room.
8. I give permission to Robert M. Goldwyn, M.D., Inc. to take still or motion clinical photographs with the understanding that such photographs remain the property of the corporation.
9. I am not known to be allergic to anything except: (list) _____

I certify that I have read the above authorization, that the explanations referred to therein were made to my satisfaction, and that I fully understand such explanations and the above authorization.

Signed _____
(Patient or person authorized to consent for patient)

Witness _____ Date _____

Robert M. Goldwyn, M.D., Inc.

Authorization for Augmentation Mammoplasty

Patient's Name

1. I authorize Robert M. Goldwyn, M.D. (the "Doctor") and his assistants to perform an operation on me (or my _____) for increasing the size of my breasts.
2. The nature and effects of the operation, the risks and complications involved, as well as alternative methods of treatment, have been fully explained to me by the Doctor and I understand them.

   The following points, among others, have been specifically made clear:
   a. The operation has been done for several years, but the end results cannot be determined for many more years.
   b. Research indicates that the material implanted in the body does not cause malignancy in human subjects.
   c. There is a possibility that my body may not tolerate these implants, thereby necessitating their removal. This event occurs in a small percentage of cases.
   d. The breasts may become firm (capsule formation and contracture). This condition may be permanent and may cause pain and discomfort.
   e. No guarantee has been given concerning size and shape of the breasts. Good results are expected but not guaranteed.
   f. In some patients the margin of the implants will be felt.
   g. The incision will heal with a scar that will be permanent.
   h. Postoperative bleeding or infection may occur around the implant, thus requiring another operation(s).
   i. After being exposed to cold temperatures (e.g., swimming in cold water), the breasts may feel cooler than surrounding body tissues.
   j. Pregnancy is not recommended for at least six (6) months after operation.
   k. Numbness or hypersensitivity of the nipple, areola, or breasts may occur following operation.
   l. The procedure is subject to the same postoperative complications as with other surgical procedures.
3. I authorize the Doctor to perform any other procedure that he may deem desirable in attempting to improve the condition stated in Paragraph 1 or any unhealthy or unforeseen condition that may be encountered during the operation.
4. I consent to the administration of anesthetics by the Doctor or under the direction of the physician responsible for this service.

Appendix

5. I understand that the practice of medicine and surgery is not an exact science and that reputable practitioners cannot guarantee results. No guarantee or assurance has been given by the Doctor or anyone else as to the results that may be obtained.
6. I understand that the two sides of the human body are not the same and can never be made the same.
7. For the purpose of advancing medical education, I consent to the admittance of authorized observers to the operating room.
8. I give permission to Robert M. Goldwyn, M.D., Inc. to take still or motion clinical photographs with the understanding that such photographs remain the property of the corporation.
9. I am not known to be allergic to anything except: (list) _____

I certify that I have read the above authorization, that the explanations referred to therein were made to my satisfaction, and that I fully understand such explanations and the above authorization.

Signed _____
(Patient or person authorized to consent for patient)

Witness _____ Date _____

Robert M. Goldwyn, M.D., Inc.

Authorization for Mastopexy (Correction of Breast Ptosis)

Patient's Name

1. I authorize Robert M. Goldwyn, M.D. (the "Doctor") and his assistants to perform on me (or my _____) the operation known as mastopexy (correction of ptotic or sagging breast[s]).
2. The nature and effects of the operation, the risks and complications involved, as well as alternative methods of treatment, have been fully explained to me by the Doctor and I understand them.

    The following points, among others, have been specifically made clear:
    a. The scars are permanent.
    b. Although having the breasts match is the surgical objective, perfect symmetry of nipples, areolae, and breasts cannot be achieved.
    c. Complications after reduction mammoplasty can be those after any surgical procedure.
    d. Bleeding and infection may occur and may require additional procedure(s) for treatment.
    e. There is a possibility that the blood supply to one or both nipples and areolae and skin of the breasts may become impaired, and necrosis (death of tissue) may result. This complication may require later reconstruction.
    f. There is decreased likelihood of breast nursing after this operation.
    g. Sensation in the nipples and areolae and breasts may be temporarily or permanently altered.
    h. As far as now known, this operation does not influence the later development of cancer.
    i. Swelling and ecchymosis (black and blue marks) may take a few weeks to disappear; several months are necessary for the breasts to assume their eventual shape, which may not be final since with time and gravity, the breast(s) may sag again.
    j. Although every attempt will be made to make each breast, including nipple and areola, as normal and pleasing in appearance as possible, this objective cannot always be attained.
3. I authorize the Doctor to perform any other procedure that he may deem desirable in attempting to improve the condition stated in Paragraph 1 or any unhealthy or unforeseen condition that may be encountered during the operation.

4. I consent to the administration of anesthetics by the Doctor or under the direction of the physician responsible for this service.
5. I understand that the practice of medicine and surgery is not an exact science and that reputable practitioners cannot guarantee results. No guarantee or assurance has been given by the Doctor or anyone else as to the results that may be obtained.
6. I understand that the two sides of the human body are not the same and can never be made the same.
7. For the purpose of advancing medical education, I consent to the admittance of authorized observers to the operating room.
8. I give permission to Robert M. Goldwyn, M.D., Inc. to take still or motion clinical photographs with the understanding that such photographs remain the property of the corporation.
9. I am not known to be allergic to anything except: (list) _____
_____

I certify that I have read the above authorization, that the explanations referred to therein were made to my satisfaction, and that I fully understand such explanations and the above authorization.

Signed _____
(Patient or person authorized to consent for patient)

Witness _____ Date _____

Robert M. Goldwyn, M.D., Inc.

Authorization for Reduction Mammoplasty

Patient's Name

1. I authorize Robert M. Goldwyn, M.D. (the "Doctor") and his assistants to perform on me (or my _____) the operation known as reduction mammoplasty (breast reduction).
2. The nature and effects of the operation, the risks and complications involved, as well as alternative methods of treatment, have been fully explained to me by the Doctor and I understand them.

    The following points, among others, have been specifically made clear:
    a. The scars are permanent.
    b. Although having the breasts match is the surgical objective, perfect symmetry of nipples, areolae, and breasts cannot be achieved.
    c. Complications after reduction mammoplasty can be those after any surgical procedure.
    d. Bleeding and infection following breast reduction may occur and may require an additional procedure(s) for treatment.
    e. There is a possibility that the blood supply to one or both nipples and areolae and skin of the breasts may become impaired, and necrosis (death of tissue) may result. This complication may require later reconstruction.
    f. There is a decreased likelihood of breast nursing after reduction mammoplasty.
    g. As far as now known, this operation does not influence the later development of breast cancer.
    h. Swelling and ecchymosis (black and blue marks) take several weeks to disappear; several months are necessary for the breasts to assume their final shape.
    i. Although every attempt will be made to make each breast, including nipple and areola, as normal and pleasing in appearance as possible, the objective cannot always be attained.
    j. Sensation to the breast, including nipple and areola, is usually altered and may be decreased permanently.
3. I authorize the Doctor to perform any other procedure that he may deem desirable in attempting to improve the condition stated in Paragraph 1 or any unhealthy or unforeseen condition that may be encountered during the operation.
4. I consent to the administration of anesthetics by the Doctor or under the direction of the physician responsible for this service.

Appendix

5. I understand that the practice of medicine and surgery is not an exact science and that reputable practitioners cannot guarantee results. No guarantee or assurance has been given by the Doctor or anyone else as to the results that may be obtained.
6. I understand that the two sides of the human body are not the same and can never be made the same.
7. For the purpose of advancing medical education, I consent to the admittance of authorized observers to the operating room.
8. I give permission to Robert M. Goldwyn, M.D., Inc. to take still or motion clinical photographs with the understanding that such photographs remain the property of the corporation.
9. I am not known to be allergic to anything except: (list) ____

I certify that I have read the above authorization, that the explanations referred to therein were made to my satisfaction, and that I fully understand such explanations and the above authorization.

Signed _____
(Patient or person authorized to consent for patient)

Witness _____ Date _____

Robert M. Goldwyn, M.D., Inc.

Authorization for Breast Reconstruction

Patient's Name

1. I authorize Robert M. Goldwyn, M.D. and his assistants to perform on me (or my _____) known as breast reconstruction.
2. The nature and effects of the operation, the risks and complications involved, as well as alternative methods of treatment, have been fully explained to me by Dr. Goldwyn and I understand them.

    The following points, among others, have been specifically made clear:

    a. Although the objective of the operation is to reconstruct the breast(s) to look as normal as possible, the final result will never be a perfectly normal-looking and normal-feeling breast.
    b. Absolute symmetry with the opposite side cannot be achieved.
    c. Swelling and ecchymosis (black and blue marks) *usually* take a few weeks to disappear. Pain and discomfort usually disappear in a few months but rarely may persist.
    d. The reconstructed breast may be excessively and uncomfortably firm.
    e. There will be permanent scarring.
    f. If an implant is used as part of the breast reconstruction, it may have to be removed because of infection, hematoma (accumulation of blood), excessive pain, and/or firmness.
    g. When skin, fat, and muscle are taken from the abdomen or back for breast reconstruction, there can be resulting tightness in the area from which it was taken. Fluid can collect (seroma) underneath the skin and can require removal by needle aspiration. The transferred tissues may turn black and not survive, or portions can undergo such changes. The use of abdominal muscles can weaken the area from which they are taken. Some people find it difficult to sit up from a lying position after this procedure.
    h. More than one operation may be necessary to achieve the goals of breast reconstruction, regardless of the particular surgical technique used.
    i. All breast reconstruction procedures are subject to complications such as bleeding, infection, pain, and poor wound healing.

3. I authorize the Doctor to perform any other procedure that he may deem desirable in attempting to improve the condition stated in Paragraph 1 or any unhealthy or unforeseen condition that may be encountered during the operation.
4. I consent to the administration of anesthetics by the Doctor or under the direction of the physician responsible for this service.
5. I understand that the practice of medicine and surgery is not an exact science and that reputable practitioners cannot guarantee results. No guarantee or assurance has been given by the Doctor or anyone else as to the results that may be obtained.
6. I understand that the two sides of the human body are not the same and can never be made the same.
7. For the purpose of advancing medical education, I consent to the admittance of authorized observers to the operating room.
8. I give permission to Robert M. Goldwyn, M.D., Inc. to take still or motion clinical photographs with the understanding that such photographs remain the property of the corporation.
9. I am not known to be allergic to anything except: (list) _____

I certify that I have read the above authorization, that the explanations referred to therein were made to my satisfaction, and that I fully understand such explanations and the above authorization.

Signed _____
(Patient or person authorized to consent for patient)

Witness _____ Date _____

Robert M. Goldwyn, M.D., Inc.

Because insurance coverage varies with different companies, I understand that I may be responsible for the hospital costs associated with any surgery undertaken to improve a result or to treat a complication.

_____
Date

_____
Signature

_____
Witness

Index

Abdominal lipectomy, authorization for, 343–344
Abdominoplasty, 211–214
　informing patient about, 212–214
　insurance coverage for, 214
　physical examination for, 212
Acne scars, dermabrasion of, 225–226
Acquiescing patient, 72–73
Acquired immunodeficiency syndrome (AIDS), patients with, rhinoplasty for, 129–131
Adiposogenital dystrophy, 188
Adolescent
　female
　　reassurance of, regarding mastectomy and reconstruction, 203
　　rhinoplasty in, 114–117
　　initial consultation with, 42
　male
　　gynecomastia correction in, 187–188
　　rhinoplasty in, 117–119
Agenesis, breast, correction of, 173–175
Aging
　double standard of, 140
　process of, 140–141
　signs of, 139
AIDS-related complex (ARC), 129–130
Alcohol-dependency, of physicians, 304
Altruism, in medicine, 13–15
American Society of Plastic and Reconstructive Surgeons, 5, 6
Antidysplasia, and esthetic surgery, 59
Apert's syndrome, 240
Appearance, enhancement of, in esthetic surgery, 55–57
Areola, altered sensation in, after breast reduction, 181
Asymmetry, breast, correction of, 173–175
Attorney
　and close family, elective treatment of, 272
　letter to, concerning scar revision, 222–223
Audiovisual aids, for informed consent, 90

349

Augmentation mammoplasty. *See* Breast augmentation
Authorization form(s), 321–322
　for abdominal lipectomy, 343–344
　for augmentation mammoplasty, 347–348
　for breast reconstruction, 327–328
　for chemical peel, 341–342
　for dermabrasion, 339–340
　for eyelidplasty, 331–332
　for facelift, 333–334
　for forehead lift, 335–336
　for liposuction, 345–346
　for mastopexy, 323–324
　personal, 329, 330
　for reduction mammoplasty, 325–326
　for rhinoplasty, 337–338
Autotransfusion, for breast reduction, 182

Basal cell carcinoma, 227–228
Behavior, negative, of physician or staff, 44
Bell's palsy, 146
Biopsy, of skin lesions, 228–229
Blepharoplasty. *See* Eyelidplasty
Blood transfusion, autologous, for breast reduction, 182
Body language, 28
Boys, young, reduction otoplasty for, 216–220
Breast
　altered sensation in, after reduction mammoplasty, 181
　facelift of. *See* Mastopexy
　opposite
　　comparison of reconstructed breast to, 199–200
　　removal of, 199
Breast agenesis
　before and after operation, 175
　correction of, 173–175
　　informing patient about, 174–175
　　physical examination for, 174
Breast asymmetry
　before and after operation, 175
　correction of, 173–175

　　informing patient about, 174–175
　　physical examination for, 174
Breast augmentation, 160–173
　authorization for, 347–348
　informing patient about, 164–173
　　ability to nurse, 167–168
　　abnormal contour, 168–169
　　altered sensation, 169–170
　　closed capsulotomy, 171–172
　　cold sensation, 169
　　firmness, 168–169
　　hematoma, 166–167
　　hypoplasia, 165–166
　　implant placement, 167
　　incisions and scars, 167
　　infection, 166–167
　　pain, 170–171
　　pectus excavatum, 166
　　possible future breast cancer, 171
　　ptosis, 165–166
　　size, 164–165
　　type of implant, 168
　instruction for patient following, 172–173
　with mastopexy, 177
　patient selection for, 160–163
　physical examination for, 163–164
Breast contour, abnormal, after augmentation, 168–169
Breast expander, patient information regarding, 196
Breast firmness, after augmentation, 168–169
Breast implant. *See also* Prosthesis
　leakage from, 172–173
　patient information regarding, 196
　placement of, 167
　rupture of, 172
　size of, 164–165
　type of, 168
Breast reconstruction, after mastectomy. *See* Mastectomy, reconstruction after
Breast reduction, 178–186
　authorization for, 325–326
　autologous transfusion for, 182
　insurance coverage for, 183

Index

mammograms prior to, 183
with mastopexy, 177
obesity and, 182
pathologic findings in, 185–186
patient selection for, 179–180
physical examination for, 180–182
postoperative care after, 183–186
Brow lift. See Forehead lift
Buttocks lift, 214–216
  informing patient about, 216
  physical examination for, 215–216

Cancellations, 262
Cancer
  breast augmentation and, 165, 171
  of head and neck. See Head and neck surgery
  oral, 235–236
  recurrence of, after mastectomy reconstruction, 206
  skin, 227–228
Capsulotomy, closed, 171–172
Care
  errors of, in emergency room, 263–264
  terminating, of patient, 265–267
Caring, quality of, 10
Chemical peel
  authorization for, 341–342
  for wrinkles, 147
Children. See also Pediatric patient(s)
  reduction otoplasty for, 216–220
Chin augmentation, rhinoplasty and, 132–134
Chin implant, with facelift, 149
Christmas disease, 301
Cold sensation, following breast augmentation, 169
Collagen injections, 159–160
Communication, 26–27
  adequate, for informed consent, 93–95
  with patient, 34–35
  with pediatric patient, 241
Competence, of physician, 14
Confidentiality, importance of, 45–46
Consent, informed, 88–95

adequate communication for, 93–95
consent forms for, 91–92
written information in, 89–91
Consent forms, 91–92
Consultation
  impartial, for scar revision, 221
  initial, 9–49
    anatomy and physiology of, 24–49
    end of, 110–112
    examination in, 41–49
    for eyelidplasty and facelift, 143–145
    face-to-face encounter in, 32–41
    physician-patient relationship in, 9–17
    primary objective of, 41
    setting for, 17–24
  for mastectomy reconstruction, 193–194
  second, for rhinoplasty, 136–137
Contour, breast, abnormal, after augmentation, 168–169
Cosmetic surgery. See also Esthetic surgery
  definition of, 52
Cross-cultural studies, 298–299

Defendant, in malpractice suit, involvement with, 273–274
Deformity, minimal, patient with, 69
Demanding patient, 65–66
Depression
  after mastectomy reconstruction, 206
  in patient, 74–75
Dermabrasion
  of acne scars, 225–226
  authorization for, 339–340
  for wrinkles, 147
Difficult patient, 259–261
  vs. dissatisfied patient, 259
Disappearing patient, 261–262
Disliked patient, 78–80
Dissatisfied patient, 82–83, 246–259
  admit reality with, 249
  future care of, 258
  make self available to, 250–251
  marshal support for, 250

Dissatisfied patient—*Continued*
  physical examination of, 256–257
  plan of action for, 249–250
  second opinion for, 252
  use of consultant with, 251–259
  vs. difficult patient, 259
Doctor-patient relationship, 9–10
  beginning of, 15–17
  differences in, 298–299
  hospitals and, 18–21
  hostility in, 49
  lack of confidentiality detrimental to, 45–46
  physician's office and, 21–24
Dressings, application of, 154
Drug-dependency, of physicians, 304
"Dry eye," 146
Dying patient, 267–270
Dystrophy, adiposogenital, 188

Ears, prominent, correction of, 216–220. *See also* Otoplasty, reduction
Elective nature, of esthetic surgery, 57–58
Embarrassment
  of esthetic surgery patient, 58–60
  of patient, 41
Emergency room, patient in, 262–264
  common errors of care in, 263–264
Enhancement of appearance, in esthetic surgery, 55–57
Epithelioma, 228
Eschemia, as complication of breast reconstruction, 200
Esthetic surgery, 53–112
  patient selection for, 64–87. *See also* Patient(s)
  special feature(s) of, 53–64
    elective nature as, 55–57
    enhancement as, 55–57
    finances as, 64
    guilt and embarrassment as, 58–60
    minimizing surgical reality as, 60–62
    objective of happiness as, 62
    pain as, 62
    physical examination as, 58
    preponderance of females as, 63
    rapid recovery and little regression as, 60
    visibility as, 54–55
Examination, physical. *See* Physical examination
Expander, breast, patient information regarding, 196
Eyelidplasty, 138–148
  authorization for, 331–332
  informing patient about 150–153
  initial consultation for, 143–145
  for malar pouches, 148
  for male patient, 142–143
  patient selection for, 138–143
  physical examination for, 145–147
  postoperative care and instructions following, 154–159
  postoperative satisfaction with, 156–159
  for wrinkling and sagging, 147–148

Facelift, 138–148
  authorization for, 333–334
  of breasts. *See* Mastopexy
  chin implant with, 149
  informing patient about, 150–153
  initial consultation for, 143–145
  for malar pouches, 148
  for male patient, 142–143
  patient selection for, 138–143
  physical examination for, 145–147
  postoperative care and instructions following, 154–159
  postoperative satisfaction with, 156–159
  for wrinkling and sagging, 147–148
Facial fracture, treatment of, 234–235
Facial peel, 147
  authorization for, 341–342
Factitious disease, patient with, 245–246
False history, patient who gives, 67–68
Family, patient's, involving, in breast reconstruction, 202–203
Fat transplantation, 159–160
Fees. *See also* Payment

financing schemes for payment of, 102–103
prepayment of, 100–101
professional courtesy, 101–102
setting of, 97–99
for surgery, 95–103
Females, preponderance of, esthetic surgery and, 63
Financing. *See also* Payment
attitudes toward, 46
Financing schemes, 102–103
Firmness, breast, after augmentation, 168–169
Flaps
breast reconstruction with, patient information concerning, 197
skin, 230
Flattery, by patient, 67
Forehead lift, 149–159
authorization for, 335–336
dressings for, application of, 154
informing patient about, 153–154
postoperative care and instructions following, 154–159
postoperative satisfaction with, 156–159
surgeon behavior during, 154
Fracture
facial, treatment of, 234–235
nasal, reduction of, 233–234
Frolich's syndrome, 188

Grafts, skin, 230–231
Guilt, of esthetic surgery patient, 58–60
Gynecomastia, correction of, 187–190
informing patient about, 188–189
patient selection for, 187–188
payment for, 189
physical examination for, 188
postoperative care following, 190
procedure for, 189–190

Happiness, as objective, in esthetic surgery, 62
Head and neck surgery, 235–240
cosmetic aspects of, 237
follow-up after, 239–240
hospital stay for, 238–239
informing patient about, 237–238
physical examination for, 236
preoperative considerations concerning, 238
Health Maintenance Organization (HMO), 4–5
Hematoma, associated with breast augmentation, 166–167
Herpes simplex infection, as complication of dermabrasion, 226
History taking, 30–31
for liposuction, 208
for mastectomy reconstruction, 193–194
from patient who gives false history, 67–68
for scar revision, 221
Hospital(s), 18–21
Hospital stay, for head and neck surgery, 238–239
for pediatric patient, 242, 243–244
Hostility, between patient and doctor, 49
Hsaio report, 96
Human immunodeficiency virus (HIV), testing for, 129
Hypoplasia, mammary, 165–166

Implant
breast. *See* Breast implant
chin, with facelift, 149
"Impression management," process of, 25–27
Incisions, for breast augmentation, 167
Indecisive patient, 68–69
Infection
associated with breast augmentation, 166–167
as complication of dermabrasion, 226
Information
patient
prior to abdominoplasty, 212–214
prior to breast augmentation, 164–173
prior to correction for breast agenesis and asymmetry, 174–175

Information—*Continued*
  prior to correction of gynecomastia, 188–189
  prior to dermabrasion of acne scars, 225–226
  prior to head and neck surgery, 237–238
  prior to liposuction, 209–211
  prior to mastectomy reconstruction, 195–198
  prior to mastopexy, 176–178
  prior to reduction otoplasty, 218–220
  prior to rhinoplasty, 120–121
  prior to scar revision, 222–223
  prior to thigh and buttocks lift, 216
  transmittal of, permission from patients for, 223
  written, in informed consent, 89–91
Informed consent, 88–95
  adequate communication for, 93–95
  consent forms for, 91–92
  written information in, 89–91
Initial consultation. *See* Consultation, initial
Injection(s), collagen, 159–160
Insurance company, letter to, concerning scar revision, 222–223
Insurance coverage
  for abdominoplasty, 214
  for breast reduction, 183
Intelligence, of patient, underestimating, 43–46
Interpersonal transactions, 25–27
Ischemic necrosis, of nipple-areola area, 181

Laryngectomy groups, 237
Latissimus dorsi flap, breast reconstruction with, patient information regarding, 197
Law, patients and, 270–274
Law suits. *See* Malpractice suits
Lesions, skin. *See* Skin lesions
Lipectomy, abdominal, authorization for, 343–344
Liposuction, 207–211
  authorization for, 345–346
  history taking for, 208
  informing patient about, 209–211
  patient selection for, 208
  physical examination for, 209

Macromastia, physical consequences of, 179
Malar pouches, treatment for, 148
Malignant melanoma, 227
Malpractice insurance, 270
Malpractice suits, 270
  involvement in, 273–274
  minimizing risks for, 271
  and patient selection, 272–273
  patient who has filed, treatment of, 272–273
  against physicians, 275–276
Mammary hypoplasia, 165–166
Mammary ptosis, 165–166
Mammograms, prior to breast reduction, 183
Mammoplasty
  augmentation. *See* Breast augmentation
  reduction. *See* Breast reduction
Mastectomy
  reconstruction after, 190–207
    attitudes toward, 190–192
    authorization for, 327–328
    complications associated with, 200
    consultation for, 193–194
    fees for, 202
    history taking for, 194
    informing patient about, 195–198
    involving patient's family and intimates in, 202–203
    limitations of, 198–199
    and opposite breast, 199–200
    other information concerning, 201
    photographs of, 201–202
    physical examination for, 194–195
    postoperative care following, 205–207
    pressures on surgeon in, 205
    psychological benefits of, 192

psychological preparation for, 204–205
timing of, 193
subcutaneous, 199
Mastopexy, 175–178
authorization for, 323–334
informing patient about, 176–178
patient selection for, 175–176
physical examination for, 176
postoperative care after, 178
Medicine, altruism and selfishness in, 13–15
Melanoma, malignant, 227
Mentoplasty, rhinoplasty and, 132–134
Moral probity, 14
Mother and daughter, rhinoplasty for, 135–136
Munchausen's syndrome, 245

Nasal fracture, reduction of, 233–234
Neck surgery. *See* Head and neck surgery
Nevus, 228–229
Nipple
altered sensation in, after breast reduction, 181
inverted, 186–187
Nipple-areola complex
ischemic necrosis of, 181
reconstruction of, patient information regarding, 197–198
Nose job. *See* Rhinoplasty
Nurse, ability to, breast augmentation and, 167–168

Obesity, and breast reduction, 182
Office, physician's, 21–24
seating arrangements in, 33–34
waiting room in, 30
Office procedure(s)
inefficiency of, 46
introduction of patient as, 32
standard, 32
Operative procedure(s)
abdominoplasty as, 211–214
for breast asymmetry or agenesis, 173–175

breast augmentation as, 160–173
collagen injection and fat transplantation as, 159–160
dermabrasion as, 225–226
eyelidplasty as, 138–148
facelift as, 138–148
chin implant with, 149
for facial fractures, 234–235
forehead lift as, 149–159
for gynecomastia correction, 187–190
for head and neck tumors, 235–240
for inverted nipple, 186–187
liposuction as, 207–211
mastopexy as, 175–178
for prominent ear correction, 216–220
reconstruction after mastectomy as, 190–207
reduction mammoplasty as, 178–186
for reduction of nasal fracture, 233–234
for removal of skin lesions, 231–232
rhinoplasty as, 114–138
for scar revision, 220–224
for skin lesions, 227–233
thigh and buttock lift as, 214–216
types of, 113–240
Oral cancer, 235–236. *See also* Head and neck surgery
Otoplasty, reduction
informing patient about, 218–220
patient selection for, 216–218
physical examination for, 218
Out-of-town patient, 80–82

Pain
associated with breast augmentation, 170–171
in esthetic surgery, 62
Palsy, Bell's, 146
Paranoid patient, 73
Paraplegic patient, 244–245
Parental support, for pediatric patient, 243
Patient(s)
acquiescing, 72–73
with acquired immunodeficiency syndrome, rhinoplasty for, 129–131

Patient(s)—*Continued*
  addressing, 33
  adolescent, 42
  from afar, 80–82
  appraising, 47–49
  attempts at communication with, 34–35
  choice of, 49
  demanding, 65–66
  depressed, 73–75
  difficult, 259–261
  disappearing, 261–262
  disliked, 78–80
  dissatisfied, 82–83, 246–259. *See also* Dissatisfied patient
  duties and rights of, 10–11
  dying, 267–270
  embarrassment of, 41
  in emergency room, 262–264
    common errors of care in, 263–264
  examination of. *See* Physical examination
  with factitious disease, 245–246
  family of, involving, in breast reconstruction, 202–203
  female
    older
      reduction otoplasty for, 216–220
      rhinoplasty for, 124–126
    preponderance of, esthetic surgery and, 63
  flattering, 67
  indecisive, 68–69
  instructions to, prior to removal of skin lesions, 232
  intelligence of, underestimating, 43–46
  and law, 270–274
  male
    eyelidplasty and facelift for, 142–143
    rhinoplasty for, 126–131
  with minimal deformity, 69
  paranoid, 73–75
  paraplegic, 244–245
  pediatric. *See* Pediatric patient(s)
  perfectionist, 70
  permission from, for transmittal of information, 223
  plasti-surgiholic, 71–72
  in psychotherapy, 75–77
  rejection of rhinoplasty for, reasons for, 131–132
  rude, 65–66
  saying "no" to, 83–86
  "shopper," 70–71
  sources of, 4–6
  "special," 78
  terminating care of, 265–267
  types of, 64–87
  unkempt, 66
  vague, 68–69
  who gives false history, 67–68
  who makes office his/her home, 66
  who refuses to be photographed, 69–70
  who refuses to undress, 69
  who writes excessively long letter, 64–65
  whose spouse says "no," 77–78
Patient awareness, during rhinoplasty, 122–123
Patient satisfaction, 62
Patient selection
  for breast augmentation, 160–163
  for correction of gynecomastia, 187–188
  for eyelidplasty and facelift, 138–143
  for liposuction, 208
  for mastopexy, 175–176
  for reduction otoplasty, 216–218
  for scar revision, 220–221
Payment. *See also* Fees; Financing
  for breast reconstruction, 202
  for cosmetic surgery, 64
  for gynecomastia correction, 189
  for rhinoplasty, 134–135
  for scar revision, 224
Pectus excavatum, 166
Pediatric patient(s), 240–244
  communication with, 241
  follow-up examination of, 242
  hospitalization of, 242, 243–244
  parental support for, 243

Perfectionist patient, 70
Personal authorization form, 329, 330
Photographs
  for breast reconstruction evaluation, 201–202
  patient who refuses, 69–70
  for rhinoplasty evaluation, 120
  for scar revision, 224
Physical examination
  for abdominoplasty, 212
  for breast agenesis and asymmetry, 174
  for breast augmentation, 163–164
  for breast reduction, 180–182
  for correction of gynecomastia, 188
  for dermabrasion of acne scars, 225
  for esthetic surgery, 58
  for eyelidplasty and facelift, 145–147
  for head and neck surgery, 236
  for liposuction, 209
  for mastectomy reconstruction, 194–195
  for mastopexy, 176
  persons present at time of, 41–42
  quality of, 42–43
  for reduction otoplasty, 218
  for rhinoplasty, in adolescent, 119–120
  for scar revision, 221–222
  for thigh and buttocks lift, 215–216
  undressing for, patient's refusal and, 69–70
Physician(s). *See also* Doctor-patient relationship
  alcohol and drug-dependency of, 304
  availability of, 250–251
  choice of, 49
  competence of, 14
  inefficiency of, 46
  law suits against, 275–276
  negative behavior of, affecting patient, 44
  office of. *See* Office, physician's
  patient trust in, 12
  preferred qualities in, 22–23
  previous experience of, 87
  professional self-image of, 6–7

referring, 109–110
responsibilities of, 12
Plaintiff, in malpractice suit, involvement with, 273–274
Plasti-surgiholic patient, 71–72
Plastic surgeon, 51
  pressures on, mastectomy patient and, 205
  professional life of, 277–305
    earliest stage in, 179–282
    last stage in, 294–298
    middle stage in, 285–294
    renewal of, 303–305
    ruminations concerning, 298–303
    second stage: early years in practice as, 282–285
  professional self-image of, 6–7
  sources of, 6
Postoperative care
  in breast reduction, 183–186
  in correction of gynecomastia, 190
  in eyelidplasty and facelift, 154–159
  in head and neck surgery, 239–240
  in mastopexy, 178
  in reconstruction after mastectomy, 205–207
  in rhinoplasty, 123–124
  in skin lesion removal, 232–233
Prepayment, 100–101
Private practice
  early years in, 282–285
  final years in, 294–298
  middle years in, 286–294
Professional courtesy, 101–102
Prosthesis. *See also* Breast implant
  in breast augmentation, 163, 164–165
  external, 191
Psychotherapy
  for mastectomy patients, 204–205
  patient in, 75–77
Ptosis, mammary, correction of, 165–166
  authorization for, 323–324

Race, and doctor-patient relationship, 29
Radiation therapy
  for head and neck tumors, 237
  for skin lesions, 228

Reconstructive surgery
  after mastectomy, 190–207. See also
    Mastectomy, reconstruction after
  definition of, 52
Recovery, rapid, from esthetic surgery, 60
Rectus abdominus flap, breast reconstruction with, patient information regarding, 197
Reduction, of nasal fracture, 233–234
Reduction mammoplasty. See Breast reduction
Reduction otoplasty. See Otoplasty, reduction
Referring physician, 109–110
Regression, less, in esthetic surgery, 60
Religion, and doctor-patient relationship, 29
Residency, in plastic surgery, 279–282
Rhinoplasty, 114–137
  in adolescent
    complications associated with, 121–122
    female, 114–117
      history of, 116–117
    informing patient of operative plans for, 120–121
    male, 117–119
    physical examination for, 119–120
    postoperative care following, 123–124
    unnecessary noise and talk during, 122–123
  authorization for, 337–338
  chin augmentation with, 132–134
  male patient for, 126–131
    acquired immunodeficiency syndrome and, 129–131
    mother and daughter combination for, 135–136
  in older woman, 124–126
  payment for, 134–135
  rejection of patient for, reasons for, 131–132
  second consultation for, 136–137
  secondary, 137–138

Rhytidectomy. See Facelift
Rude patient, 65–66

Sagging, treatment for, 147–148
Scar revision, 220–224
  informing patient about, 223
  and letter to attorney or insurance company, 222–223
  patient permission for transmittal of information, 223
  patient selection for, 220–221
  payment for, 224
  photographs for, 224
  physical examination for, 221–222
  when to operate, 224
Scars
  acne, dermabrasion of, 225–226
  from breast augmentation, 167
Scheduling, for surgery, 103–108
Secondary rhinoplasty, 137–138
Selfishness, in medicine, 13–15
Seniority, of surgeons, 295
Sensation
  altered
    following breast augmentation, 169–170
    following breast reduction, 181
  cold, following breast augmentation, 169
"Shopper" patient, 70–71
Skin cancer, 227–228
Skin flaps, 230
Skin grafts, 230–231
Skin lesions
  biopsy of, 228–229
  instructions to patient, 231
  operative procedures, 231–232
  postoperative care, 232–233
  preoperative considerations concerning, 229–231
  underestimating problem of, 229–231
Socioeconomic status, and doctor-patient relationship, 29
Spouse, reluctant, 77–78
Squamous cell carcinoma, 227
Staff, negative behavior of, affecting patient, 44

Surgeon(s)
  "ghost," 17
  incomplete, 113
  older, 296–298
  plastic. *See* Plastic surgeon
  previous experience of, 87
  professional self-image of, 6–7
  seniority of, 295
Surgery
  cosmetic, definition of, 52
  esthetic. *See* Esthetic surgery
  fees for, 95–103
  informed consent for, 88–95
  prospective, persons consulted about, 108–110
  reconstructive, definition of, 52
  scheduling for, 103–108
Surgical reality, minimizing, in esthetic surgery, 60–62

Teenager. *See* Adolescent
Thigh lift, 214–216
  informing patient about, 216
  physical examination for, 215–216
Timing, of mastectomy reconstruction, 193
Transactions, interpersonal, 25–27
Transfusion, autologous, for breast reduction, 182
Transplantation, fat, 159–160
Trust, between patient and physician, 12
"Tummy tuck." *See* Abdominoplasty
Tumors, of head and neck, surgery for, 235–240. *See also* Head and neck surgery
"Two-party contract," in doctor-patient relationship, 10

Unkempt patient, 66

Vague patient, 68–69
Vanity, and esthetic surgery, 59
VIP patient, 78
Visibility, in esthetic surgery, 54–55

Waiting room, 30
Wrinkles, treatment for, 147–148
Written information, in informed consent, 89–91

Zygomatic fracture, treatment of, 234

RD 119 .G58 1991
Goldwyn, Robert M.
The patient and the plastic surgeon